Essentials for
Speech-Language Pathologists

Dedication

*This book is respectfully and lovingly dedicated
to my family for their support and patience with me
during the course of this project.*

Essentials for
Speech-Language Pathologists

Betsy P. Vinson, M.M.Sc., CCC/SLP

Clinical Assistant Professor
Director of Clinical Education
University of Florida

SINGULAR
THOMSON LEARNING ™

Australia Canada Mexico Singapore Spain United Kingdom United States

NOTICE TO THE READER

Singular Staff:
Business Unit Director: William Brottmiller
Acquisitions Editor: Marie Linvill
Developmental Editor: Kristin Banach
Editorial Assistant: Cara Jenkins
Executive Marketing Manager: Dawn F. Gerrain
Channel Manager: Kathryn Bamberger
Project Editor: Patricia Gillivan
Production Coordinator: Anne Sherman
Art/Design Coordinator: Timothy J. Conners

Printed in Canada
1 2 3 4 5 6 7 8 9 10 XXX 05 04 03 02 01 00

For more information, contact Singular Publishing Group, 401 West "A" Street, Suite 325, San Diego, CA 92101-7904; or find us on the World Wide Web at http://www.singpub.com

Library of Congress Cataloging-in-Publication Data

Vinson, Betsy Partin.
    Essentials for speech-language pathologists / author, Betsy P. Vinson
        p. ; cm
    Includes bibliographical references and index.
    ISBN 0-7693-0071-5
    1. Speech therapy.   2. Speech therapy—Practice.   I. Title.
    [DNLM: 1. Language Disorders—United States.   2. Delivery of Health Care—United States—Legislation.   3. Speech-Language Pathology—United States.   4. Teaching—United States—Legislation. WL 340.2 V788e 2001]
    RCA423.V558 2001
    616.8'55—dc21   00-63483

CONTENTS

SECTION III: DISORDERS

APPENDICES

REFERENCES

INDEX

Essentials for Speech-Language Pathologists was written in an effort to provide new professionals with a quick reference for the many disorders we face in our workplaces. It is a practical-application book; there is little theory in this book, as was the request of the originator of the idea for this book, Dr. Sadanad Singh.

The book addresses three primary areas. Chapters 1 and 2 constitute the first area. Chapter 1 consists of Professional Issues that reflect day-to-day interactions that have nothing to do with the disorders we treat. This includes information related to documentation, health care reform, critical pathways, home health care, forms of payment, malpractice, standards of care, support personnel, and behavior management. Also included in Chapter 1 are the ASHA Code of Ethics, and statement of Practices and Procedures.

Chapter 2 addresses Counseling. Counseling is a critical component of our job, but typically the one in which we are least trained. This chapter provides an overview of couseling techniques, the grief process, and listening techniques.

The second primary area of this book is composed of Section II, addressing case law and legislation that affect service delivery in speech-language pathology. Section II is divided into 3 chapters: (1) Education-Related Laws and Legislation, (2) Health Care Legislation, and (3) Public Laws Affecting Employment of Persons with Disabilities. Case law and federal legislation are presented, including Brown vs the Board of Education, which lay the foundation for so much of the non-discriminatory legislation subsequently passed for the handicapped.

The third area of *Essentials for Speech-Language Pathologists* is dedicated to the disorders. This area consists of 18 chapters addressing disorders, a chapter on multicultural issues in assessment and treatment, and a chapter on frequently seen syndromes. Each disorders chapter is divided into four major areas: (1) Definition/Description, (2) DSM Criteria (where applicable), (3) Assessment, and (4) Treatment. This area of the book offers a review of the defining characteristics of each disorder and why speech-language pathologists are involved in the assessment and treatment of persons with the specific disorder. The assessment portion of each chapter reviews basic testing protocol related to the disorder. In some cases, the names of published tests are provided, as well as informal procedures that can be used to assess clients with the discussed disorder. The treatment portion of each chapter contains information on techniques that have been proven by research to be successful with the specified disorder, although if one is looking for a "cookbook" on treatment there will be some disappointment!

Finally, there are two Appendices at the end of the book. The first one contains the standard reading passages used for a variety of assessments (The Grandfather Passage, The Rainbow

Passage, and the Declaration of Independence). The second Appendix consists of a variety of resources including websites, addresses and telephone numbers of numerous professional and client-oriented organizations, ordering information for AAC devices and laryngectomy equipment, and the names, addresses, and telephone numbers of various companies that offer assessment and therapy materials.

It has been a learning experience writing this book. I began by asking CFY clinicians across the State of Florida what information they needed starting out in the profession that was not completely covered in graduate school. The number one response dealt with legislation and case law governing the provision of our services, and a close second was on counseling information. Some clinicians wished to know more about the changing health care climate, so this was also included. Finally, the disorders section was designed to provide a "one-stop" shop to review the essentials of each disorder. The reader is referred to the extensive reference list at the end of the book for sources of additional information on each topic. I hope the reader will gain as much from using this book as I did in writing it.

SECTION ONE
Professional Issues in Speech-Language Pathology

CHAPTER ONE

Professional Issues

There are many issues with which the speech-language pathologist must deal during the course of a professional lifetime. The purpose of this section is to provide an overview of some of these issues, definitions, and practices for the purpose of having an easy reference.

DEFINITIONS OF IMPAIRMENT, DISABILITY, AND HANDICAP AS THEY RELATE TO COMMUNICATION DISORDERS

The World Health Organization's International Classification of Impairments, Disabilities, and Handicaps (ICIDH), currently has two classifications in development. According to Frattali, the ICIDH "has evolved from a biomedical model focused on causation and cure, to an integrated biopsychosocial model of human functioning and disablement that extends its focus to removing barriers that interfere with activities of daily living and quality of life." (Frattali, 1999, pp. 32–33).

The definitions of impairment, disability, and handicap are as follows:

Impairment: "specific speech, language, swallowing, or cognitive deficits" (Frattali, 1999, p. 32);

Disability: "the effects of the impairment(s) on everyday communication or eating activities" (Frattali, 1999, p. 32);

Handicap: "a range of social effects as defined by the work place or school system, family relationships, community roles, etc." (Frattali, 1999, p. 32).

A modification of the original ICIDH codes has been made to reflect a new social understanding of disability and describe the dimensions of functioning and disablement at three levels: the body, the person, and society. Definitions of these levels of functioning are:

Impairment: a loss or abnormality of body structure or of a physiological or psychological function (for example, loss of speech, loss of vision);

Activity: the nature and extent of functioning at the level of the person (such as taking care of oneself, communication activities, activities required of a job); activities may be limited in nature, duration, and quality;

Participation: the nature and extent of a person's involvement in life situations in relation to impairment, activities, health conditions, and contextual factors (such as being employed, participating in community events, ability to do both). Participation may be restricted in nature, duration, and quality. (Frattali, 1999, p. 32)

Disabilities, regardless of whether they are chronic or sudden in nature, typically have a negative impact on body image, self-concept, ego, and identity. Therefore, when determining the impact of disability, it is important to understand patient and family dynamics and their emotional states because it may affect how one interprets the progress of the patient during and after rehabilitation (Dikengil, 1998).

It is important to assist the patient's progression through the grief process by empowering the patient (and family) to take advantage of their assets, and to maximize the capabilities of the patient (Davidhizar, 1997). Family roles, changes in relationships with spouses, children, and friends are all impacted by disability. The speech-language pathologist can help by offering empathy and acting as a role model for family members to interact with the family member who has an impairment. The patient and family members should be referred to support groups, and it is best if the patient goes to a separate support group from the family members. The clinician can provide reading materials at an appropriate information level for the patient and family members. However, the most important thing a clinician can do to help a family cope with impending disability is to actively involve the family in the rehabilitation process (Dikengil, 1998).

DEFINITIONS RELATED TO ASHA

The following definitions refer to statements issued by ASHA. The definitions are found in Cornett & Davidson (1999, p. 74).

Preferred practice patterns: "statements that define universally applicable characteristics of activities directed toward individual patients/clients, and that address structural requisites of the practice, processes to be carried out, and expected outcomes."

Position statements: "Statements that specify ASHA's policy and stance on a matter that is important not only to the membership but also to other outside agencies or groups."

Practice guidelines: "A recommended set of procedures for a specific area of practice, based on research findings and current practice that details the knowledge, skills, and/or competencies needed to perform the procedures effectively."

DOCUMENTATION

Documentation of health care serves as a health management document, a business document, and a legal document. "The primary purpose of patient care documentation is to communicate vital information about a patient's health status to other health care providers concurrently caring for that patient and having an imminent need to know the information contained therein" (Scott, 2000, p. 31). Documentation also serves as a method for planning intervention and continuity of care as in, for example, when a patient is discharged from a hospital to home care. Another reason for documentation is to provide a historical progression of the patient's health which may be of vital interest in future instances of the patient's needing medical intervention.

Maintenance of quality of care is also a vital purpose of documentation. Agencies such as the Joint Commission on the Accreditation of Healthcare Organizations (JCAHO), the Commission on Accreditation of Rehabilitation Facilities (CARF), the National Committee on Quality Assurance (NCQA), and other local, state, and federal accrediting agencies require proof of quality management programs. In these cases, documentation serves "as a basis for monitoring and evaluating the quality of care rendered to patients as part of a quality management program" (Scott, 2000, p. 32).

Documentation also serves to fulfill some very functional, practical needs. For example, patient documentation can be used to formulate a database for monitoring patient care, and for extracting information for research purposes. It can be used to evaluate resource management, to insure that resources (human and nonhuman) are being utilized in an effective and efficient manner. Deficiencies and training needs can also be realized through patient documentation (Scott, 2000).

On a practical note, patient documentation serves as a business document whereby the health care provider is reimbursed for his or her services. "The patient care record is also evaluated by governmental third-party payer entities such as Medicare, Medicaid, TriCare (for military beneficiaries), state and local governmental entities, and by insurance companies and other payers to determine levels of reimbursement for patient care" (Scott, 2000, p. 32). In other words, documentation serves as the primary means by which reimbursement for services is justified.

In the event that a malpractice suit is filed, patient documentation can serve as substantive and relatively objective evidence of the management of the patient's health care. Expert witnesses can use the documentation as a basis from which to attest to whether the individual adhered to the professional and legal standards of care. Legally, documentation can also serve to uphold a patient's wishes with regard to informed consent, advanced directives, and personal autonomy. It can also serve as evidentiary documentation in cases of workman's compensation cases (Scott, 2000).

Flowsheets and Pathway Documentation

Flowsheets are seen most commonly at bedside, and they usually span 24 hours with cells for various parameters. Care pathways "are 'maps' of the case plan for particular diagnoses or conditions spanning the entire event of care from admission . . . through the projected day of dismissal" (Golper, 1998, p. 41). Care or clinical pathways used for treatment in a rehabilitation center will outline or map out the expected course of treatment from admission to discharge, and expected outcomes from the intervention received in the rehabilitation center.

Source Oriented or Source Indexed Medical Records

Source Oriented (SO) or Source Indexed (SI) medical records are usually written in a narrative format. Separate sections for various areas of assessment and care are included. SO/SI medical records include the popular SOAP and SOAPIE formats.

SOAP/SOAPIE

SOAP is an acronym for a report that includes four sections: Subjective/Objective/Assessment/Plan. Frequently, the SOAP and SOAPIE formats are used for progress notes.

The subjective section is used to record the clinician's subjective observations of the patient, such as "The patient is doing better than yesterday." It can also be used to record the patient's history and to summarize the patient's own analysis of his status.

The objective section includes objective observations made by the clinician based on testing, data collection during treatment, or instrumental evaluation. Assessment is based on analysis and formulation by the clinician. This analysis and formulation is, primarily, an interpretation of the objective and subjective sections of the report. In the SOAP format, the final section is for the Plan in which the clinician outlines future intervention strategies. In the SOAPIE format, the "P" section is for Problems, and provides a section to list problems the patient is exhibiting. The final two sections are Interventions, which is equivalent to the Plan section of the SOAP format, and Evaluation in which the clinician evaluates the efficacy and outcomes of the interventions (Golper, 1998). Others may add a Goals section (S-O-A-P-G) to the standard SOAP format (Scott, 2000).

Problem-Oriented Medical Records

POMRs are based on the patient's "problem list" with complaints listed and numbered. They usually include an Introductory section, also known as the Data Base; a Problem List; the Initial Plan; and "Progress Notes" (Golper, 1998). The progress notes are keyed to the problem list by problem number and name. They can be presented either in narrative form or flow sheets. "Flow sheets are used to record those aspects of client progress that are easily summarized by recording measurements . . . or by recording aspects of progress that lend themselves to some kind of scaling" (Flower, 1984, p. 149).

Problem-oriented medical records also call for discharge and interim summaries. Discharge summaries are completed when a client is leaving a facility, or when treatment is terminated. Interim summaries are completed at regular intervals (e.g., monthly, bimonthly, every 2 weeks, etc.) established by the appropriate agency (Flower, 1984).

Adapting the POMR System for Use by Speech-Language Pathologists

A listing of the client's conditions should be at the beginning of a POMR. This helps to identify any contributing factors to the speech, language, and/or hearing deficit. It also helps to create a data base that can serve as a foundation for clinical research. According to Weed (1972), there are six categories of data base information that can be used:

1. Chief complaint: This can be recorded based on the report from the client and/or his family and caregivers. The complaint is the reason the individual is seeking out the services of the speech-language pathologist. In some cases, a client may be following through on a referral, even though he has no particular concerns or complaints. This, too, should be documented under "chief complaint."

2. Client profile: The client profile includes information such as the client's level of education, social activity, and vocational information.

3. Present communication disorder or disorders: This is a summary of the client's complaints and previous diagnoses.

4. Past history: The past history should take into account factors relating to the onset of the communication disorder, associated disorders, previous evaluations and treatment, and social and economic factors.

5. Initial evaluation: Documentation of tests given and their results and interpretation should be listed in the initial evaluation.

6. Progress notes: Progress notes provide an ongoing evaluation of the client's performance in therapy.

Standards-Based Documentation or Documentation by Exception

In Standards-based documentation or documentation by exception, symbols and abbreviations are used to make notations referring to predefined norms, protocols, and standards of care. Like pathways and flowsheets, these are typically in a 24-hour format. Standards-based documentation or documentation by exception may be accompanied by focus notes which are one or two phrase narrative notes. The narrative notes are used to denote any variations in the typical plan or in the patient's response.

Chronologic Records

Chronologic records are frequently used in outpatient clinics where the patient is being followed for one problem. All information in chronologic records is filed sequentially, hence the name (Golper, 1998).

Computerized Flowsheets and Electronic Data or Order Entries

Although highly convenient, these types of documentation are plagued by breakdown and expense. However, there is increased "legibility, standardization of information and data base development," and increased confidentiality (Golper, 1998, p. 44).

Common Problems, Errors, and Suggestions

Scott (2000, pp. 40–42) delineates 25 common problems, errors, and suggestions related to patient care documentation:

Problems

1. Illegible notation;

2. Use of multiple or inconsistent documentation formats by providers in a facility;

3. Pen runs out of ink midway through a patient care record entry;

4. Line spacing in patient care record entries;

5. Signing patient care record entries;

6. Error correction;

7. Physician orders: transcription problems; examining and intervening on behalf of patients without written orders where legally required;

8. Failing to delineate patient care rendered or identify clinical information supplied by another provider.

Errors

9. Failure to identify (or correctly identify) the patient under care;

10. Failure to annotate the date (and time, depending on customary practice) of patient care activities;

11. Failure to use an indelible instrument to record examination, evaluation, diagnostic, prognostic, intervention, or outcome data about a patient under care;

12. Unauthorized abbreviations;

13. Use of improper spelling, grammar, and the use of extraneous verbage not affecting patient care;

14. Untimely documentation of patient care activities;

15. Identifying or filing an incident report in the patient care record;

16. Blaming or disparaging another provider in the patient care record;

17. Expressing personal feelings about a patient or patient family member or significant other in the patient care record;

18. Recording hearsay ("second-hand" input) as fact;

19. Failure to document a patient's informed consent to examination and intervention.

Suggestions

20. Document observations and findings objectively;

21. Document with specificity;

22. Exercise special caution when countersigning another provider's, student's, or intern's patient care notation;

23. Document thoroughly patient's/family's/significant other's understanding of, and safe compliance with, discharge, home care, and follow-up instructions;

24. Carefully document a patient's noncompliance with provider directives or recommendations;

25. Carefully document a patient's or family member's/significant other's possible contributory negligence related to alleged patient injuries or lack of progress.

HEALTH CARE REFORM

According to Griffin and Fazen (1993), managed care

> is a system that integrates the financing and delivery of appropriate health care services. Managed care programs have certain common elements: First of all, arrangements are made with selected providers to furnish comprehensive

health care services to covered persons. In some programs, this limits the choice of providers to whom the patient can go for services. Secondly, fees and rates which are lower than the normal price of services are negotiated with the selected providers. On most bills, there is an "amount charged" and the prenegotiated "amount allowed" column. Thirdly, formal programs exist for ongoing quality improvement and utilization review. A fourth characteristic is that significant financial incentives are offered for covered persons to use providers and procedures covered by the managed care plan. (p. 1)

There are five types of managed care organizations (MCOs).

1. Managed indemnity insurance programs: Also known as fee-for-service, participants in this type of MCO pay a monthly premium, and are reimbursed based on the billed charges. Participants may choose any licensed provider, "although the plans specify the services and types of providers that are covered" (Griffin & Fazen, 1993, p. 2).

2. Preferred provider organizations (PPOs): In PPOs, the provider or insurer negotiates a lower rate with a network of selected group of providers. Enrollees can opt to go to a non-preferred provider, although they will pay a higher fee, and may be limited in the service options.

3. Health maintenance organizations (HMOs): "HMOs provide a defined, comprehensive set of health services to a voluntarily enrolled population within a specified geographic service area" (Griffin & Fazen, 1993, p. 2). Members are required to seek services within the provider network. The providers are reimbursed based on a capitated amount that is pre-negotiated. There are four main types of HMOs:

   • Staff model HMO: The HMO owns a central facility (or facilities), and the health care providers are all salaried employees.

   • Group model: The HMO contracts with multispecialty physician group practices to provide care either in a company-owned facility or in their own offices (ASHA, 1993).

   • Independent practice associations (IPAs): In IPAs, the physicians see the patients in their own offices, and are reimbursed under a variety of plans. The patient sees a health practitioner who has a contract with the HMO to provide services.

   • Network: Designed to serve a large population of HMO members, the network consists of a contract between the HMO and both multispecialty groups and independent practitioners in a large geographic area (ASHA, 1993).

4. Point of service plan (POS): This is also known as the open-ended HMO. Members have the option of seeing providers who are not in the plan. However, "there is a strong financial incentive to use the affiliated providers" (Griffin & Fazen, 1993, p. 2).

5. Physician hospital organization (PHO): The PHO contracts with the MCOs to provide physician and hospital services to enrollees. All decisions are made within the network, so there is no third-party. The PHO is organized by the physician community and hospital.

Carol Frattali outlines six influences that are currently and presently shaping "a consumer-directed approach to care": The first influence is a social definition of quality care. Excessive care is expensive and unethical. In today's health care climate, providing excessive care to one patient may, in the long run, be denying care to another patient. One must think of the impact of one's service delivery system not only on current patients, but on future patients as well.

Secondly, there is increased specialization in health care. As clinical and scientific knowledge expands, there is a tendency to define increased specialization which, over time, leads to fragmentation of health care. Third-party providers see increased specialization as more expensive, thus the patient suffers because benefits for specialized tests and care are denied.

Regulatory reforms constitute a third influence. The use of clinical competence standards instead of credentials has led to dramatic changes in staffing patterns based on regulation agencies' standards. Clinicians must "both define and document their competencies to accreditation agencies and payers" (Frattali , 1998, p. 243). Those who do not do this are subject to having their competencies defined by the medical staff and/or outside agencies for whom they work.

Lack of convincing treatment data is a fourth influence. Much has been said in recent years about the need for valid and reliable outcome data which can document the effectiveness of treatment methodology employed by speech-language pathologists. It is critical that we prove that lower cost treatment alternatives result in less satisfactory outcomes both clinically and economically.

Emerging models of care are another characteristic of the consumer-driven approach to health care. "New models based on an integration of social science (e.g., the patient's perception of health, functional status, quality of life) rather than medical science paradigms (diagnosis and cure) are just recently gaining the attention of the health care community and are predicted to influence approaches to service delivery" (Frattali, 1998, p. 243). The emphasis is predicted to continue a shift toward functional outcomes, for example, dealing with useful communication tools instead of underlying language processes.

Finally, consumer choice and satisfaction drive the current health care system. Consumers have more options than ever with regard to selecting a health care plan. Thus, if they are not satisfied, they can elect to change to a different carrier. Even though many of the changes are the result of federal mandates, the market is consumer driven.

Managed Care Plans

Managed care plans may be variously referred to as health maintenance organizations (HMOs), preferred provider organizations (PPOs), and independent practice associations (IPAs). "The most sweeping changes in health care involve managed care in all its hybrid forms. Generally, managed care describes a cost-effective system that integrates both the financing and delivery of health care services. It is defined by the American Association of Health Plans (American Managed Care and Review Association, 1995), the national trade association representing managed care organizations, as a comprehensive approach to health care delivery that encompasses planning and coordination of care, patient and provider education, monitoring of care quality, and cost control" (Frattali, 1998, p. 244).

Henri and Hallowell (1999) state that there are three goals of managed care. The first is to assure the quality and coordination of care, and the second is to create access to medical care for people who need it. However, with time, goals one and two have fallen by the wayside in favor of the third goal which is cost control. The impacts of HMOs and MCOs is felt in fee-for-service medicine as well as in Medicaid and Medicare. Henri and Hallowell (1999) state the situation as follows:

> These mechanisms include increasingly stringent utilization review; pre-admission certification for hospital stays; required preauthorization for services; negotiated reduced reimbursement rates; designation of a restricted list of preferred providers; the designation of physicians as "gatekeepers" of patients' access to health care services; salaried employment of physicians by payer organizations; incentives for physicians not to refer patients to specialty services (such as rehabilitation services); use of red-flag diagnostic or treatment categories to deny reimbursement; and restrictions on frequency, intensity, and duration of care. (p. 4)

One of the primary features of managed care is the use of a "gatekeeper" who coordinates a patient's care. The gatekeeper is typically the primary care physician who must make the decisions regarding the scope and intensity of managed care. For example, a patient who is seeking speech-language therapy services would need to make the request through his/her primary care physician who would then, if he deemed it appropriate, refer the patient for therapy (Frattali, 1998).

A second feature is utilization review (UR) which refers to the monitoring of a patient's use of health care services and resources. This would include "second opinions, precertifications, treatment authorizations, discharge planning, and chart reviews" (Frattali, 1998, p. 245).

A third common feature of managed care systems is authorization of services. Authorization is a management technique that helps to facilitate compliance with the Federal HMO Act of 1973.

Managed care has had a tremendous impact on rehabilitation services. In the last fifteen years, there has been an increase in subacute facilities to bridge the gap between acute care hospitals and nursing facilities. Patients are discharged from acute care settings more rapidly than in previous times, necessitating the development of facilities designed to provide intermediate care and rehabilitation before a patient is discharged to a long-term care facility or home. Home health agencies also have proliferated to accommodate those patients discharged to home (frequently due to caps on medical coverage).

According to Henri and Hallowell (1999), managed care challenges in speech-language pathology and audiology can be divided into five categories:

The first is **consumers' access to services**: There has been a decrease in the number of referrals from "gatekeepers" who tend to focus more on acute care. There has been an increase in lack of coverage due to clauses related to pre-existing conditions that reduce or negate the payment for rehabilitation services. Also, there is a demand from managed care organizations for consistent improvement that may not be evident in elderly patients and patients with chronic disability, multiple disabilities, or degenerative conditions. Others who have less access to services include minorities and low income individuals, since they are typically not in jobs with employee health plans. In addition, some managed care organizations state that services that are provided must meet specific criteria with regard to medical necessity. Perkins and Olson (1998) define medical necessity as follows:

1. "To prevent the onset or worsening of an illness, condition, or disability";

2. "To establish a diagnosis";

3. "To provide palliative, curative, or restorative treatment for physical and/or mental health conditions";

4. "To assist the individual to achieve or maintain maximum functional capacity in performing daily activities, taking into account both the functional capacity of the individual and those functional capacities that are appropriate for individuals of the same age" (Henri & Hallowell, 1999, p. 20).

Since many rehabilitation services are not considered to be medically necessary, they may not be covered under some HMOs/MCOs. (Henri & Hallowell, 1999). Kahan et al. (1994, pp. 357–359) provide some "helpful direction in supporting the medical necessity of clinical services. They present the following four criteria:

1. The procedure must be appropriate (that is, its benefits must sufficiently outweigh its risks to make it worth performing, and it must do at least as well as the next-best available procedure);

2. It would be improper care not to recommend this service;

3. There is a reasonable chance that the procedure will benefit the patient;

4. The benefit to the patient is not small" (Henri & Hallowell, p. 19).

The second category relates to the **quality, intensity, duration, and frequency of care that is provided.** Based on a particular diagnosis, the number of treatment sessions may be predetermined, with the number being restricted within a given period of time. In some cases, duration of therapy is limited to six visits in acute stages, and 60 days during rehabilitation as opposed to the more traditional 12 to 18 months for CVAs, TBIs, and those with degenerative nervous system disorders. "These restrictions also create the possibility of a circular process; when little progress is made because few visits are permitted, the insurer denies further care because little progress was made" (Henri & Hallowell, 1999, p. 7). There also may be delays in the initiation of treatment while waiting for authorization or reauthorization for services. Treatment sessions are shorter, usually lasting 30–45 minutes instead of the traditional 60 minutes. It is also becoming more common for insurance companies to intervene with goal writing, treatment planning, scheduling, determining progress, and selecting augmentative/alternative communication devices (Henri & Hallowell, 1999).

The **fiscal stability of service providing agencies** is the third category of managed care challenges for the speech-language pathologist or audiologist. Tied in with this is the fourth category of challenge which is the **livelihood of professionals in the field**. Slow processing of claims, and reduced coverage (sometimes up to 80% reduction in rates to members of some HMOs/MCOs) have led to reduced coverage of services and reductions in the number of staff. Some clinicians are hiring more assistants and aides as a lower cost method of providing coverage in therapy. While trained paraprofessionals can help with some tasks, some HMOs/MCOs will not pay unless services are provided by the highest quality provider. Some clinicians use trained volunteers and family members to assist with generalization and maintenance. There is also increased competition between agencies to become providers for specific HMOs/MCOs (Henri & Hallowell, 1999).

Approximately 30% of submissions for authorization of diagnosis and treatment are denied, although approximately 90% of the appeals result in overturning the original refusal. To appeal, the clinician needs to submit "a written request for authorization by the primary care physician or additional supporting documentation resulting from the evalua- tion or treatment" (Henri & Hallowell, 1999, p. 23). The patient can also file a complaint with the human resources department where he is employed. He should also submit a copy sent to the insurer. It is prudent to file a complaint with the state insurance commissioner if the appeal is not upheld. Wherever the complaint is filed, it is helpful to be cooperative, not adversarial, and to always be a patient advocate (Henri & Hallowell, 1999).

The **maintenance of professional integrity** is the fifth category of challenges. Members of the American Speech-Language-Hearing Association are bound by a Code of Ethics (1994) (Appendix 1–A) that helps to define and shape the reputation and worthiness of the pro- fession. The increased use of paraprofessionals and the increased emphasis on multiskilling are direct threats to our professional integrity. The role of HMOs/MCOs in the decision-making process removes some of the professional autonomy which has long been a standard for ASHA members. Furthermore, the demand for cost-effective treatment, reducing costs, and increasing the productivity frequently puts clinicians in an ethical and moral bind. Also at issue is the provision of care to patients who cannot reasonably benefit from services in order to meet productivity requirements. The compromising of care to meet arbitrary standards set by the health care industry also has a negative impact on our profession.

These challenges dictate the need for our profession to develop outcome measures that can be used to justify decision making related to the provision of diagnostic and therapeutic interventions. Donabedian (1980) defines the term "outcome" as "a change in a patient's current and future health status that can be attributed to antecedent health care." Typically, outcomes have emphasized the physical and physiological aspects of performance. However, in the new health care environment, outcomes need to reflect changes in the social and psychological functioning of the patient as well. Other components of health which merit consideration include the patient's attitudes, his satisfaction with the services he is receiving, his health-related knowledge, and the behavioral changes that come about as a result of his knowledge and attitude.

The National Outcomes Measurement System (NOMS) is based on the Functional Communication Measures which is a seven-point scale used to determine a patient's abilities at the time he is admitted into therapy, and at the time of discharge. It is hoped that the clinicians can use the data as measured by the Functional Communication Measures to validate their services, improve the quality of their services, and make adjustments in the practice patterns as needed (Henri & Hallowell, 1999). Frattali (1999) suggests three guid- ing questions when choosing outcome measures:

1. Has the client's speech improved?

2. Is he or she a more functional communicator as a result?

3. Does the client feel better about himself/herself and less socially stigmatized? (p. 36)

ASHA has pointed out the need to collect state and national outcomes data in order to effectively lobby legislators to allocate a portion of the health care dollars to rehabilitation

TABLE I-I Treatment outcomes	
Type of Outcome	**Examples**
Clinically derived	Ability to sustain phonation Accuracy in naming Type & frequency of disfluencies in a speech sample Integrity of the swallowing mechanism
Functional	Ability to communicate basic needs Ability to use the telephone Ability to read the newspaper Ability to eat independently
Social	Employability Ability to learn reintegration in community
Patient-defined	Satisfaction with treatment Quality of life
Administrative	Patient referral patterns Average length of stay Rate of missed sessions Productivity level in direct patient care
Financial	Cost-effective care Cost benefit of care Rate of rehospitalizations Discharge destination

From "Measuring and Managing Outcomes," by C.M. Frattali, 1999, in *Clinical Practice Management for Speech-Language Pathologists* by B.S. Cornett, Gaithersburg, MD: Aspen Publishers, Inc. Copyright 1999 by Aspen Publishers, Inc. Reprinted with permission.

services such as speech-language pathology. With increased dollars come increased access for those in need of speech-language pathology and audiology services. There is also a need to compare state performances to the national averages as a "benchmark of quality of care" (Frattali, 1999, p. 37).

Frattali (1999) points out that clinical intervention can result in a variety of different outcomes as described and delineated in Table 1–1.

One also must consider the temporal aspects of outcomes.

> Intermediate outcomes determine, from session to session, whether treatment is benefiting the client. . . . Instrumental outcomes activate the learning process. These are outcomes that, when reached, trigger the ultimate outcome . . . Ultimate outcomes demonstrate the social or ecological validity of interventions, such as functional communication, reemployability, community reintegration, and individually defined quality of life. (Frattali, 1999, p. 39)

The Agency for Health Care Policy and Research (AHCPR) has, in the near past, worked on the development of nationally recognized clinical practice guidelines, but has recently redirected its efforts to establish "evidence-based practice centers." The purpose of these centers is to "provide extensive literature review on assigned topics and to produce 'evidence reports' or technology assessments so that clinicians can make critical health care decisions based upon the latest and most comprehensive scientific knowledge" (Cornett & Davidson, 1999, p. 57).

Spath (1994) suggests that clinicians should concentrate on the elements outlined in Table 1–2 to achieve outcomes management.

TABLE 1–2 Elements of outcomes management	
Element	**Description**
Outcomes specification	Define expected outcomes and measures to assess achievement of results
Outcomes measurement	Design valid and reliable assessment tools
Information systems	Design automated or manual information systems to support data collection, input, retrieval, and analysis
Process improvement	Design continuous quality improvement techniques to improve the processes of care

From "Structuring Clinical Practice: Guidelines, Pathways, and Protocols," by B. S. Cornett and T. L. Davidson, 1999, in *Clinical Practice Management for Speech-Language Pathologists* by B.S. Cornett, Gaithersburg, MD: Aspen Publishers, Inc. Copyright 1999 by Aspen Publishers, Inc. Reprinted with permission.

Documentation should be brief and concise. It should include a brief history and a description of the presenting problem. A summary of formal and informal assessment procedures should follow. Outcome-oriented, long-range goals should be included in the report, as well as a diagnosis and prognostic statement and, if possible, the estimated duration of treatment also should be included. Session by session progress notes documenting any change of goals (including justifications), and progress toward goals in that particular session also should be noted (Henri & Hallowell, 1999).

CRITICAL PATHWAYS

Critical pathways are guidelines for evaluation and treatment based on a particular diagnosis. They are used to "maintain quality care within limited timeframes" (Dikengil, 1998, p. 9). The concept of critical pathways originated at Boston's New England Medical Center in the 1980s in an attempt to address four core questions:

1. What is required by each discipline to bring patients with similar diagnoses to realistic outcomes?

2. What is the best way to produce that work?

3 Who is accountable for those outcomes?

4. How can we restructure care so that this happens more consistently? (Dikengil, 1998, p. 9)

Critical pathways are designed to account for all the steps in a patient's care from the time he is admitted until he is discharged. Their primary purpose is to "provide a framework for describing clinical treatment protocols and outcomes that a health care facility expects to deliver to a patient population during a preset number of days" (Dikengil, 1998, p. 9). They are a critical component in negotiating contracts with managed care organizations. They provide structure to treatment goals and standardization of the service delivery process by encompassing guidelines for how and when care should be provided. As expected, some patients will not conform to the guidelines, so clinicians must be prepared to explain the variance and advocate for increased or different services.

McRury (1998) recommends the following steps in pathway development:

1. Establish a multidisciplinary team. It is important to include key physicians and a representative of each profession that is defined in the critical pathway. McRury also recommends that the team choose its project leader(s) wisely. Teams may want to have cochairs in addition to a physician sponsor or leader.

2. Decide on a beginning and end point of care segments along the way.

3. Gather baseline data (such as current length of stay, patient satisfaction survey data, outcomes measures, costs, charges, and reimbursements).

4. Determine available resources (existing guidelines, other pathways, protocols, benchmark data, and evidence in the literature).

5. Identify outcomes to be achieved (patient-focused, measurable).

6. Specify level of detail desired in content of document (Henri & Hallowell, 1999, p. 73).

A critical pathways reference and resource list is available from the ASHA Health Services Division. The phone number is (301)897-5700 ext. 235.

HOME HEALTH CARE

Home health care is one of the fastest growing segments of the health care industry. In 1963, there were 1100 agencies providing home health care. In 1995, there were 17,500 providers of home health care serving seven million patients in the home. The increase was in response to efforts to decrease health care costs which expanded from being 5.3% of the U.S. Gross National Product in 1960 to 16% in 1994. It is estimated that $52 billion dollars were spent on home health services in 1997 (Dikengil, 1998).

Why use home health care? Home health care came about as a product of changes in the allocation of funding to Medicare and Medicaid, the advent of managed care, and health care reform. Simply put, home health care was cost effective when compared to hospital care. Also, patients expressed a desire to be seen in the comfort of their own home instead of a hospital. It is easier to involve the family and friends in facilitating recuperation in the home, and there is a belief that patients are more motivated to become independent. Thus, they achieve functional outcomes in shorter periods of time.

Historically, payment has been based on fee-for-service with unlimited visits and the patient and/or insurance company paying for the services as they were rendered. Now, with regard to home health care, there are two primary systems of payment through health maintenance organizations (HMOs):

1. Insurance companies predetermine a limited number of visits as a measure of cost containment;

2. Insurance companies offer a set amount of money per member per month, and the providers decide how to disburse the payments.

Two terms frequently associated with home health care are "gatekeeper" and "capitation." The gatekeeper is usually a registered nurse (RN), who serves as the case manager at an insurance company. This individual "determines the extent of the coverage and provides preauthorization for treatment, generally for a specific period of time" (Dikengil, p. 7). With regard to capitation, managed care organizations have decreased health care costs, which was a primary goal for MCOs. However, physicians now are restricted in the amount of time they can spend with a patient and still be reimbursed. In other words, the payment is capped per patient.

Capitation poses some ethical dilemmas. With capitation, services are delivered based on reimbursement dictates instead of on patient needs. The average number of funded visits under a Medicare HMO is 10, versus 76 for fee-for-service patients. (Dikengil, 1998). This has resulted in a compromising of the quality of services for some patients. The phrase "medically necessary" is applied to services and results in dilemmas for the service providers. Speech-language pathologists need to "have an impact on these changes and assist in formulating reasonable changes so that communication disorders don't end up being perceived as unnecessary to treat or of low priority on the health care continuum" (Dikengil, 1998, p. 8).

Obviously, managed care has posed some challenges for the speech-language pathologist. The question is, "How do we meet those challenges?" One way is to make a paradigm shift "from the traditional service delivery model of reducing the patient's impairment over time, to providing functional approaches that focus on the disability and handicap that the impairment causes the patient" (Dikengil, 1998, p. 9). One way to do this is to increase the family involvement in recovery through prioritizing and achieving goals. Clinicians need to be proactive in establishing critical pathways to meet the needs of their patients.

Another way to meet the challenge is to initiate interaction between providers and payers. Provide inservice training to payers to inform them about the patient's needs, the patient's potential, and justification for continued services. Also, hold off initiating treatment until the patient is medically stable. With shorter acute care stays, patients are being sent home before they are ready to withstand the rigors of therapeutic intervention. Thus, delaying treatment until the patient is more able to benefit from the intervention is a wise move on the part of the clinician.

Speech-language pathologists must justify their services. One way to do this is to have out-come data when negotiating for contracts. Payers want to know how long it will take to treat the patient, how much it will cost, and if the intervention will make a difference. Three instruments that can be used to measure outcomes are as follows:

1. ASHA's Functional Assessment of Communication Skills for Adults (ASHA FACS);

2. ASHA's Functional Communication Measure (FCM);

3. Beaumont Outcome Software System (BOSS).

Outcome measures should include follow-up information at three and six months post treatment to determine the adequacy and effectiveness of the therapy.

Another important piece of data is gleaned from patient satisfaction measures. Including reports from patients regarding their level of satisfaction with the services provided and the outcomes achieved can lend further support to justifying the provision of intervention.

Criteria for Defining the Home Care Patient

The pediatric home care patient is one who has dysphagia, is failing to thrive, or exhibits developmental delay. Geriatric home care patients are those who have suffered strokes, craniotomies, traumatic brain injury, tumors, progressive neurological disease, or cancer. The Beacon Health Corporation has set up the following criteria to determine if a patient qualifies for home health care:

1. Is the patient confined to home?

2. Is the confinement related to a medical or physical condition?

3. What if the patient does leave home?

   • medical absences (absences to receive medical care that cannot be provided in the home);

   • Social (nonmedical) absences (day care, respite care, once a month visits to the barber, etc.).

If the patient leaves home once a week or more on a regular basis, he does not qualify for homebound services.

The Role of the Speech-Language Pathologist in Home Health Care

Dikengil (1998) presents the following list based on ASHA's description of the role of the speech-language pathologist in home health care:

1. Conducting speech, language, and/or oral pharyngeal evaluations;

2. Developing and recommending appropriate individual treatment/education programs;

3. Providing treatment;

4. Referring to other health professionals;

5. Instructing and counseling family members, nurses, and other members of the home care team;

6. Providing referral and follow-up with other community resources;

7. Recommending prosthetic and augmentative communication devices;

8. Conducting hearing screenings;

9. Providing aural rehabilitation in consultation with an audiologist;

10. Participating in admission/discharge planning;

11. Providing appropriate documentation;

12. Supervising peers, clinical fellows, supportive personnel, and students in training;

13. Providing inservice training to agency staff;

14. Providing public education;

15. Conducting research;

16. Developing and participating in prevention activities;

17. Directing and administering home care services;

18. Maintaining a quality control. (p. 26–27)

FORMS OF PAYMENT

There are many different forms of payment in today's health care system. Two of the most common, "discounted fee for service" and "capitation," are discussed in this section.

Discounted Fee for Service

The managed care organization negotiates a discount from the typical fee the provider charges, and is subsequently reimbursed based on this discounted fee. This was established as a cost-containment maneuver, but has, for the most part, failed. The reason it has failed is that the providers simply raised their rates so that the discounted amount met their original fee. For example, the therapist may have originally charged $90.00 per hour of therapy, which may have been reimbursed as $50.00 an hour. The negotiated discount may only permit the charging of $90.00 per hour. Thus, to get the desired $90.00 per hour, the therapist may raise his/her rates to $130.00 per hour. The provider agrees to accept this discounted rate in order to continue as a provider for that particular MCO.

Capitation

Capitation is a predetermined, "fixed amount of money set by contract between a managed care organization (MCO) and the provider, to be paid on a per-person (per capita) basis regardless of the number of services rendered or costs incurred" (Frattali, 1998, p. 246). Instead of having the payment based on the actual service rendered, the payment is based on cost units referred to as "per member per month (PMPM)." The use of capitation has the effect of limiting the number of special services a patient receives, including testing and hospitalizations. This is because the physician (or gatekeeper) receives a set fee per patient regardless of the number of tests performed, hospitalizations required, or special services (such as rehabilitation) he recommends (Frattali, 1998).

A table depicting the payment systems for medical rehabilitation services is in Table 1–3.

TABLE 1-3 Payment systems for medical rehabilitation services

Payment System	Level of Care	Description
Diagnosis-related groups (DRGs)	In-patient hospital	A prospectively based reimbursement system, in place since 1983, that classifies hospital in-patients into groups, codified by principal diagnosis, and assigns a predetermined flat fee for the costs associated with hospitalization. The prospective payment system (PPS) has resulted in shorter lengths of hospital stay, delayed (or decreased) referrals to rehab practitioners, and a general reduction in utilization of services. As a result of PPS, the SLP's case mix in hospitals has changed notably, with dysphagia becoming the primary diagnosis treated. In some cases, SLPs report that 90% of the caseload in in-patient acute hospitals consists of patients with dysphagia.
Function-related groups (FRGs)	In-patient rehabilitation	A prospectively based reimbursement system that was developed for in-patient rehabilitation, which classifies patients into function-related groups (on the basis of Functional Independence Measure [FIM] scores), and assigns a predetermined flat fee for the costs associated with in-patient rehab services.
Medicare salary equivalency	Contracted services	In the fall of 1996, proposed regulations were written for the implementation of hourly reimbursement limits for Medicare contracted services, effective mid-1997 at the earliest . . . . Payment applies to the time in a facility, not just treatment time . . . Large rehabilitation organizations that provide contractual services as well as private practices have felt the effects. Cost-saving maneuvers were implemented including cutting expenses by reducing middle management.
Ambulatory patient groups (APGs)	Out-patient services	Since 1990, Congress has been funding research for the design of a Medicare PPS for hospital out-patient services. Health Care Financing Administration (HCFA) was under pressure to develop a system that could be implemented by 2002. This is another prospectively based reimbursement system that assigns a patient to one or more ambulatory patient groups and is also based on measurements of functional status. "Speech-language treatment" is one of the 297 APGs used to describe patient services . . .
Resource utilization groups (RUGs)	Nursing facility care	Since the early 90s, Congress has been funding research in the hopes of establishing a PPS in nursing homes for Medicare as well as Medicaid (since medicaid pays 50% of the nation's nursing home bills) . . . The PPS allows annual payments to SNFs for SLP, audiology, PT, and OT based on a combination of: 1. A facility's average monthly rehab payments from a previous 12 month period; and

continued

TABLE I–3 continued		
Payment System	*Level of Care*	*Description*
		2. **The national average Medicare SNF payment amount for rehab services, adjusted for number of discharges.**
		When monthly allotment of rehabilitation funds runs out or is nearing depletion, the SLP must present a convincing case to the facility administrator for seeking priority over PT and OT services.
Prospective payment	Home health care	**. . .The prospectively determined fees for rehabilitation will be based on scores from a functional status measure.**

Adapted from "Clinical Care in a Changing Health System," by C. M. Frattali, 1998, in *Approaches to the Treatment of Aphasia* (pp. 262–263), by N. Helm-Estabrooks and A. Holland, San Diego, CA: Singular Publishing Group. Copyright 1998 by Singular Publishing Group. Adapted with permission.

MALPRACTICE

There are two approaches to defining malpractice in the health care professions. Traditionally, malpractice referred to conduct that constitutes professional negligence. The broader definition which fits with today's atmosphere more completely is as follows:

Any potential legal basis for imposition of liability, including:

- Professional negligence;

- Breach of a patient-professional contractual promise;

- Liability for defective care-related equipment or products that injure patients or clients;

- Strict liability (absolute liability without regard for fault) for abnormally dangerous care-related professional activities;

- Intentional care-related provider misconduct conduct. (Scott, 2000, p. 4)

Negligence is the "delivery of patient care that falls below the standards expected of ordinary, reasonable practitioners of the same profession acting under the same or similar circumstances" (Scott, 2000, p. 5). Should a patient file a complaint of malpractice, he must prove four requisite elements:

1. The provider owed the patient a special duty of due care;

2. The provider violated the special duty owed;

3. As a result, the patient was injured; and

4. The patient is entitled to legally recognized money damages. (Scott, 2000, p. 6)

Rowland (1988) wrote that

> Malpractice is not limited to the negligent (unintentional) infliction or creation of pain during evaluation or management of a disorder. Malpractice can include: (1) misdiagnosis; (2) failure to reveal alternative remediations; (3) improper or substandard remediation techniques; (4) failure to refer when not competent to manage; (5) referral to an inferior system for management; (6) breach of an actual warranty (for service or for a product); (7) breach of an implied warranty; (8) release of information to unauthorized persons (including "loose talk") or failure to release information to authorized persons; (9) failure to properly instruct in the use of a potentially hazardous product; (10) failure to warn of a potential hazard or harm. (1988, p. 45)

He defined malpractice as existing "anytime a physical or mental injury or economic loss results from an action or omission which falls within a recognized standard of care" (Rowland, 1988, p. 45).

ASHA also has a few cases of malpractice reported annually. Typically, these complaints are related to deceitful and/or misleading advertising, and insurance fraud. Other areas of complaint include license fraud; general practice fraud; unprofessional conduct; low standards of care; unethical practices; refusal of services; inadequate record keeping (Trace & Breske, 1993).

To file a complaint of malpractice with ASHA, the complainer must file the complaint in writing, and it must be signed by the individual filing the grievance. The complainant also signs a waiver of confidentiality. The complaint is sent to the violator, who has 45 days to respond. The Ethical Practices Board convenes and either dismisses or adjudicates the complaint (Appendix 1–B). The Board informs the parties of their decision and, when appropriate, cites the specific code infringement, and the proposed sanction. The violator can request an appearance before the Board, and take counsel if so desired. ASHA typically has three forms of retribution: the reprimand, censure, and revocation of membership and/or certification. The reprimand is a private "slap on the wrist," while censure is a public "slap on the wrist." Revocation of membership and/or certification takes away the rights of the person as a member of ASHA to continue practicing as a speech-language pathologist.

Malpractice vs. Liability

Liability is the state of being responsible for the professional treatment of one's patients and to the ASHA Code of Ethics, and is the result of malpractice. Professional liability occurs when the speech-language pathologist's conduct is negligent during the course of assessing or treating a patient, and this negligence results in injury to the patient. It is difficult to define malpractice, but any treatment that causes injury to a patient, or that can be interpreted as harmful, unprofessional, or neglectful could be defined as malpractice. In essence, malpractice is the action of conduct that is unprofessional, and liability is the result.

Negligence law covers compensation of individuals who have been accidentally harmed by another. It is based on the principle of reasonable care: if your failure to use reasonable care in the treatment of your patient results in harm to that person, potentially, you could be legally liable.

It is advisable for speech-language pathologists to carry liability insurance. The Albert H. Wohlers Company is recommended by ASHA as a source for liability insurance. The address is:

Albert H. Wohlers and Company
1440 N. Northeast Highway
Park Ridge, IL 60068-1400.

Strategies to Avoid Being the Subject of a Complaint

One of the most important strategies to avoid being the subject of a complaint is to establish positive relationships with patients and their families. This includes returning phone calls, not neglecting appointments, adhering to schedules, maintaining a pleasant attitude, and addressing the needs and concerns of the patient.

It is also helpful to educate the patient and his family about the disorder or illness, and to help them establish realistic goals for the patient.

Finally, documentation is absolutely critical in avoiding becoming a violator. Documentation should include the following:

1. Date and time seen;
2. Patient concerns/complaints;
3. Description of visits/comments/feedback;
4. Specific language regarding the disorder or illness;
5. Appropriately marking errors (Trace & Breske, 1993).

Appropriately marked errors are those that have a single line drawn through the error, are labeled as an error, and have the date and the clinician's signature. Never use correction fluid on a legal document.

Being Served a Summons

If you are served with a summons, the first course of action should be to notify your supervisor and/or legal counsel and discuss the reason for the summons. If a malpractice suit is filed, you should also contact your insurance carrier.

In order to avoid a default judgment, immediately file a response to the summons. Your attorney should file the response. Typically, there is a time limit of 30 days in which the alleged violator has to file his/her response, although this can vary from state to state.

You should work closely with your attorney and take an active role in your response and defense. This is especially critical in health care cases in which the lawyer may need some guidance in understanding the specific circumstances surrounding the alleged violation. You should review the patient's medical records, and educate your attorney accordingly.

It is advisable to attend the patient's deposition. Also, as a witness, you should explain terminology (to help gain the jury's respect) and use demonstrative aids such as videos and audiotapes to explain the type of service being provided to the patient (Trace & Breske, 1993).

STANDARDS OF CARE

Standards are a consumer protection device used to ensure quality services and quality products. ASHA sets three types of standards for the following:

1. The provision of services by individuals to persons with communication disorders;

2. The provision of services by programs to persons with communication disorders;

3. The graduate education of persons providing the services.

Standards are needed to help consumers determine the quality of services and products. It is better to develop standards internally as much as possible. Otherwise, external groups may develop the standards without having adequate understanding of all the issues involved in developing standards that are in the best interest of the consumer, and standards that place reasonable requirements on the service provider.

Standards include policies and procedures. A policy is defined as "broad, current, comprehensive, inviolate, (statements) written to specify responsibility for action" (Bureau of Business Practices, 1988). Procedures are sequences of steps needed to complete a specified activity. Procedures may change frequently; policies are more long-term in nature. A policy and procedure manual is a "consistent guide to be followed under a given set of circumstances" (Rao & Goldsmith, p. 233). The manual serves as a framework for management and staff decision making. It organizes and centralizes the policies and procedures. The content of a policy and procedure manual in a speech-language pathology practice should follow the eight areas of review for accreditation by the Professional Services Board.

In the American Speech-Language-Hearing Association, standards are developed by two councils: the Council on Professional Standards in Speech-Language Pathology and Audiology, an autonomous board appointed by the ASHA Executive Board; and the Standards Council of ASHA. The Standards Council develops standards for the certification of individuals, the accreditation of graduate programs, and the accreditation of professional service delivery programs. They are implemented by three boards:

1. The Clinical Certification Board (review applications for individuals seeking the CCC/SLP or CCC/A);

2. Education Standards Board (accreditation of master's programs in speech-language pathology and audiology);

3. Professional Services Board (accreditation of professional service programs in speech-language pathology and audiology).

Implementation of standards is the responsibility of the operating boards. Implementation includes the development of indexes by which standards may be met and the development of policies and procedures for reviewing applications. (Madell, 1994, p. 53)

Accreditation of graduate programs by the Educational Standards Board is based on a review of five areas: (1) administration, (2) instructional staff, (3) curriculum, (4) clinical education, and (5) program self-analysis.

Accreditation of service programs by the Professional Standards Board is based on eight mandatory standards:

1. Missions, goals, and objectives;

2. Nature and quality of services;

3. Quality improvement and program evaluation (effectiveness and efficiency of services provided);

4. Administration (licensure, leave, federal, state, and local regulations);

5. Financial resources and management;

6. Human resources (continuing education);

7. Physical facilities and program environment;

8. Equipment and materials.

In addition, there are state and federal standards which must be met by various organizations to maintain accreditation.

The Joint Commission on the Accreditation of Healthcare Organizations (JCAHO) is responsible for setting the standards for acute care hospitals, psychiatric facilities, substance abuse and rehabilitation facilities, home health care, hospice services, long-term care facilities, and group homes. The Commission on Accreditation of Rehabilitation Facilities (CARF) sets the standards for rehabilitation organizations including speech-language pathology, occupational therapy, physical therapy, music therapy, vocational therapy, psychological counseling, and recreation therapy programs. They look at the organization, accessibility, safety, and self-evaluation systems. The contact information for JCAHO is as follows:

Joint Commission on the Accreditation of Healthcare Organizations
One Renaissance Boulevard
Oakbrook Terrace, IL 60181
(708) 916-5400.

The contact information for CARF is as follows:

Commission on Accreditation of Rehabilitation Facilities
101 North Wilmot Road
Suite 500
Tucson, AZ 85711
(602) 748-1212.

As a professional speech-language pathologist, you are expected to exercise *more* than reasonable care, and this is defined by ASHA's standard of accepted professional practice. Standards of care can be defined by statutory laws, common law, and professional codes of ethics. Standards of care defined by statutory laws are those created by federal, state, or local legislative bodies. Licensure laws and laws defining the scope of practice fall under the jurisdiction of statutory laws.

Standards of care defined by common law include those that are created as the result of principles that are established through the resolution of prior legal actions. Finally, standards of care defined by the ASHA Code of Ethics define such things as proper evaluation, proper treatment, and appropriate referrals.

ASHA publishes standards of care which outline the reasonable measures that should be taken in the care of patients of speech-language pathologists and audiologists. According to Scott (2000), there are three formulations for the legal standard of care for health care professionals:

1. Traditional rule: Compare defendant with peers in the same community;

2. Modern majority rule: Compare defendant with peers in the same community or in similar communities, state- or nationwide;

3. Trend: Compare defendant with any or all peers, state- or nationwide, acting under the same or similar circumstances (p. 8).

Standards of care are defined nationally by various accrediting agencies, as well as locally by the facilities serving the patients. The speech-language pathologist is responsible for knowing the standards of care that are in effect in any facility in which he/she works.

SUPPORT PERSONNEL

The use of support personnel has emerged as one way to handle the rising costs of health care. However, even though trained paraprofessionals can provide assistance in generalization and maintenance programs, some HMOs/MCOs will not pay unless services are provided by the highest qualified provider. In addition to the use of support personnel, there has been increased need for family involvement since rehab stays are shorter and outpatient services are curtailed. It is critical that the professional identify factors in a family that will minimize or maximize follow-through at home.

In November, 1994, ASHA adopted a position statement on the use of support personnel in speech-language pathology, stressing it supports the use of support personnel, but reminds the speech-language pathologist that "the communication needs and protection of the consumer must be held paramount at all times" (p. 21). ASHA defined support personnel as "people who, following academic and/or on-the-job training, perform tasks as prescribed, directed, and supervised by certified speech-language pathologists" (ASHA, 1995, p. 2; Kayser, 1994, p. 289). The use of support personnel enables a speech-language pathologist to increase the efficiency, availability, and frequency of services provided as long as the personnel are well-trained and well-supervised. However, it should be made clear to a client when a paraprofessional is providing the services, that the speech-language pathologist "retains legal and ethical responsibility for all services provided or omitted" (ASHA, 1995, p. 3). A paraprofessional can conduct speech, language, and/or hearing screenings after having been trained by the supervising clinician. He/she can also provide intervention services that are designed by the supervising clinician, and that do not require any clinical decision making. They can also assist in maintaining clinical records, chart recording, and preparation of clinical materials. In no way, however, should a paraprofessional be involved in clinical decision making, determining eligibility for services, assessing and diagnosing clients, interpreting data, writing assessment or intervention reports, or transmitting clinical information to other professionals (Kayser, 1994).

ASHA recommend that a paraprofessional have an associates degree, or its equivalent. Aides or paraprofessionals in school settings may have different qualifications and scopes of practice depending on the district in which they are hired. A speech-language pathologist should not supervise support personnel until the speech-language pathologist "has completed the ASHA certification examination, the Clinical Fellowship, and two additional years of clinical experience after receiving the Certificate of Clinical Competence in Speech-Language Pathology from ASHA" (ASHA, 1995, p. 42).

ASHA recommends that support personnel be supervised for 30% of their first 90 days of employment, with at least 20% of that 30% being direct supervision. Following the first 90 days, supervision should be at a 20% level with at least 10% being direct. Direct supervision is defined as "on-site, in-view observation and guidance by a speech-language pathologist while an assigned activity is performed by support personnel" (ASHA, 1995, p. 4). Indirect supervision includes demonstrations, review of audio and or videotapes, chart reviews, and/or interactive television. They further recommend that each supervisor should supervise no more than three assistants at one time.

Some school-based clinicians train their paraprofessionals to run computer intervention programs, and to assist in providing classroom-based intervention. However, the supervising clinician should adhere to the ASHA description, particularly with regard to scope of practice, as closely as possible.

Some support personnel fulfill the role of translator or interpreter for students who have limited English skills. They can assist the clinician in providing therapy in their first language if there is a language or speech disorder, or they can serve to facilitate the learning of English as a second language.

Suggested competencies for speech-language pathology assistants include interpersonal skills, personal qualities, and technical assistance skills. Skills related to screening and treatment are also suggested. These are summarized in Table 1–4.

TABLE I-4 Suggested competencies for SLP assistants

  I. Interpersonal Skills (communicates honestly, clearly, accurately, coherently, and concisely)
- A. Deals effectively with attitudes and behaviors of the clients
- B. Uses appropriate language (written and oral) in dealing with clients and others
- C. Deals effectively with supervisor

  II. Personal Qualities
- A. Manages time effectively
- B. Demonstrates appropriate conduct

  III. Technical-Assistance Skills
- A. Maintains a facilitating environment for assigned tasks
- B. Selects, prepares, and presents materials effectively
- C. Maintains documentation
- D. Provides assistance as needed

  IV. Screening
- A. Demonstrates knowledge and use of a variety of screening tools and protocols
- B. Demonstrates appropriate administration and scoring of screening tools
- C. Manages screenings and documentation
- D. Communicates screening results and all supplemental information to supervisor

  V. Treatment
- A. Performs tasks as outlined and instructed by the supervisor
- B. Demonstrates skills in managing behavior and treatment program
- C. Demonstrates knowledge of treatment objectives and plan

From "Guidelines for the Training, Credentialing, Use, and Supervision of Speech-Language Pathology Assistants" by the ASHA Task Force on Support Personnel, December 1995. Reprinted with permission.

BEHAVIOR MANAGEMENT

Operant conditioning through the use of a stimulus-response-contingency paradigm is at the core of the principles of therapy. In using operant conditioning, the clinician is attempting to change a voluntary behavior. To do so, the clinician must understand the relationship between the stimulus and the response, and the response and the contingencies in order to conduct effective and efficient therapy. The contingencies are often referred to as either a reinforcer or a punisher. A matrix to help differentiate between the two is in Table 1–5.

Reinforcement

The presentation of a positive stimulus is positive reinforcement. Positive reinforcement can be in the form of primary reinforcement or secondary reinforcement. Primary reinforcement

TABLE I-5 Behavioral Contingencies Matrix

	Aversive Stimuli	*Positive Stimuli*
Presentation	Punishment I	Positive Reinforcement
Withdrawal	Negative Reinforcement	Punishment II

Adapted from *Clinical Skills for Speech-Language Pathologists* by S. A. Goldberg. 1997, p. 126, San Diego: Singular Publishing Group. Copyright 1997 by Singular Publishing Group. Adapted and reprinted with permission.

encompasses food and/or drink. It can be used to establish a behavior quickly. However, once withdrawn, the behavior frequently extinguishes. Therefore, primary reinforcement should be paired with secondary reinforcement, which is more social in nature. Clapping one's hands, stickers, verbal praise, and a pat on the back are examples of secondary, or social, reinforcement. If secondary reinforcement is paired with primary reinforcement, the primary reinforcement can gradually be withdrawn and the behavior will not extinguish. The clinician is advised to vary the verbal reinforcer, or the words will become essentially meaningless when heard repeatedly. A list of 65 ways to offer a verbal reinforcer is delineated in Table 1–6.

Negative reinforcement is the withdrawal of a negative reinforcer. In the classic behavioral experiments, this could be a low grade electrical shock that would interrupt when the mouse tapped a lever. In the educational setting, this could be the removal of a teacher's stern look or negative body language when the child presents the desired response. With both negative reinforcement and positive reinforcement, the goal is to increase a desired behavior.

The goal is for the therapy activities to become intrinsically reinforcing in and of themselves, so that, gradually, most reinforcers can be removed. That is to say, the activities should be "pleasurable enough so that the individual would engage in it just out of the sheer enjoyment the activity causes" (Goldberg, 1997, p. 126). This is in opposition to extrinsic reinforcement. In this case, reinforcement is found in the completion of the activity. "When the completion of an activity is reinforcing, regardless of the reinforcing quality of the activity itself, the activity is extrinsically reinforcing" (Goldberg, 1997, p. 130).

TABLE 1–6 Words that can be used for social reinforcement

A+ job	Hurray for you	That's incredible
Awesome	I knew you could do it	That's correct
Beautiful sharing	I'm proud of you	That's the best
Beautiful work	Looking good	Way to go
Beautiful	Magnificent	Well done
Bingo	Marvelous	What a good listener
Bravo	Neat	Wow
Creative job	Nice work	You learned it right
Dynamite	Nice job	You tried hard
Excellent	Nothing can stop you now	You're a real trooper
Exceptional performance	Now you're flying	You're a winner
Fantastic	Now you've got it	You're spectacular
Fantastic job	Outstanding performance	You're sensational
Good job	Outstanding	You're beautiful
Good for you	Phenomenal	You're on top of it
Good	Remarkable job	You're on your way
Great discovery	Remarkable	You're on target
Great	Spectacular	You're fantastic
Hip hip hurray	Super	You're incredible
Hot dog	Super job	You're catching on
How nice	Super work	You've discovered the secret
How smart	Terrific	

From *Clinical Skills for Speech-Language Pathologists* by S. A. Goldberg. 1997, p. 126, San Diego: Singular Publishing Group. Copyright 1997 by Singular Publishing Group. Reprinted with permission.

Extraneous reinforcement is a reinforcer that has no relationship to the activity, nor to its completion. It is used to increase and maintain a desired response. Extraneous reinforcers include verbal praise and tokens. A token economy system is one in which the client receives tokens that can be exchanged for a reinforcer of value to the client. The tokens themselves hold no value; the items for which they can be exchanged make them worthwhile. A token economy system can easily be paired with response cost in that a token can be removed if the desired behaviors or responses are not forthcoming.

A frequent activity in therapy with children is the use of a board game in which the child rolls the die or spins a wheel to determine how many places to move his marker. Goldberg (1997) warns that the sequencing of these activities is of critical concern. If the child is allowed to spin the wheel and move his marker prior to giving the correct response, there is no motivation to produce the desired response. Rather, the opportunity to spin the wheel (or roll the die) should be the reinforcing event for giving the desired response. Whether using a game, verbal praise, or a token of some kind, it is critical that the timing of the presentation of the reinforcer be immediately following the desired response. Otherwise, undesired behaviors or responses may inadvertently be reinforced. If the clinician gives an extraneous reinforcer at the end of the session, he/she should take care to let the client know that the reinforcer is for "all the good responses" or "all the fine effort," so there is no confusion as to why the reinforcement is being delivered.

Goldberg (1997) states that, ideally, a therapy activity will involve intrinsic, extrinsic, and extraneous reinforcers. Ideally, the clinician should "first design an intervention program that is intrinsically reinforcing. Then have the completion of the activity be extrinsically reinforcing. Finally, have an extraneous reinforcer available if all else fails" (Goldberg, 1997, p. 132).

Punishment

Punishment is used to reduce or eliminate a behavior. Alberto and Troutman (1986) write that a punishment is a consequent stimulus that:

1. Decreases the future rate and/or probability of occurrence of behavior;

2. Is administered contingently upon the production of an undesired or inappropriate behavior;

3. Is administered immediately following the production of the undesired or inappropriate behavior. (p. 245)

Punishment can take two forms: Punishment I and Punishment II. Punishment I is the presentation of an aversive stimulus. In most educational and therapeutic situations, many forms of Punishment I are not permitted. However, the clinician's saying "No" in a firm voice could be considered the presentation of an aversive stimulus. Punishment II is the same as response cost. Response cost is the withdrawal of a positive reinforcer. This could include time-out, because the child is removed from the opportunity to be reinforced. An example of response cost is the removal of a token from a child due to an incorrect response or an undesired behavior.

Setting Behavioral Goals

Writing Behavioral Objectives

Behavioral objectives are written for three reasons. First, the clinician needs behavioral objectives as a "roadmap toward remediation." Behavioral objectives help to state clearly what is expected with regard to client accomplishment as a result of the therapeutic process. Second, they become a standard against which to determine client progress in therapy. Behavioral objectives help bridge the gap between the results of the assessment and the beginning of therapy by summarizing the client's strengths and weaknesses to provide a focus for therapy. Behavioral objectives form a basis of continuing assessment for the measurement of improvement by the client. Finally, they are written to communicate to the client exactly what is expected. The client and/or his family needs to participate in deciding what goals are most important, which ones should be addressed first, and which goals will have the most dramatic impact on improving communication (Meyer, 1998).

Behavioral objectives consist of four parts: who is performing the behavior, what is to be done (the performance), how it is to be done (condition), and the criteria. This is true regardless of whether or not one is writing a short-term objective, or a long-term objective. Short-term objectives are written to define the small steps needed to accomplish the long-term goals. For each short-term objective, procedures for obtaining those objectives must be specified. Typically, the short-term objectives paired with the procedures define a lesson plan. Following is an example of a long-term objective and accompanying short-term objectives.

Long Term Objective: Sam will correctly produce the phoneme /t/ in the initial position in conversation with 90–100% accuracy.

Short-Term Objectives:

1. Sam will correctly produce the phoneme /t/ in isolation with 90–95% accuracy following a model;

2. Sam will correctly produce the phoneme /t/ in isolation with 90–95% accuracy spontaneously;

3. Sam will correctly produce the phoneme /t/ in the initial position of single-syllable words with 90–95% accuracy following a model;

4. Sam will independently correctly produce the phoneme /t/ in the initial position of single-syllable words with 90–95% accuracy spontaneously.

When setting behavioral change goals, the clinician should keep in mind the following factors:

1. The necessity for stating goals in objective, measurable terms;

2. The assurance that achieving the goal will benefit the (client) more than the school or institution;

3. A reasonable degree of certainty that achieving the goal is realistic for the (client);

4. The assurance that the program will help the (client) develop appropriate behaviors, not just suppress inappropriate ones;

5. The certainty that a behavior to be changed is not one which is protected by (clients') constitutional rights. (Alberto & Troutman, p. 47)

A behavioral goal consists of 4 parts:

1. Who;

2. What behavior is to be targeted;

3. Under what conditions the behavior will occur;

4. The criteria.

An example of a short-term objective (or goal) is, "Joe will produce /r/ in the postvocalic position without a model with 80–90% accuracy on 20 trials for 3 consecutive sessions." It is best to write discrete goals; that is, only one behavior should be addressed per short-term goal.

Setting Criteria for Responses

Criteria can be set in one of four ways:

1. Percentage of correct responses;

2. Number of consecutive correct responses;

3. Percentage of time;

4. Absolute amount of time.

The percentage of correct responses should always be reported in terms of the percentage and the number of trials (Goldberg, 1997). Achieving 80% accuracy on five trials is therapeutically different from maintaining 80% accuracy over twenty trials. Criterion for success typically should be around 90%. It is probably best to put a range of acceptable response levels, such as 80–90% for two or more consecutive sessions. By specifying two or more consecutive sessions, the clinician can be reassured that the new skill is truly incorporated into the client's repertoire of behaviors. By specifying a range, the clinician allows for individual variability from day to day.

Criteria based on the number of consecutive correct responses does not have data in the literature to support its use (Goldberg, 1997). The primary question to be asked is what criteria to set. How many consecutive responses are needed to insure mastery? There is no answer for this question.

Percentage of time is primarily used to measure either attending behavior or in-seat behaviors. A more efficient type of treatment would be to modify the activities so there would be a concomitant decrease in the behaviors that contribute to lack of attending, or lack of in-seat behaviors. However, another use of percentage of time could be in stuttering therapy. The clinician may wish to measure the percentage of time during a session in which a client is fluent.

Also known as duration recording (Alberto & Troutman, 1986), the absolute amount of time refers to the length of time within the session that the client engages in a specified behavior. This type of data is most useful when measuring discrete behaviors that have a clearly defined onset and conclusion.

APPENDIX I-A: ASHA CODE OF ETHICS

Preamble

The preservation of the highest standards of integrity and ethical principles is vital to the responsible discharge of obligations in the professions of speech-language pathology and audiology. This Code of Ethics sets forth the fundamental principles and rules considered essential to this purpose.

Every individual who is (a) a member of the American Speech-Language-Hearing Association, whether certified or not, (b) a nonmember holding the Certificate of Clinical Competence from the Association, (c) an applicant for membership or certification, or (d) a Clinical Fellow seeking to fulfill standards for certification shall abide by this Code of Ethics.

Any action that violates the spirit and purpose of this Code shall be considered unethical. Failure to specify any particular responsibility or practice in this Code of Ethics shall not be construed as denial of the existence of such responsibilities or practices.

The fundamentals of ethical conduct are described by Principles of Ethics and by Rules of Ethics as they relate to responsibility to persons served, to the public, and to the professions of speech-language pathology and audiology.

Principles of Ethics, aspirational and inspirational in nature, form the underlying moral basis for the Code of Ethics. Individuals shall observe these principles as affirmative obligations under all conditions of professional activity.

Rules of Ethics are specific statements of minimally acceptable professional conduct or of prohibitions and are applicable to all individuals.

Principles of Ethics I

Individuals shall honor their responsibility to hold paramount the welfare of persons they serve professionally.

Rules of Ethics

A. Individuals shall provide all services competently.

B. Individuals shall use every resource, including referral when appropriate, to ensure that high-quality service is provided.

C. Individuals shall not discriminate in the delivery of professional services on the basis of race or ethnicity, gender, age, religion, national origin, sexual orientation, or disability.

D. Individuals shall fully inform the persons they serve of the nature and possible effects of services rendered and products dispensed.

E. Individuals shall evaluate the effectiveness of services rendered and of products dispensed and shall provide services or dispense products only when benefit can reasonably be expected.

F. Individuals shall not guarantee the results of any treatment or procedure, directly or by implication; however, they may make a reasonable statement of prognosis.

G. Individuals shall not evaluate or treat speech, language, or hearing disorders solely by correspondence.

H. Individuals shall maintain adequate records of professional services rendered and products dispensed and shall allow access to these records when appropriately authorized.

I. Individuals shall not reveal, without authorization, any professional or personal information about the person served professionally, unless required by law to do so, or unless doing so is necessary to protect the welfare of the person or of the community.

J. Individuals shall not charge for services not rendered, nor shall they misrepresent,[1] in any fashion, services rendered or products dispensed.

K. Individuals shall use persons in research or as subjects of teaching demonstrations only with their informed consent.

L. Individuals whose professional services are adversely affected by substance abuse or other health-related conditions shall seek professional assistance and, where appropriate, withdraw from the affected areas of practice.

Principle of Ethics II

Individuals shall honor their responsibility to achieve and maintain the highest level of professional competence.

Rules of Ethics

A. Individuals shall engage in the provision of clinical services only when they hold the appropriate Certificate of Clinical Competence or when they are in the certification process and are supervised by an individual who holds the appropriate Certificate of Clinical Competence.

B. Individuals shall engage in only those aspects of the professions that are within the scope of their competence, considering their level of education, training, and experience.

C. Individuals shall continue their professional development throughout their careers.

D. Individuals shall delegate the provision of clinical services only to persons who are certified or to persons in the education or certification process who are appropriately supervised. The provision of support services may be delegated to persons who are neither certified nor in the certification process only when a certificate holder provides appropriate supervision.

E. Individuals shall prohibit any of their professional staff from providing services that exceed the staff member's competence, considering the staff member's level of education, training, and experience.

---

[1]For purposes of this Code of Ethics, misrepresentation includes any untrue statements or statements that are likely to mislead. Misrepresentation also includes the failure to state any information that is material and that ought, in fairness, to be considered.

F.   Individuals shall ensure that all equipment used in the provision of services is in proper working order and is properly calibrated.

Principle of Ethics III

Individuals shall honor their responsibility to the public by promoting public understanding of the professions, by supporting the development of services designed to fulfill the unmet needs of the public, and by providing accurate information in all communications involving any aspect of the professions.

Rules of Ethics

A.   Individuals shall not misrepresent their credentials, competence, education, training, or experience.

B.   Individuals shall not participate in professional activities that constitute a conflict of interest.

C.   Individuals shall not misrepresent diagnostic information, services rendered, or products dispensed or engage in any scheme or artifice to defraud in connection with obtaining payment or reimbursement for such services or products.

D.   Individuals' statements to the public shall provide accurate information about the nature and management of communication disorders, about the professions, and about professional services.

E.   Individuals' statements to the public—advertising, announcing, and marketing their professional services, reporting research results, and promoting products—shall adhere to prevailing professional standards and shall not contain misrepresentations.

Principle of Ethics IV

Individuals shall honor their responsibilities to the professions and their relationships with colleagues, students, and members of allied professions. Individuals shall uphold the dignity and autonomy of the professions, maintain harmonious interprofessional and intraprofessional relationships, and accept the professions' self-imposed standards.

Rules of Ethics

A.   Individuals shall prohibit anyone under their supervision from engaging in any practice that violates the Code of Ethics.

B.   Individuals shall not engage in dishonesty, fraud, deceit, misrepresentation, or any form of conduct that adversely reflects on the profession's or on the individual's fitness to serve persons professionally.

C.   Individuals shall assign credit only to those who have contributed to a publication, presentation, or product. Credit shall be assigned in proportion to the contribution and only with the contributor's consent.

D. Individuals' statements to colleagues about professional services, research results, and products shall adhere to prevailing professional standards and shall contain no misrepresentations.

E. Individuals shall not provide professional services without exercising independent professional judgment, regardless of referral source or prescription.

F. Individuals shall not discriminate in their relationships with colleagues, students, and members of allied professions on the basis of race or ethnicity, gender, age, religion, national origin, sexual orientation, or disability.

G. Individuals who have reason to believe that the Code of Ethics has been violated shall inform the Ethical Practice Board.

H. Individuals shall cooperate fully with the Ethical Practice Board in its investigation and adjudication of matters related to this Code of Ethics.

APPENDIX 1-B: STATEMENT OF PRACTICES AND PROCEDURES

The Ethical Practice Board (EPB) is charged by the Bylaws of the American Speech-Language-Hearing Association with the responsibility to interpret, administer, and enforce the Code of Ethics of the Association. Accordingly, the EPB hereby adopts the following practices and procedures to be followed in administering and enforcing that Code.

A fundamental precept that guides the EPB in the discharge of its responsibility is that an effective Code of Ethics requires an orderly and fair administration and enforcement of its terms and requires full compliance by all members of the Association and all holders of Certificates of Clinical Competence. The EPB recognizes that each case must be judged on an individual basis, and that no two cases are likely to be identical. Thus, the EPB has the responsibility to exercise its judgment on the merits of each case and on its interpretation of the Code.

A. Definitions of Terms:

1. EPB: Ethical Practice Board;

2. Association: American Speech-Language-Hearing Association;

3. Code: Code of Ethics of the Association;

4. Certificate(s): Certificate(s) of Clinical Competence;

5. Respondent: The alleged offender;

6. Complainant(s): The person(s) alleging that a violation occurred;

7. Initial Determination: Initial Determination by the EPB, subject to Further Consideration and appeal, of the (a) finding, (b) proposed sanction, and (c) extent of disclosure;

8. Sanction(s): Penalties imposed by the EPB;

9. Disclosure: Announcement of the final EPB Decision to other than Respondent;

10. Further Consideration: Further consideration by the EPB of its Initial Determination;

11. EPB Decision: Final decision of the EPB after: (a) Further Consideration; or (b) 30 days from the date of notice on the Initial Determination by the EPB if no request for Further Consideration is received;

12. Appeal: Written request from Respondent to EPB alleging error in the EPB Decision and asking that it be reversed in whole or in part by the Executive Board.

B. Investigative Procedures

1. Alleged violations shall be reviewed by the EPB in such manner as the EPB may, in its discretion, deem necessary and proper. If, after review, the EPB elects to investigate the allegation, the EPB shall notify Respondent of the alleged offense in writing and shall advise Respondent that Respondent's answer to the allegation shall be in writing and must be received by the EPB no later than 45 days after the date of the EPB notice to

Respondent. Voluntary resignation of membership and/or voluntary surrender of the Certificate(s) shall not preclude the EPB from continuing to process the alleged violation to conclusion, and the notice from the EPB to Respondent requesting an answer shall so advise Respondent.

2. At the discretion of the EPB, the Director of the Professional Affairs Department of the Association's National Office may be informed that Respondent is under investigation by the EPB for alleged violation of the Code and may be instructed that no change in membership and/or certification status shall be permitted without approval of the EPB.

3. The EPB shall consider all information secured from its investigation, including Respondent's answer to the allegation, and shall base its Initial Determination on that information.

4. If the EPB finds that there is not sufficient evidence to warrant further proceedings, Respondent and Complainant(s) shall be so advised and the investigation shall be terminated.

5. If the EPB finds that there is sufficient evidence to warrant further proceedings, the EPB shall make an Initial Determination, which includes (a) the finding of violation, (b) the proposed sanction, and (c) the proposed extent of disclosure. In this regard, the final decision of any State, Federal, regulatory, or judicial body may be considered sufficient evidence that the Code was violated.

6. The EPB may, as part of its Initial Determination, order that the Respondent cease and desist from any practice found to be a violation of the Code. Failure to comply with such a Cease and Desist Order is, itself, a violation of the Code, and shall normally result in Revocation of Membership and/or Revocation of Certificate(s).

7. The EPB shall give Respondent notice of its Initial Determination. The notice shall also advise Respondent of the right to request Further Consideration by the EPB and of the right, after Further Consideration, to request an appeal to the Executive Board. The procedures to be followed in exercising those rights are described in Sections F and G of this statement.

C. Notices and Answers

All notices and answers shall be in writing and considered to be given or furnished (a) to the Respondent when sent—Certified Mail, Addressee Only, Return Receipt Requested—to the address then listed in the ASHA membership records, and (b) to the EPB when received by the EPB.

D. Sanctions

Sanctions shall consist of one or more of the following: Reprimand; Censure; Withhold, Suspend, or Revoke Membership; Withhold, Suspend, or Revoke the Certificate(s); or other measures determined by the EPB at its discretion.

E. Disclosure

1. The EPB Decision, upon becoming final, shall be published in the journal *Asha* unless the sanction is Reprimand. In the case of Reprimand, the EPB Decision normally shall be disclosed only to Respondent, Respondent's counsel, Complainant(s), witnesses at the EPB Further Consideration hearing, staff, and Association counsel, each of whom shall be advised that the decision is strictly confidential and that any breach of that confidentiality by any party who is a member and/or certificate holder of the Association is, itself, a violation of the Code.

2. In appropriate cases, including when the sanction is Reprimand, the EPB may also determine that its Decision shall be disclosed to aggrieved parties and/or other appropriate individuals, bodies, or agencies.

F. Further Consideration by the EPB of the Initial Determination

1. When the notice of Initial Determination from the EPB states that Respondent has violated the Code and announces a proposed sanction and extent of disclosure, the Respondent may request that the EPB give Further Consideration to the Initial Determination.

2. Respondent's request for Further Consideration shall be in writing and must be *received* by the EPB Chair no later than 30 days after the date of notice of Initial Determination. *The request for Further Consideration must specify in what respects the Initial Determination was allegedly wrong and why.* In the absence of a timely request for Further Consideration, the Initial Determination shall be the EPB Decision, which decision shall be final: There shall be no further right of appeal to the Executive Board.

3. If Respondent submits a timely request for Further Consideration by the EPB, the EPB shall schedule a hearing and notify Respondent. At the hearing, Respondent shall be entitled to submit a written brief or to appear personally to present evidence and to be accompanied by counsel. The proceeding shall be informal; strict adherence to the rules of evidence shall not be observed, but all evidence shall be accorded such weight as it deserves. As an alternative to personal appearance at the hearing, the EPB shall afford Respondent the opportunity to make a presentation to the EPB and to respond to questions from the EPB via a conference telephone call placed to Respondent by the EPB. All personal costs in connection with the Further Consideration hearing, including travel and lodging costs incurred by Respondent and Respondent's counsel and witnesses, and counsel and other fees, shall be Respondent's sole responsibility. The hearing shall be transcribed in full, and, upon request, a copy of the transcript shall be made available to Respondent at Respondent's sole expense.

4. After the Further Consideration Hearing, the EPB shall render its decision and notify Respondent. If evidence presented at the hearing warrants, the EPB may modify the finding, increase or decrease the severity of the sanction, and/or modify the extent of disclosure that was announced to Respondent in the Initial Determination. This decision shall be the EPB Decision, and, in the absence of a timely appeal to the Executive Board, the EPB Decision shall be final.

G. Appeal of EPB Decision to Executive Board

1. Respondent may appeal the EPB Decision to the Executive Board when that decision requires revocation of membership and/or certification or when the decision requires disclosure of the sanction in the journal *Asha*. The request for appeal shall be in writing and must be received by the EPB Chair no later than 30 days after the date of notice of the EPB Decision. *The request for appeal shall specify in what respects the EPB Decision was allegedly wrong and why.*

2. The procedures for a hearing before the Executive Board are described in the *Executive Board Statement of Practices and Procedures for Appeals of Decisions of the Ethical Practice Board.*

H. Reinstatement

Persons whose membership or certification has been revoked may, upon application therefore, be reinstated after one year upon a two-thirds vote of the EPB. If the application is received five years or more after revocation, current membership or certification requirements must also be met.

In all cases, the applicant bears the burden of demonstrating with appropriate documentation that conditions that led to revocation have been rectified and that, upon reinstatement, applicant will abide by the Code. The EPB's deliberations will be guided by the premise that reinstatement is in the best interest of the Association and of persons served professionally.

I. Amendment

This *Statement of Practices and Procedures* may be amended upon recommendation of the EPB and a vote of the Executive Board. All such changes will be given appropriate publicity.

CHAPTER TWO
Counseling

Counseling is an important part of the assessment, diagnostic, and intervention aspects of speech-language pathology. However, it remains one of the most undertaught skills in our profession. This chapter will address the definition and role of counseling, determining a patient's status, and three types of counseling interviews.

DEFINITION AND ROLE OF COUNSELING

ASHA's Preferred Practice Patterns delineate the specific purpose of counseling as "to provide patients/clients and their families with information and support, make appropriate referrals to other professionals, and help patients/clients to develop problem-solving strategies to enhance the (re)habilitation process" (ASHA, 1993, p. 19). Also, according to ASHA, the expected outcome of counseling is

> to develop appropriate goals for recovery from, adjustment to, or prevention of a communication or related disorder by facilitating change and growth in which patients/clients become more autonomous, more self-directing, and more responsible for achieving their potential and realizing their goals to communicate more effectively (ASHA, 1993, p. 19).

The primary role of counseling is to match the client's perceptions with external reality. It is important when the client's impairment has reached a point of being a handicap or a disability. Disability can cause tension, anxiety, loss of self-esteem, and a lowered quality of life. These aspects of one's coping strategies, as well as the client's perception of problematic/ disordered speech vs. non-problematic differences can be assisted through counseling (Crowe, 1997).

There are times when counseling is not within the realm of the speech-language pathologist's training. For example, if the primary problem is something other than the speech, language, and/or hearing deficit, the client should be referred to another more appropriate counselor, such as a psychiatrist or a psychologist. Emotional problems that eclipse the communication problems, and the presence of mental disorders that are unrelated to the communication disorder, should also be referred. Certainly, there are professional boundaries that should not be crossed in a relationship between a client and the speech-language pathologist. For example, if the client presents with sexual or relationship problems related to the communication disorder, and counseling takes prevalence over the communication disorder, this individual should be referred for other types of counseling (Crowe, 1997).

There is a distinct difference between counseling and psychotherapy. The goal of psychotherapy, which is often long-term, is to recognize the person's conflicts within himself (severe anxiety, clinical depression, persistent guilt, etc.) and is accomplished by a trained counselor or psychologist. Psychotherapy attempts to restructure the personality, especially in terms of a particular theoretical orientation about the nature and dynamics of personality. In psychotherapy, the patient is generally viewed as being ill and, as a result, searches for the cause or etiology of a person's problems. Counseling, on the other hand, deals with the present, with here-and-now strategies for coping with life, decision making, and current problems. Instead of a medical illness approach, a learning model is employed whereby the counselor helps clients to become aware of themselves, of what they believe and feel, and of how these things affect what they do and how they interact with society. Counseling is often related to specific types of situations, such as the onset of a communication disorder (Shames, 2000).

Counseling by the speech-language pathologist is appropriate when it is part of a holistic approach. Self-reliant clinicians and clients focus on the present and on those changes that can be made now in the pursuit of personal growth. Growth can only occur when the client feels the control and power of the present and challenges a perceived negative or stagnant self-image. Although the clinician may employ counseling techniques in the treatment of any communication disorder, it is particularly important in the treatment of voice and fluency disorders, and in the treatment of clients with lifelong and/or life threatening illnesses, such as ALS and cancer. Counseling with the client and his/her family and caregivers is necessary when one reaches the generalization and maintenance stages of therapy. Care must be taken during the cognitive stages of therapy not to make the client too dependent on the clinician-client relationship in order to succeed. Another problem that affects generalization and maintenance is when the client is struggling with disabling emotions, that is, he may be getting more out of being disabled than being healed.

It is important that the client's self-concept be addressed throughout therapy. The clinician must take into account the question, "Is my client's self concept altered by the presence or absence of the communication disorder?" Do the disabling emotions continue even after the communication disorder is resolved? Therapy should address the cognitive and affective components of the client's self-concept. Clients should be taught that it takes less personal strength to support coping behaviors than to support defensive, resigning, and/or withdrawing behaviors. Occasionally, the speech-language pathologist may be faced with a client who has a psychogenic communication disorder. In these cases, it is necessary to demonstrate didactically that therapy is not needed. It is important in these cases to address the client's fears and concerns, and not to dismiss their concerns too quickly. This is because the perceived disorders are very real to the client. It may become necessary to refer these clients for further professional help from a psychiatrist or psychologist.

INTERPERSONAL NATURE OF COMMUNICATION

When counseling a client with a communication disorder, the speech-language pathologist has to consider the client's actual ability to communicate. Is the client able to express his thoughts and feelings adequately, or does he depend on someone else to speak for him? If so, how can we know that the caregiver is adequately expressing the client's concerns? It is also important to observe the client's and family members' attitudes toward communication. Attitudes may vary depending on the setting and the people with whom the client is attempting to communicate. Thus, through counseling, one hopes to obtain an improvement in an individual's quality of life through a decrease in the negative physical and psychological effects of the communication disorder.

In counseling situations, the clinician is often dealing with a client and/or his family at a time when they are quite vulnerable. In the case of parents with a newborn child with birth defects, there are shattered dreams as to what they had imagined their child would be. A spouse may bemoan his or her shattered dreams when his loved one suffers an event that leads to impaired communication. Similarly, the client goes through a period of shattered dreams with regard to what he had envisioned for the remainder of his life. Yet, at a time when these individuals are most vulnerable, we are asking them to embrace a whole new way of learning.

It is important to develop a dialogue with the client. The aim of dialogue is not to give opinions, but to provide the client with guidance in developing coping strategies. Dialogue is a form of communication that imposes certain duties upon the questioner. The questioner has a duty to listen to all responses, and to be responsive to would-be answers. Through the use of critical questions, the listener should be sure he/she fully understands and assesses the responses. The responder in a dialogue has a responsibility to act responsibly, and to recognize and accept the responsibility to explain, clarify, and, if need be, defend one's responses before the one asking the questions (Zaner, 1993).

It is critical that the problem be clarified. A problem can denote either a shelter under which one hides from reality, or an obstacle that keeps one from reaching desired goals. Whether a shelter or an obstacle, it is a disturbance that needs to be resolved. Sometimes, an impasse is reached. The impasses themselves call for choices and decisions. As an appeal for a response, each situation is tied to specific circumstances, even though these and the problems they pose may not have been clearly understood or recognized as such. But the problems are present and pressing even as a person fails or refuses to acknowledge them (Zaner, 1993).

A critical question is, "Is the client's self-concept altered by the presence or absence of the communication disorder?" According to Zaner (1993), we need to look at things from the point of view of the person with the impairment. People who have an impairment not only want to know what is wrong, why they are hurting, what can be expected, and what can and should be done about it, but they also want to know whether anybody *cares*, and whether the people to *take care of* them also *care for* them.

Empathy

Clients may perceive that the speech-language pathologist is the "only person who understands their travail and is the only person in whom they can confide their fears and concerns about living life as persons with communicative disorders. If clinicians counsel with their clients about these concerns, mainly by being empathic listeners, their clients might not only resolve their fears but in the process also take responsibility and find direction to correct their communicative disorders" (Crowe, 1997, p. 24). Thus, the clinician needs to create an environment in which the patient can take charge of his life.

Empathy is not the same as sympathy. According to the Random House Dictionary of the English Language, empathy is "the intellectual identification with or vicarious experiencing of the feelings, thoughts, or attitudes of another person" (p. 433). On the other hand, sympathy is defined as "a quality of mutual relations between people or things whereby whatever affects one also affects the other," and "the ability to share the feelings of another, especially in sorrow or trouble; compassion or commiseration." While we can experience the pain of a communication disorder, we cannot specifically feel the feelings that the affected person and/or his family members are feeling. The clinician should never say, "I know how you feel" because an impairment or disability affects everyone differently. Therefore, based on our experience, we can understand the feelings of the affected person, but we cannot know how they feel.

Awareness Levels

Clients and their family members are typically at one of three levels of awareness with regard to the communication disorder. The first level is minimal awareness. The client at this level refuses to recognize the abnormalities. They may look for other causes, frequently unfounded, to explain the symptoms. They believe that treatment will cure the problem, and that life will not be affected by the communication disorder.

The second level of awareness is the level of partial awareness. The individual at the level of partial awareness describes the symptoms they have observed, and asks questions about their etiology. They hope for improvement, but have a nagging fear that it will not come. They also question their ability to cope. As professionals, we feel that the client (or family member) has some awareness of the true problem and is on his way to the third level of awareness.

Considerable awareness is the third level of awareness. The individual at this level will blatantly state that he or his family member has an impairment or a disability. He recognizes the limitations of treatment, but hopes that some improvement will result from intervention. This individual will request information about appropriate treatment, education, etc.

The levels of awareness also parallel the steps of the grief process which most clients and/or their family members will experience at the onset of an illness or impairment.

THE GRIEF PROCESS

The clinician's interaction with the grieving client can significantly impact the client's ultimate acceptance of the impairment, and also affect his motivation and desire for intervention. It is critical that the clinician understands the grief process because interruption of the process can reduce the client's motivation for therapy. It can also interfere with the client-clinician relationship. Short and long-term goals can be altered and/or postponed when the grief process is interrupted. The interference can also lead to the maintenance of counter-productive measures (Tanner, 1980).

The grieving process lets the client "buy time to find the inner strength needed to deal with" the loss (McFarlane, Fujiki, & Brinton, 1984, p. 7). Since grieving is a natural and necessary process, it makes sense that the grieving individual needs acceptance, not judgment, as they experience the components of the grief process. He needs to know that it is all right to have the emotions that he is experiencing. If clients "are allowed to share these feelings without being patronized or judged, most will eventually emerge capable of dealing with the problem. However, if such feelings are repressed, this emergence may be significantly delayed" (McFarlane et al., 1984, p. 7).

Clinicians should also be aware that there is not always a linear progression through the grief process, and that individuals vary in how long they take to work through the entire process. Sometimes a client may plateau at one of the stages. Sometimes he may regress to a previous stage, although it typically takes less time to re-emerge from a stage when it is being revisited.

Denial

The first stage of the grief process is denial. Denial is typically experienced at the onset of the impairment, or delayed until the realization that the condition is permanent, or that no cures exist. Denial also occurs when the client realizes he cannot ignore the disability or dismiss it as temporary. Denial is a double-edged sword because it "provides the needed hope that helps you get through many difficult days, but if maintained too long can eventually interfere with realistic efforts at community integration" (DiLima, 1995, p. 19). According to Crowe (1997), denial is a primitive defense used to reject the existence of a painful or frightening reality.

Kubler-Ross (1969) identified three factors that might influence the existence and recalcitrance of denial in grieving:

1. The accuracy and completeness of information about the illness or disorder determine if and for how long an individual will express denial. If accurate and full insight emerge only after considerable time, denial might also extend over time and acceptance be delayed.

2. The time an individual needs to resolve grief might affect duration and intensity of denial. A patient facing imminent death has only a short time to work through the grief stages, so he may be feeling the pressure of time and the need to come to terms with fate before confronting it. Others may see the inevitablity of fate with so much dread that they become fixated in denial, or any, stages of grief. On the other hand, those who are experiencing a long-term illness or disability may not feel they are in any hurry to come out of denial. Others with long-term problems may very quickly decide that the problems are real, that they are not going to go away, but that they intend to lead productive lives regardless of the impairment. These individuals are anxious to work through the grief and proceed with therapy.

3. An individual's premorbid tendency to rely on denial as a defense against life's pressures increases the probability and intensity of its presence with illness or disability. If a client used denial as a buffer against bad news prior to the onset of the communication disorder, he is likely to stay in the denial stage longer after the onset. In fact, for many of these individuals, denial is the most prominent stage of the grief process.

The client's grieving may continue for some time after therapy has begun, but it should progressively show signs of weakening and yielding to other defenses that do not interfere as much with the intervention process.

Anger

Anger is the second stage of the grief process. Clients in the anger stage exhibit passive-aggressive behaiors. They ask the question, "Why me?" When clients ask this question, it is important for the clinician to realize how the client understands his problems, and how that understanding is related to his mechanisms.

The individual in the anger stage may resent the clinician and caregivers, and may be a difficult individual with whom to deal. Anger may be misdirected at the clinician, but the clinician needs to remember that the anger is a consequence of the loss, and not a reaction to intervention (Tanner, 1999). The degree of anger may depend, to some degree, on the potential for the diagnosis to be disabling, and on its prognosis. Individuals who have an organic etiology may feel more anger because of the potential for the diagnosis to be more debilitating. There may be secondary crises associated with the diagnosis, including role reversals, financial problems, job-related consequences, mental health problems, relationship issues, and self-concept issues (Crowe, 1997).

Subtle signs of unexpresed anger include vocal and nonvocal displacement behaviors directed toward clinicians and/or family members. Little enthusiasm for therapy, a high frustration level, and intattention may also be signs of unexpressed anger. The clinician needs to recognize these signs and help the client work through his anger so that it no longer remains an interfering factor in treatment.

To help the client cope with his anger, the clinician should remain nonjudgmental and offer strong, consistent reinforcement of the client's attempts to achieve his goals in therapy. Continued counseling can help the client examine and express his anger and channel it in productive directions. Strong support from family members and significant others is critical in extending the comfort of therapy into the client's natural environments. Early success in therapy can also help to abate the anger (Crowe, 1997).

Bargaining

Bargaining is a universal and life-sustaining behavior that we learn from childhood. Bargaining helps the client to set and achieve goals by bargaining with himself through self-reinforcement. It helps the client to gradually accept the shock of the disability or impairment by creating a middle-ground when interpersonal disputes occur (Crowe, 1997).

According to Tanner, the individual who is at the bargaining stage is trying to delay the loss or reduce the effects of the loss in the only way he knows how to (Tanner, 1999). The client at this stage is often highly motivated and enthusiastic regarding the prospects of therapy because he may believe that, if he does what the clinician requests, he will get his communication abilities restored. Bargaining is the point in the "grieving process where the stage can be set for therapy success or failure. Clients who believe in their bargaining potency are eager to initiate therapy and negotiate therapy contracts with their clinicians" (Crowe, 1997, p. 37).

Depression

The fourth stage of the grief process is depression. Depression may be characterized by irritability, loss of appetite, and a poor sleep-wake cycle. Depression occurs "when a client realizes that denial, anger, and bargaining were to no avail and that he or she is left with no course other than to accept the facts of an illness or disability" (Crowe, 1997, p. 37).

Depression can be a good or bad sign. As a good sign, it heralds the arrival of acceptance. However, if it becomes self-perpetuating, it can become a major barrier to progress in therapy (Crowe, 1997).

Kubler-Ross (1969) distinguishes between two types of depression:

1. Reactive depression: This is a reaction to the associated events of the loss. It may include reactions over the cost of hospital care and pharmaceuticals, isolation, and the loss of attractiveness. The client with reactive depression may exaggerate the significance of the loss.

2. Preparatory depression: Preparatory depression occurs in the terminally ill client who is preparing for his final separation from this world. Attempts to cheer up the client with preparatory depression devalue the significance of the loss.

Wohlman (1989) notes that "depression is differentiated from terms such as sadness, unhappiness, and sorrow because depression, unlike those emotions, involves feelings of helplessness, and a personal sense of guilt for being helpless" (Crowe, 1997, p. 38). The client who has depression may give up on therapy and lose his hope for improvement. A downward emotional spiral can be created when the client assumes self-blame that leads to a loss of self-esteem. The loss of self-esteem may lead to increased guilt which, in turn, deepens the sense of depression. The client who is in the throes of depression will make little progress in therapy. An individual with severe depression should be referred to a psychologist or psychiatrist for further counseling.

Crowe (1997) points out that depression is the reverse feeling of anger. The individual who is angry becomes aggressive toward all those who are perceived to be involved with his loss. However, the person with depression becomes passive, although there may be a increase in anxiety, with the development of obsessive behaviors and thoughts. How long the depression lasts may depend on the actual disabling potential of the loss, and the client's perceptions of difference, disorder, and handicap. Since an organic loss has a poorer prognosis, depression may last longer in those cases than in those with a functional loss. Finally, the prognosis for correction or compensation for the loss also affects the duration of the depression stage (Crowe, 1997).

Acceptance

Once the client reaches the stage of acceptance, he no longer needs to expend energy on the psychological resolution of his loss, and he can channel all his energies toward rehabilitation (Tanner, 1999). "Acceptance symbolizes a client's conscious awareness of the reality that he or she is and may always be a person with a communicative disorder until an earnest attempt is made to do something about it" (Crowe, 1997, p. 39). Acceptance symbolizes resolution of the loss, and an acceptance of the situation (but not necessarily its limits) (Tanner, 1999).

Crowe (1997) points out the need to differentiate between resignation and acceptance. Resignation indicates that the individual has accepted his fate and feels helpless to do anything about the future. Acceptance, on the other hand, is the result of acknowledgment of the realities of one's fate. We can help clients remain at a level of acceptance by explaining to them, carefully and in detail, evaluation results, prognosis, and therapy procedures and rationales. However, the clinician should remain vigilant to his/her client's level of motivation and not assume that, because the client has reached the level of acceptance, motivation is not longer a concern. Remember, that a client can regress to any stage of the grief process at any time. For example, if progress is not as rapid as the client had hoped, he may regress to the anger or depression stage (Crowe, 1997).

CLINICAL INTERVIEWING

An interview is an interpersonal and efficient way of obtaining and providing information. Even though one may have a case history completed by the client before the first meeting, "new information can emerge about the origin, course, and present state of the problem as well as the informant's and/or client's feelings and attitudes" (Shipley, 1992, p. 7). An interview also helps to clarify and elaborate on information received in the case history, and to give information about the client's thoughts and beliefs, which typically are not fully expressed on a case history form.

An interview is defined by as "a communicative event between someone with specific knowledge or expertise in an area and someone who would presumably benefit from that expertise" (Shipley, 1992, p. 7). It typically involves a dyadic exchange. There are four functions of an interview:

1. Amplify: if information provided is insufficient or irrelevant

2. Clarify: if information is vague, ambiguous, or inconsistent

3. Verify: if information received is unreliable (e.g., if there are inconsistencies in verbal behaviors and responses). One can typically get more information from the verbal exchange by listening for what is not said as well as to what is said. The clinician should look for inconsistencies and gaps. For example, do the client's words express concern, but not his voice and other mannerisms.

4. To influence someone's behavior and/or attitudes. (Shipley, 1992).

THREE TYPES OF INTERVIEWS

There are three types of interviews which a speech-language pathologist typically uses: information-getting interviews, information-giving interviews, and counseling interviews.

Information-Getting Interviews

The information-getting interview should be a routine part of the diagnostic process because the information gained can be a crucial determinant in diagnosis and planning remediation. In an information-getting interview, the clinician obtains objective information, such as dates, specific conditions, and events that preceded the problem. He/she also seeks subjective information, such as attitudes and feelings about the problems being experienced.

Important questions to ask in an information-getting interview include the following:

1. When and how did the problem develop?

2. Has the problem changed since it was first noticed?

3. Are there times the problem varies, or circumstances that create fluctuations in the difficulties?

4. How do the client, family members, and/or caregivers react to the communicative problem?

5. Where else has the client been seen? What did the other professionals find or suggest?

6. How have the client, family members, or caregivers tried to help?

7. Can the interviewee describe the specific communicative difficulty?

Information-Giving Interviews

Information-giving interviews are used to convey test results, diagnostic impressions, suggestions and recommendations. In this type of interview, the clinician provides information about the nature of the communication difficulty, the proposed plan for case management, and various prognostic implications. Information-giving interviews occur throughout the course of treatment sessions. However, one should be cognizant of what the client brings to the first information-giving interview that typically follows the first diagnostic session. At that point, the client is concerned about both the diagnosis and the prognosis. He may have questions as to the validity of the testing; the clinician should not have a defensive posturing to these questions but rather inform the client as to why the tests used were chosen, and why he/she believes the testing is an accurate reflection of the client's abilities. At this meeting, the client may have feelings of concern, fear, and anxiety.

As the assessing clinician, you also have the responsibility for conducting the post-assessment interview. The clinician brings a body of knowledge gathered from the pre-assessment interview/case history, and from the individual's performance on the various tests that were administered. At this point, the clinician should also have an idea of what the client, family member, and/or caregivers expect from him/her. One of the most important aspects of the information-giving interview is the empowerment of the family to be a part of the diagnostic process; the clinician should elicit their help in this process.

How does the clinician convey the information to the patient? The clinician should tell the client and his significant others the name of the tests used, what they were designed to assess, why they were chosen. Test scores and their interpretation should also be shared at this conference. However, more important than the scores is a review of the items missed or passed. The clinician should question the family members and/or caregivers as to whether this is an accurate reflection of the client's typical abilities. For example, the clinician may say, "Let me tell you some of the things I saw in the evaluation, and you can tell me if they fit in with what you have observed at home."

The clinician should also review factors that may have affected test outcome. Following the information-giving, the clinician should ask the client and his significant others, "What do you need to know at this point?" Their answer to this question will guide you as to how much information they are willing and able to receive. Also, you should keep in mind that the value of the diagnostic session may very well depend on the quality of the post-assessment conference.

A problem-solving approach is the best one to assume in an information-giving interview. Remember, your best procedures are worthless if you cannot make them meaningful to the family. If they seem to deny or not accept the test results as reported, show them the forms and demonstrate the family member's responses. Then, given all this information and the client's reaction to it, is therapy warranted? The decision to pursue therapy should be a team decision with the family's desires as important as the clinician's recommendation. At this interview, what many patients want is not advice, but confirmation. If the client and/or family members and caregivers are having a difficult time making the decision, the clinician can use a "counter question" ("What do you want to do?") to force the person to reveal his position.

If therapy will be pursued, work through the test results to determine, as a team, appropriate goals for therapy. Stress to clients that even though they have no choice about having the communication disorder, they do have a choice as to how they are going to let it (disability/handicap) affect their lives.

There are several interpersonal factors which need to guide the interview:

1. Do not intimidate the patient; do not give more information than he can easily handle;

2. Keep focused;

3. Maintain flexibility—be ready for various reactions (including hostility or lack of trust);

4. Do not permit expression of your own subjective feelings—maintain objectivity;

5. Do just as much listening as talking (if not more); Give the patient opportunities to express his feelings. Statements such as "Some patients feel like they are walking in someone else's nightmare" or "Some patients feel like they have been hit by a Mack truck" sometimes open the door for parents/family members to share their feelings;

6. Reflective listening (paraphrasing, restating, etc.): You convey your willingness to care through your willingness to listen and be responsive;

7. Other suggestions:

   - If more than three to five important points need to be made, consider alternative methods for conveying the information.

   - Try to sandwich your negative points between more positive observations

   - Keep your language simple and appropriate

   - Avoid relying on test names and protocols

   - Continuously watch for signs of misunderstanding or resistance

   - Accept emotional responses professionally and supportively (Shipley, 1992).

Counseling Interviews

A counseling interview is one that is used to influence someone's attitudes and/or behaviors. It provides both release and support for the interviewee(s). In a counseling interview, the clinician should provide the client, family members, and/or caregivers with support and direction, and encourage them to express their feelings and attitudes about their difficulties (Shipley, 1992). This is also the time to "modify their methods of interaction, to assist in the treatment, or to understand and correct the ways they may be hindering the client's progress" (Shipley, 1992, p. 10).

Depending on the length of time between the onset of the disorder and the information-giving interview, the client and/or his family members may express a variety of emotions. These include anger caused by fear, a feeling of being threatened, and frustration. There may be an underlying sense of vulnerability, pain, and anxiety. The interviewees may express defensive reactions, of which there are six types:

1. Reaction formation: The client and/or family members immerse themselves in activities in order to appear supportive and hide the resentment;

2. Suppression: The client and/or family members keep their true feelings to themselves;

3. Repression: Consciously, for this person, the problem is non-existent, therefore it does not need to be addressed;

4. Rationalization: The individual using rationalization focuses on the positive actions that need to be accomplished and forgets the actions that did not get done, because he will continue to rationalize about what has not gotten done;

5. Displacement: The person using displacement may express his anger by slamming doors or creating scapegoats;

6. Projection: Through projection, the client and/or his family members transfer blame, excuse failures, and minimize their own weaknesses. (Shipley, 1992)

CONDITIONS THAT FACILITATE COMMUNICATION

Sensitivity

The client's feelings and personal perceptions about a subject will influence his thinking about and receptivity toward that subject as a topic of discussion. The clinician should be sensitive to the client's interests in and levels of concern about their problems. Being sensitive toward the client's and family member's level of knowledge (i.e., avoid technical jargon) is also important.

Respect

Respect is defined by as "having regard for and showing appropriate courtesy to the other party" (Shipley, 1992, p. 36). Respect is conveyed through words, actions, and behaviors. Respect can be used to help individuals face the positive aspects of any information that is difficult to accept and to help them move ahead in a constructive manner. Also, the clinician should be aware that every question may have an underlying concern, so he/she should be forthright, courteous, and respectful in answering the interviewee's questions.

Empathy

"Empathy is built upon the knowledge and understanding of an individual's circumstances" (Shipley, 1992, p. 37). Empathy encompasses learning about and attempting to understand the individual. The clinician should be careful not to sympathize with a client, and he/she should be aware of his/her own attitudes and beliefs since they can engender feelings and reactions and create an impression on the client and/or his family members.

Objectivity

The clinician must remain objective in his/her clinical roles. Being objective does not mean being impersonal, unfriendly, or insensitive. Rather, it means that the clinician does not let personal emotions inappropriately influence the situation. The clinician should maintain a realistic and practical point of view, and use good listening skills.

Listening Skills

Four critical factors determine the effectiveness of listening:

1. Concentration: requires hearing what is said, having patience, and removing any distractions from the interaction;

2. Active participation: requires that the clinician's mind remain ready, alert, open, flexible, and free from distraction;

3. Comprehension: involves hearing the underlying meanings as well as the surface messages expressed by the words;

4. Objectivity: requires that the clinician avoid imposing personal feelings and attitudes upon interviewees and what they may be expressing (Shipley, 1992, p. 38).

There are three approaches to listening:

1. Listening for comprehension: this involves receiving content that requires little feedback from the listener. The listener should remain objective instead of critically analyzing or responding to the other person's comments;

2. Listening with empathy: empathy can be used to convey understanding of what the client may be experiencing emotionally. It involves providing comfort, warmth, and reassurance to the client, his family members, and/or caregivers. Although the clinician cannot "feel what the client feels," he/she can try to convey an understanding of his feelings and attitudes.

3. Listening for evaluation: when listening for evaluation, the clinician attempts to use the information that has been accrued in all three types of interviews to reach an evaluative conclusion on what needs to be done (Shipley, 1992).

Concentration

The speech-language pathologist should avoid becoming overstimulated by or emotionally involved with what the interviewee says. The "clinician should work to identify and recognize the types of words, attitudes, and positions that affect her emotionally so that their impact will be reduced when they are encountered in interview sessions" (Shipley, 1992, p. 41). When the clinician has his/her own emotions under control, he/she should be able to pay careful attention to what the interviewee is saying, particularly when the information is difficult and/or hard to deal with. If the clinician does not understand what the interviewee is trying to convey, he/she should ask for clarification, in order to avoid any misinterpretations of the client's beliefs, attitudes, and feelings.

Motivation

Van Riper (1979) said "perhaps the most important of all clinical skills required for effective therapy is the clinician's ability to motivate his clients" (p. 82). When the client and the clinician work together to develop the same goals, the client's motivation to achieve those goals is greatly enhanced by the shared effort and responsibility. Also, both the interviewee(s) and the clinician benefit when everyone is "aware of the purposes of the interaction, how any information shared will be used, and what is expected of the participants" (Shipley, 1992, p. 45). Furthermore, motivation will be greater if the clinician is more concerned about the implementation of the therapy procedures and activities than simply focusing on the goals.

Rapport

When rapport is established between a client and the clinician, there is a sense of trust and confidence present in the interactions. However, the clinician is warned that the establishment of rapport with a client and his family members is an ongoing process.

Types Of Questions

Open-Ended Questions

Open-ended questions are general, relatively nonspecific requests for information. They are, by far, the most productive types of questions to use in all three types of interviews. Open-ended questions require that the interviewee be "actively involved in the interview process and to organize and structure their thoughts before responding" (Shipley, 1992, p. 75). Examples of open-ended questions include statements such as "Tell me about . . ." and "What are . . ." questions. The clinician can also repeat key words used by the interviewee as a method of securing additional information.

Closed Questions

Closed questions typically yield the least amount of information, particularly with regard to the client's thoughts, attitudes, and beliefs. Questions can be moderately closed ("How often does your child stutter?"), highly closed ("Do you stutter all the time, frequently, or only occasionally?"), or bipolar (yes/no questions).

Primary vs. Secondary Questions

Primary questions introduce new topics or new areas within a topic, while secondary questions are follow-up questions to elicit more specific or detailed information (Shipley, 1992).

Who, What, When, Where, How, and Why Questions

Who questions address the client, family, and caregivers. *What* questions are designed to yield specific details of the situation. *What* questions most often lead to facts. *When* questions are used to identify when the problem started and any related events. *Where* questions are used to facilitate the client's telling in what situations/contexts the communication problems exist. The answers to *how* questions convey how the client and/or family members react and feel about the problem. These questions typically lead to discussion about processes, sequences, feelings. Finally, *why* questions help a clinician find out why a problem occurs, and lead to discussion of reasons behind the communication disorder.

Neutral vs. Leading Questions

Neutral questions allow the respondent to choose his answers without being influenced by the clinician. They are unbiased questions that allow the respondent to answer within his own frames of reference. Neutral questions could be worded as "How do you feel about . . ." or "Tell me about . . . ".

Leading questions make honesty difficult because the client is likely to answer in the way he expects you want him to respond.

Types of Responses

Summary Statements and Reflections

Summary statements are used to echo essential elements of client's comments. They facilitate communication by signaling that the information has been heard and understood. This signaling is through mirroring the messages, attitudes, and feelings that the client has expressed. Summaries facilitate discussion by encouraging the client to explore attitudes, beliefs, feelings, and topics in greater detail (Shipley, 1992).

In summary statements, the clinician uses his/her own words to make the clients understand that he/she accepts them and their feelings. They can also be used to wrap up or terminate discussion. When using the summary to end a discussion, it is helpful to highlight the key points of the discussion and convey to the interviewee that he has accomplished a purpose.

"Reflections are like summaries, but they stick more closely to the very words that the interviewee has used to express feelings and ideas" (Shipley, 1992, p. 88). Reflections are used to mirror the content of the client's message and the feelings that the client has expressed about the content. Another method of reflection is called accentuation. In accentuation, the clinician restates key words or phrases as questions.

Clarifications

Clarifications are used to specify an area of confusion and to more fully understand the client and the client's difficulties. They can be used to find out more about specific behaviors or to exchange perceptions regarding what has been said. Examples of clarification responses are, "Did I understand you correctly when you said . . . " and "Tell me more about . . . ".

Repetitions

"The clinician should not assume that the interviewee's complete attention can be maintained at all times—the attention may drift periodically" (Shipley, 1992, p. 89). Especially when a client is being told information for the first time, the use of repetitions can help the client and/or his family members to understand the basic message even if they miss some of the specific comments made by the clinician. By varying the wordings and giving bits of additional information, the clinician can help to achieve clarity and emphasis, making it easier for the client to comprehend the information (Shipley, 1992).

Pauses

Pauses in the conversation allow the interviewee to ponder and reflect on what has been said. One of the best interviewing tools available is the ability of the clinician to wait silently for the client's responses or comments. There is no need to fill every moment with talking.

Confrontations

Confrontations are also among the most useful techniques available for a clinician. Confrontation can enable the client and/or his family members "to face and deal with realities, situations, and behaviors that they are inclined to avoid or deny" (Shipley, 1992, p. 89). A confrontation should never be used to punish a client, or to express hostility or anger. Rather, the clinician should use an accepting tone of voice to convey empathy with the client's situation. An example of a confrontation would be if a client is not using his stutter-free techniques, and the clinician might say, "You say you do not want to stutter, yet you don't use the techniques we have discussed in therapy" (Shipley, 1992).

SUMMARY

The quality of the assessment portion may well rest on the quality of the information-getting interview, and the quality of the complete diagnostic process may rest on the quality of the information-giving interview. Thus, the speech-language pathologist should hone his/her interviewing skills in anticipation of using them throughout the diagnostic and treatment phases. The ability to motivate the client and to involve the family are critical components of counseling, and the success of therapy may ride on the skills of the clinician as a counselor.

The speech-language pathologist needs to understand the stages of the grief process and recognize the stages in his/her clients. The clinician can help the client work through the grief process by creating an accepting and nonjudgmental clinical setting, and by being an empathetic listener. Nondirective counseling techniques are of the greatest benefit to an individual working through the grief process. Allowing clients to remain in control of their progress throughout the grief process will help them to progress through the various stages in a healthy and productive manner. "By allowing patients to be involved in decision-making in therapy, the patient may regain control of some aspects of his or her life and may alleviate feelings of helplessness" (Dikengil, 1998, p. 59).

"The American Speech-Language-Hearing Association includes counseling in the scope of practice of speech-language pathologists and audiologists and in its preferred practice patterns (American Speech-Language-Hearing Association, 1993). Even so, clinicians should be careful not to exceed their professional boundaries in counseling with clients, nor attempt to employ helping skills that they do not fully comprehend how and when to use" (Crowe, 1997, p. 26).

SECTION TWO
Case Law and Legislation

LEGISLATION AFFECTING SERVICE DELIVERY IN SPEECH-LANGUAGE PATHOLOGY

Case law, local, and federal legislation often serve as the foundations upon which decisions are made regarding the delivery of services in speech-language pathology. This section will address legislation affecting service delivery in educational settings, medical settings, and vocational settings.

CHAPTER THREE
Education-Related Laws and Legislation

BROWN VS. BOARD OF EDUCATION (1954)

Brown versus Board of Education was handed down as a Supreme Court ruling in 1954. Brown vs. Board of Education is a reversal of the 1896 U. S. Supreme Court Ruling in Plessey vs. Ferguson, which upheld the laws of segregation as constitutional.

Actually, Brown vs. Board of Education is a consolidated opinion based on cases from Kansas, South Carolina, Virginia, and Delaware. In his decision, Chief Justice Earl Warren wrote that (1)"separate but equal isn't equal with regards to education,"due to stigma associated with the lack of cross-cultural interaction (Rothstein, 1990, p. 12); and (2) it was also stated in the decision that desegregation in the schools must occur with "all deliberate speed" (Fischer & Sorenson, 1985, p. 236).

During the implementation stages of the ruling, riots and demonstrations halted the desegregation process. Examples of these disruptions are listed in Table 3–1.

TABLE 3–I	Incidents during implementation of Brown vs. Board of Education
YEAR	**INCIDENT**
1957	President Dwight Eisenhower sent Federal troops to Central High School in Little Rock, Arkansas to enforce the decision and to restore peace in the public high school; nine blacks had been admitted which provoked riots and temporarily closed the schools
1962	In New Orleans, a federal judge ruled to end segregation
1962	In Oxford, Mississippi, James Meredith tried to enroll at the University of Mississippi. President John Kennedy ordered in Federal troops to enforce the decision and defuse the situation
1963	The second black student enrolled at the University of Mississippi
1963	A black student enrolled at the University of Alabama which meant that there was one integrated public school in every state
1963	The New Jersey Commission of Education ruled to correct racial imbalances in the schools; the racial imbalances were created by customs and housing patterns
1964	A federal statute, the 1964 Civil Rights Act/Title VI, was passed. It stated that any program receiving federal aid could not discriminate based on race, color, or national origin

THE CIVIL RIGHTS ACT OF 1964

The Civil Rights Act of 1964 stated that federal funds could not go to programs that discriminated based on race, color, or national origin. Some schools, upon realizing that their funding would soon be cut, changed into private schools, thus giving up the money in order to retain segregation. With the passage of time, this law was extended to include non-discrimination against the handicapped as well.

PUBLIC LAW 91-230 (1970)

Public Law 91-230 was passed by Congress on April 13, 1970 as an extension of the Elementary and Secondary Education Act of 1965. The law authorized and provided federal funding as grants to states to encourage special education programming by creating services and centers to meet the special needs of the handicapped. The funding included the training of personnel (including "Speech Correctionists") to work with handicapped children in educational settings. Public Law 91-230 expressed a moral commitment to children with disabilities, and established that individuals who have disabilities are guaranteed the same constitutional rights as non-disabled people (Fischer & Sorenson, 1985).

PENNSYLVANIA ASSOCIATION FOR RETARDED CITIZENS (PARC) VS. THE COMMONWEALTH OF PENNSYLVANIA (1971)

This case was an extension of Brown vs. Board of Education and concerned the rights of handicapped children to an appropriate education. The right to an education for all children is a civil right. The PARC case was filed on behalf of 13 children with mental retardation against the Pennsylvania Board of Education. The case had three goals:

1. Establish the right to a free education for retarded children. The goal was to add the specification of "handicapped" to the Civil Rights specifications of race, color, and national origin;

2. A second goal was to mandate school accountability. Parents wanted their children to have access to a guaranteed education that would involve both the parents and the children;

3. The third major goal of the case was to insure that the handicapped had equal access to due process under the law, as well as legal protection.

PARC was successful in procuring a "free and appropriate" public education. Although Pennsylvania previously had established programs for the handicapped, several loopholes existed that resulted in the denial of a free and appropriate education to many children with handicapping conditions. The victory for PARC in this case led to the establishment of Public Law 94-142, the Education for All Handicapped Children Act of 1975.

MILLS VS. BOARD OF EDUCATION (1972)

In light of the victory in PARC vs. The Commonwealth of Pennsylvania, a suit was brought against Washington D.C., the Department of Human Services, and the mayor by the parents and guardians of seven handicapped children in the District of Columbia. The parents and guardians claimed that all children were not being provided a free public education, and that the children were being denied equal protection and due process under the 14th Amendment of the United States Constitution.

The plaintiffs won the case, and the defendants were ordered to provide all children with free education and to also provide a list of all children being denied education within one month of the ruling. The judge also decreed that any child being denied an education was being denied his rights of due process and equal protection under the law. The Mills ruling created a procedural framework that was incorporated into Public Law 94-142 based on the precedent that all children, regardless of their handicapping condition, have the right to free and appropriate education. The framework defined what due process would entail, stating that it included labeling, placement, and exclusionary stages of decision-making. Specifically, it included (1) the right to a hearing with representation, (2) the right to appeal, (3) the right to have access to records, and (4) the right to written notices at all stages of the process. The ruling also stated that funds should be distributed in an equitable manner between programs for regular education, and programs of special education.

THE REHABILITATION ACT OF 1973

The Rehabilitation Act of 1973 is a non-discrimination statute signed into law on September 26, 1973 by President Richard Nixon. Section 504 provided for non-discrimination under federal grants by stating that "no otherwise qualified handicapped individual in the United States as defined in Section 7(6), shall, solely by reason of his handicap, be excluded from the participation in, be denied the benefits of, or be subjected to discrimination under any program receiving Federal financial assistance" (School Law Register). The term "handicapped" included such diseases or conditions as speech, hearing, visual, and orthopedic impairments; cerebral palsy, epilepsy, muscular dystrophy, multiple sclerosis, cancer, diabetes, heart disease, mental retardation, emotional illness; and specific learning disabilities, such as perceptual handicaps, dyslexia, minimal brain dysfunction, and developmental aphasia (Hagerty & Howard, 1978).

Along with Public Law 94-142, Section 504 of Public Law 93-112 is considered to be the most important federal law related to the rights of handicapped persons, and in particular, students with handicaps. Section 504 serves as backup legislation to Public Law 94-142 to help insure that handicapped individuals are not discriminated against in educational pursuits. Section 504 has additional, wide-ranging implications because of its mandates that buildings and facilities must be accessible and that employers not discriminate against disabled job applicants. The force of the two laws has allowed for significant and continuous change in educational, vocational, and social opportunities for persons with handicaps (Lombana, 1982).

If a parent believes a violation has occurred, he has 180 days from the time of the supposed violation to file a complaint with the federal Department of Education. The Department of Education will investigate and/or hold a hearing to determine if a violation has occurred. It is important to note that this usually will not resolve that particular child's case; rather, there is simply a determination of whether or not a violation has occurred, and if any punishments are warranted.

Since states have the responsibility of developing their regulations to comply with federal laws, most school-related cases are heard in the state courts. Most states have a three-tiered system of courts similar to the three-tiered system in the federal courts: Trial Court, where facts are established and legal principles are applied to the facts; Appellate Court, a court of appeals where the case is reviewed and it is determined if the legal principles were applied judiciously and correctly; and Highest State Court, the final authority unless there is a federal law on the same matter.

If the matter is not resolved to the satisfaction of all parties, the matter may be taken to the United States Supreme Court if the complaint is based on a violation of the Constitution, its amendments, or other federal statutes.

Administrative hearings are often used in school-related cases before they go to trial court. An administrative hearing is an impartial hearing, and regulations establishing its use were developed in an effort to expedite school-related cases, and to reduce the costs of a trial. Findings in an administrative hearing are subject to review by the State Education Agency, then by a state or federal court. If a satisfactory resolution cannot be achieved, the case then goes to either a state trial court or a federal district court.

The Rehabilitation Act Amendments of 1986 "placed considerable emphasis on the provision of technology to assist individuals with disabilities in entering and maintaining employment" (Ourand & Gray, 1997, p. 343). In 1992, the Rehabilitation Act was again amended to add new state plan requirements to the states' vocational rehabilitation plans. Specifically, states are now required to:

- Describe how a broad range of rehabilitation technology services will be provided at each stage of the rehabilitation process. [Sec. 101(a)(5)(C)(i)]

- Describe how a broad range of rehabilitation technology services will be provided on a statewide basis. [Sec. 101(a)(5)(C)(ii)]

- Describe the training that will be provided to vocational rehabilitation counselors, client assistance personnel, and other related services personnel. [Sec. 101(a)(5)(C)(iii)]

- Describe the manner in which assistive technology devices and services will be provided, or worksite assessments for determining eligibility and vocational rehabilitation needs of an individual. [Sec 101(a)(31)] (Ourand & Gray, 1997, p. 343).

Adults receiving services in the Vocational Rehabilitation system must have an Individualized Written Rehabilitation Program (IWRP). The IWRP "describes specific services and equipment that will be provided, with vocational goals tied to the provision of assistive technology. Without a written signed IWRP, no AAC services or equipment can be provided" (Ourand & Gray, 1997, p. 344).

The 1992 Amendments also address transitional services to help students make the transition from school to the workplace under Vocational Rehabilitation. These services may be provided to students 14 years of age and older.

PUBLIC LAW 93-380: EDUCATION AMENDMENTS OF 1974

Public Law 93-380 was signed into law by President Gerald Ford in 1974. It increased federal funding for educational programs for children with handicaps. It also established procedures to insure that handicapped children were educated with non-handicapped children, unless stated that by the nature or severity of the handicap mainstreaming would not be satisfactory. However, the most important aspect of Public Law 93-380 was in the area of parental rights.

Section 513 (Family Education Rights and Privacy Act or FERPA), known as the Buckley Amendment, provided children with handicaps and their parents procedural safeguards in matters concerning identification, evaluation, and educational placement of the child. This set forth an educational philosophy that acknowledged the right of parents (and students 18 or over) to be involved in the educational process. This involvement included having access to educational records, challenging the accuracy of those records, and having some control over their dissemination. In other words, the law dealt with the issues of access to and accuracy of educational records. In 1975, Public Law 94-142 extended this to include issues of cost and destruction of educational records.

Section 438 of Public Law 93-380 declared that parents must give their written permission for the release of confidential information regarding their child. Section 612 addressed the concept of least restrictive environment, mandating that children with handicaps be educated in the "mainstream" with non-handicapped children, unless the nature and severity of the handicapping condition was such that participation in a regular classroom could not be achieved satisfactorily.

EQUAL EDUCATIONAL OPPORTUNITIES ACT OF 1974 (EEOA)

This federal law was based on the findings of the Lau vs. Nichols case in which it was ruled that Chinese children were being discriminated against and overrepresented in special education classes due to the fact that English was their second language. It was also based on the 14th Amendment of the United States Constitution, which guarantees equal protection of all individuals under the law. The EEOA determined that states may not deny an equal education opportunity to an individual due to the failure by that educational agency to take appropriate action to overcome existing language barriers that impede equal participation by its students. Thus, the schools are obligated to provide language assistance to each non-native speaker who demonstrates a need (Fischer & Sorenson, 1985).

PUBLIC LAW 94-142: THE EDUCATION FOR ALL HANDICAPPED CHILDREN ACT OF 1975

General Information

Public Law 94-142 was passed in 1975 and enacted on October 1, 1977. The primary purpose of this law was to guarantee funding for the implementation of previous legislation related to education of handicapped children. Technically, it was an amendment to the Education for the Handicapped Act (Public Law 91-230), which was passed in 1970 and had provided grants to states offering special education. Public Law 94-142 authorized the expenditure of federal funds to subsidize special education provided by individual states. As in the Brown vs. Board of Education case, this law was founded on the Constitutional principles of equal protection and due process. The amendment included procedural safeguards, integration, non-discriminatory testing, and evaluation materials and procedures.

Basic Fundamental Principles

The foundation of the law was that all handicapped children who meet age eligibility must be given an education. Specifically, a free and appropriate education must be provided to children aged 6–18 years. In addition, children aged 3–5 and 19–21 also should have an education provided if non-handicapped children in those age brackets were also served. Public Law 94-142 included a mainstreaming mandate that dictated that children with handicaps should be served in the least restrictive environment that could be achieved while still providing an appropriate education.

A third fundamental of the law was that education of children with handicaps be individualized and appropriate to the child's unique needs. Every child was to have an Individualized Education Plan (I.E.P.) that detailed the services to be provided, the current level of functioning, the long-term objectives and short-term goals. Information as to how progress would be measured was to be included in the I.E.P.

The fourth dictate of the law was that the education was to be provided free of charge to the families of the children with handicapping conditions. In other words, handicapped children would have equal access to public education as non-handicapped children.

The law delineated several procedural protections to ensure that the requirements and intent of the law have been met. These procedural protections included four major features:

1. Due process: Parents who believe their child is not being provided with a free and appropriate education in the least restrictive environment have a right to challenge the decisions of the educational institution in court. The 14th Amendment to the United States Constitution contains equal protection and due process clauses which provide a basis to challenge unequal treatment in the educational process. "Section 1983 of the Civil Rights Act is the statutory basis through which constitutional and federal statutory violations can be redressed" (Rothstein, 1990, p. 219). Complaints under Section 504/1983 must be filed within 180 days of the violation and contain the following information: identifying information of complaining party; basis for the complaint; who has been

affected; identifying information of (alleged) discriminatory agency; approximate date of violation; brief description of the event; and signature of the complaining party.

2. Least restrictive environment: Children are to be served in the least restrictive environment. School systems must provide a continuum of alternative placements to benefit all handicapped students.

3. Non-discriminatory testing: Children are to be tested using standardized measures that were standardized on children with handicaps.

4. Child find: Each educational area is to provide a means of educating the public about the services that are available to children with handicaps, and to have a system of identifying and evaluating those children.

Speech-Language Pathologist's Roles and Obligations as Defined by Public Law 94-142

The speech-language pathologist had five roles and obligations defined by Public Law 94-142: (1) Identification of children with speech or language disorders; (2) Diagnosis and appraisal of specific speech or language disorders; (3) Referral for medical or other professional attention necessary for the rehabilitation of speech or language disorders; (4) Provision of speech and language services for the rehabilitation or prevention of communicative disorders; (5) Counseling and guidance of parents, children, and teachers regarding speech and language disorders.

Related Services vs. Special Education

The law distinguished between related services and special education services. "Related services" refers to developmental, corrective, or other supportive services as required to assist a handicapped child to benefit from special education. "Special education" refers to the primary service being provided for the child. Speech-language pathology can be a related service or a special education service. For example, if a child has a placement in a special education classroom based on a physical and/or mental handicap, and the child receives speech-language pathology services, that child's therapy would be considered as a related service because it is a supportive service to his primary placement. If, on the other hand, a child's only handicapping condition is his or her speech and the child spends his or her day in a regular education setting, the service would be a special education service because it would be the primary service provided.

Issues Related to Parent Notification

Some of the procedural safeguards included the fact that parents must be informed in writing of any changes in their child's educational plan. Specifically, written permission must be obtained prior to testing any child. It is not required for screening, but is mandatory for testing. In addition, parents are to be notified in advance of an I.E.P. meeting and given an invitation to attend. Anytime a child's I.E.P. is changed, the parent is to be notified in writing and invited to attend the meeting at which the change is to be documented.

Due Process

The 14th Amendment to the United States Constitution contains equal protection and due process clauses, which provide a basis to challenge unequal treatment in the educational process."Section 1983 of the Civil Rights Act is the statutory basis through which constitutional and federal statutory violations can be redressed. It provides that individuals deprived of rights, privileges, or immunities of the Constitution or federal laws may bring action in court" (Rothstein, 1990, p. 219).

Complaints under section 504/1983 must be filed within 180 days of the violation. The complaint is filed with the Office for Civil Rights of the Department of Education, and must contain the name, address, and phone number of the complaining party; the basis for the complaint; who has been affected by the discrimination (may be a group or individual); the name and address of the discriminating agency; the approximate date the discrimination occurred; a brief description of the event; the signature of the complaining party.

Public Law 99-372 was passed in 1986 to address the issue of the recovery of attorney's fees incurred during due process procedures.

Parents' Rights

> The parents in special education situations have important rights and an essential role. Their rights include a right to a hearing and an opportunity to challenge the school's proposal decisions. With that right comes an important role—that of being a participant at almost all stages of the development of an appropriate program and deciding on an appropriate placement for the child. These rights and roles are unique to special education. In no other aspect of public education do parents have such an important role and such significant rights. (Rothstein, 1990, p. 49)

Educational Records

There are four major issues related to educational records:

1. Accuracy: There are stigma associated with inaccurate information. Also, inaccurate information could jeopardize federal funding.

2. Access: Protective procedures are needed to protect files from misuse and indiscrete communications. State laws regulate access to medical information other than when used for placement decisions.

3. Cost: Reasonable costs may be assessed to parents for copies of records. The school must waive the fee if the cost prevents the family from obtaining copies of the records of their child.

4. Destruction: Individual states have regulations regarding the destruction of records. In some states, records must be kept for up to seven years beyond the child's dismissal from the educational system.

The Individualized Education Plan (I.E.P.)

Every child in a special education placement must have an Individualized Education Plan. A minimum of three professionals should attend the I.E.P. meeting. The I.E.P. includes long-term goals, short-term objectives, how, when, and by whom the objectives will be addressed and measured, related services being provided to the student, and the percentage of time the child spends in regular education, special education, and related services. I.E.P.s are written annually, and the child must be re-evaluated every three years. Parents are asked to sign the I.E.P., as are the professionals involved in its creation.

Funding Sources and Issues

Funding under Public Law 94-142 is based on a count of handicapped children receiving special education and related services. The Education for All Handicapped Children Act "defines a handicapped child as one who is mentally retarded, hard of hearing, deaf, speech impaired, visually handicapped, orthopedically impaired, or other health impaired . . . or with specific learning disabilities, who by reason/of the handicap require(s) special education and related services" (Rothstein, 1990, p. 41). The amount of funding is derived by a formula that is based on the average cost of educating a handicapped child. It does not take into account the wide range of disabilities and handicaps represented in the public schools.

THE ANN ARBOR DECISION (1979)

The parents of the black children at an elementary school in Ann Arbor, Michigan were concerned that their children's dialect created a barrier to their educational progress, particularly in learning to read. The case addressed the issue, and subsequently proved, that teacher rejection to the "home language" causes student rejection of efforts in learning, and that these students did poorly and/or failed at school (Battle, 1983). The court held that, indeed, children were being discriminated against due to their dialect. The court ordered the Ann Arbor schools to develop a plan to help teachers identify speakers of Black English. It also required a plan to teach standard English to dialect speakers, and to make teachers more sensitive to dialectal variations. The case established a legal precedent for other schools and hoped that these schools would also recognize the linguistic validity of social dialects. In many schools, the speech-language pathologists were responsible for developing a plan for honoring the "home language" while teaching standard English to speakers of other dialects. (Bountress, 1987)

PUBLIC LAW 99-457: THE EDUCATION FOR ALL HANDICAPPED CHILDREN ACT AMENDMENTS OF 1986

Public Law 99-457 amends Public Law 94-142 by creating a new mandate for state education agencies to serve all three, four, and five year old handicapped children. Known as Part H (the Handicapped Infants and Toddlers Act), the services had to be in place by the 1990–1991 school year, or the state risked losing federal funding for education of handicapped children. It also included provisions for "at risk" children between the ages of birth and six years.

Public Law 99-457 had three primary purposes: (1) to increase a handicapped infant's development by increasing the family's ability to serve its child; (2) to decrease the possibility of institutionalization of the child with the handicap(s); and (3) to minimize the need for special education once the child attains school age.

Public Law 99-457 also reauthorized other Education of the Handicapped Act's discretionary programs, which included training for parents of handicapped children.

Individualized Family Service Plan (I.F.S.P.)

Similar to the I.E.P., an I.F.S.P. must be written for all children whose education is funded through Public Law 99-457. The I.F.S.P. must be reviewed every six months, and rewritten annually. Many of the children are served through homebound services, with a focus on teaching the family how to provide intervention and environmental enhancement for their child who is handicapped.

Funding Sources

Funding sources for Public Law 99-457 included preschool grant funds, all Public Law 94-142 dollars that were generated by the three- to five-year-old population, and all grants and contracts related to preschool special education funded under the Education of the Handicapped Discretionary program.

PUBLIC LAW 101-476: THE INDIVIDUALS WITH DISABILITIES EDUCATION ACT (IDEA)

Passed in 1990, IDEA is another amendment of Public Law 94-142. IDEA reinforces that "all eligible preschool and school-aged children and youth with disabilities are entitled to receive a free appropriate public education, including special education and related services. Under IDEA, eligibility for school-age services is determined according to 13 disability areas: autism, deaf-blindness, deafness, hearing impairment, mental retardation, multiple disabilities, orthopedic impairment, other health impaired, serious emotional disturbance, learning disability, speech or language impairment, traumatic brain injury, and visual impairment (Ourand & Gray, 1997).

In addition, IDEA ensures that the rights of children and youth with disabilities and their parents are protected, assists states and localities in the provision of services, and evaluates and ensures the effectiveness of programs. (ASHA, 1994). The major change that came about as a result of the passing of IDEA was to add transition as a service area to be addressed on the I.E.P. Schools are requested to define what they are doing to help children in transition into school from home, and into the workplace from school. It is required that transition be addressed in all I.E.P.s for students aged 16 and older; it is encouraged that it be addressed on I.E.P.s of children younger than 16 years of age.

Transition services are defined as a coordinated set of activities for a student that are designed with an outcome-oriented process, and that promote movement from school to post-school activities. The activities must be based on (1) the student's needs; and (2) needed activities in the areas of instruction, community experiences, the development of employment and other postschool adult living objectives, and if appropriate, the acquisition of daily living skills and functional vocational evaluation.

CHAPTER FOUR
Health Care Legislation

Most legislation which relates to health care settings is based on issues related to reimbursement. Other issues of primary concern are those related to liability and malpractice.

THE SOCIAL SECURITY ACT OF 1935

This act was passed during the Depression, and represented the first major entrance of the federal government into the area of health care insurance. Eventually, the Social Security Act of 1935 formed the basis for the current Medicaid and Medicare programs. Specifically, the act provides a system for federal benefits for aged persons, blind persons, dependent and disabled children, maternal and child welfare, public health, and unemployment compensation laws.

SOCIAL SECURITY ACT AMENDMENTS OF 1965

Title XVIII of the Social Security Act Amendments of 1965 established Medicare (national health insurance for the aged). Part A provides hospital insurance benefits for hospital costs and related post hospital outpatient services.

Part B provides supplemental medical insurance benefits. Part B is a voluntary program. The benefits are financed by the participant with matching funds from general revenues. This program includes physicians' services, lab tests, X-rays, supplies and equipment, and home health care.

Audiology is included under the umbrella of speech-language pathology and is covered under Part A and Part B. The benefits cover nearly everything related to audiology, except for hearing aids and hearing aid evaluations. Also, the participant must have prescription/authorization from a physician for the audiology services in order to be eligible for Medicare reimbursement.

Title XIX of the Social Security Act Amendments of 1965 initiated Medicaid which established federally supported and state administered programs of health insurance for recipients of public assistance. It also provides benefits to medically indigent persons not on welfare. It is up to individual states as to which services will be provided within the following six categories: inpatient hospital services; outpatient hospital services; laboratory and X-ray services; skilled nursing facility services; physicians services; and other services as allowed by state (including SLP and Audiology).

SOCIAL SECURITY ACT AMENDMENTS OF 1972

In 1972, another set of Social Security Act Amendments was passed by the Congress. The 1972 revisions added speech-language pathology services as part of outpatient physical therapy services. Under Part B, speech-language pathologists can get their own provider number if they meet the requirements for designation as a rehabilitation agency.

The 1972 Amendments also established the Early and Periodic Screening, Diagnosis, and Treatment Program under Medicaid which provides child health screening (including SLP/hearing); hearing aids; and augmentative devices and follow-up treatment for families receiving aid for dependent children.

SOCIAL SECURITY ACT AMENDMENTS OF 1982

The Social Security Act Amendments of 1982 changed reimbursement procedures as a direct result of the Tax Equity and Fiscal Responsibility Act (TEFRA). Previously, hospitals were reimbursed according to actual reported costs of care. Following the 1982 Amendments, hospitals were paid a fixed payment or discharge limit for all hospital related costs, including speech-language pathology and audiology services. This was done to encourage cost containment.

The 1982 Amendments also added reimbursement for hospice care, including speech-language pathology services for terminally ill patients if services are offered in a manner consistent with accepted standards of practice.

SOCIAL SECURITY ACT AMENDMENTS OF 1983

The Social Security Act Amendments of 1983 reinforced TEFRA by creating PPS (Prospective Payment System). This established reimbursement caps based on a patient's diagnosis or diagnosis-related group (DRG). Arguably, PPS has led to compromises in the quality of care provided by members of medical and allied health professionals.

MEDICARE COMMUNICATION DISORDERS AND SERVICES ACT (1984)

The Medicare Communication Disorders and Services Act provided for independent provider status for speech-language pathologists, and coverage for aural rehabilitation services provided by an audiologist. It also permitted the removal of complex eligibility requirements for patients to qualify for audiology services, and provided coverage for individuals who need assistive and augmentative communication devices.

Actually, this Act failed to pass in 1992 and 1993, but in 1994 the technical portions dealing with speech-language pathology and audiology were passed as part of the Social Security Act Amendments of 1994.

MEDICAID REFORM

Medicaid reform proposals being considered include capping annual growth of federal Medicaid spending at 5–7%, which would negatively affect Medicaid and SSI recipients. The effort to have a balanced budget by 2002 includes caps on several federal entitlement programs including Aid to Families with Dependent Children, Supplemental Security Income (SSI), and Medicaid.

It is also necessary to keep an eye on the Individuals with Disabilities Education Act (IDEA) and Americans with Disabilities Act (ADA) funding in spite of the fact that there are amendments that protect these civil rights statutes.

U.S. PUBLIC HEALTH SERVICE ACT (1944)

The U.S. Public Health Service Act (1944) was passed for the sole purpose of consolidating all legislation relating to national public health services. Subsequent amendments affecting speech language pathologists are as follows:

Title XIII: Health Maintenance Organization Act of 1973

This Act creates the provision of basic medical services under a fixed periodic payment community rating system, including physician services; inpatient and outpatient services; medically necessary emergency health services; short-term outpatient evaluation services; and crisis intervention mental health services (limited to 20 visits).

In addition, patients can contract for supplemental health services, including intermediate and long-term care; vision care; dental and mental health services; and prescription drugs.

With regard to authorization for medical services, the Federal HMO Act of 1973 reads as follows:

> Federally qualified HMOs must provide or arrange for outpatient service and inpatient hospital services which shall include short-term rehabilitation and physical therapy, the provision of which the HMO determines can be expected to result in the significant improvement of a member's condition within a period of two months. (Code of Federal Regulations, Title 42, Section 110.102 [1990])

Unfortunately, the period of two months is most frequently interpreted as meaning a maximum of two months, instead of a minimum of two months as was the intention of the act (Frattali, 1998).

The Social Security Act Amendments of 1976

The Social Security Act Amendments in 1976 were less stringent than those of previous years. If the Health Maintenance Organization (HMO) is receiving Medicare/Medicaid reimbursement, it must be federally qualified. These Amendments also limited speech-language pathology and audiology services by saying that the HMO can determine the conditions under which improvement is expected in two months.

Technology-Related Assistance for Individuals with Disabilities Act of 1988

This act was passed to increase availability and funding for assistive technology.

Numerous Omnibus Budget Reconciliation Acts

The Omnibus Budget Reconciliation Acts were developed to instruct authorizing committees to cut spending in health programs.

The years 1980, 1985, 1986, 1987, 1989, 1990 are significant for speech-language pathology and/or audiology because they contained provisions that related directly to the delivery of speech-language pathology and audiology services. The 1980 act, which became effective on January 1, 1981, enabled speech-language pathologists to write their own treatment plans for Medicare beneficiaries. In 1987, the act increased access to speech-language pathology services for residents in nursing facilities.

PUBLIC LAW 101-518: SECTION 4206 (PATIENT SELF-DETERMINATION ACT OF 1990)

Section 4206 of Public Law 101-518 states that "all Medicare and Medicaid provider organizations such as hospitals, nursing homes, and home health agencies must: (a) provide information to patients regarding the right to refuse medical treatment and to formulate advance directives, (b) maintain documentation and records of advance directives, (c) review advance directives periodically, (d) comply with directives as dictated by state law, and (e) educate staff and the community on issues concerning advance directives" (Sabatino & Gottlich, 1991). According to Sabatino and Gottlich (1991), the primary goals of the Patient Self-Determination Act were to encourage patient autonomy and to give patients the legal right to execute advance directives. In addition, the act sought to "eliminate problems associated with terminating life-sustaining treatment for incompetent patients by mandating increased communication about patients' rights between patients and their health care providers" (Mulholland, 1991, p. 616).

Applebaum and Grisso (1998) put forth four categories of legal standards that should be taken into consideration and evaluated when determining an individual's competence:

1. Ability to communicate choices consistently;

2. Ability to understand relevant information about a treatment decision;

3. Ability to comprehend a situation and its probable consequences;

4. Ability to use logical reasoning to compare benefits and risks of treatment options.

They further maintain that competent patients should have the right to refuse any type of treatment, regardless of the consequences. In addition, the court ruled that incompetent patients lose the right to refuse treatment, and decisions are made for them (Landes, 1999).

CRUZAN VS. DIRECTOR, MISSOURI DEPARTMENT OF HEALTH (1990)

Cruzan vs. Director, Missouri Department of Health (1990) was a critical case in decision-making about life-sustaining treatment. The plaintiffs were the parents of a 25-year-old woman who had sustained a significant head injury in a car accident. Cruzan was subsequently diagnosed as being in a chronic vegetative state with essentially no chance of regaining her mental abilities. Cruzan did not leave any advance directives regarding the use of life-sustaining measures. Her parents requested that artificial nutrition and hydration be discontinued, but the hospital refused to do so without a court order. The local court's approval was overturned by the Missouri Supreme Court and eventually upheld by the United States Supreme Court. The ruling of the Missouri Supreme Court "took an important first step by guaranteeing the right of a competent person to refuse unwanted medical treatment" (Gottlich, 1990, p. 633). The ruling of the United States Supreme Court was slightly different in that it ruled that, under certain circumstances, it extended the right to refuse treatment to incompetent persons. However, since Nancy Cruzan had left no instructions regarding her wishes, the United States Supreme Court upheld the ruling of the lower court. This ruling led to the development of advance directives, the establishment of surrogate status (allowing a competent person designated by the individual to make decisions should the individual become incompetent), additional safeguards, and the establishment of a Guardian ad Litem to act on the patient's behalf.

CHAPTER FIVE

Public Laws Affecting Employment of Persons with Disabilities

PUBLIC LAW 101-336: AMERICANS WITH DISABILITIES ACT (ADA)

Signed into law on July 26, 1990, Public Law 101-336 was modeled after previous civil rights legislation. "Major provisions of the law provide comprehensive civil rights protection to persons with disabilities, and prohibit state and local governments from refusing to allow a person with a disability to participate in a service, program, or activity simply because the person has a disability" (Ourand & Gray, 1997, p. 345). Disability refers to physical and/or mental impairments that interfere with or limit major life activities. This includes speech and language impairments and specific learning disabilities.

The law addresses access to public facilities, transportation, employment, telecommunications, and state and local government services. The law does not address funding or provision of services. The primary focus is on access. "Employers with more than 15 employees are required to provide reasonable accommodations for employees with disabilities to enable qualified employees to carry out their jobs, unless the accommodations cause undue hardship on the employer" (Ourand & Gray, 1997, p. 345). Reasonable accommodations include the provision of AAC and other assistive technology when so indicated. The implementation dates were July 26, 1992 for agencies with 25 or more employees, and July 26, 1994 for agencies with 15 or more employees.

Additional information on ADA is available in a booklet entitled "The Americans with Disabilities Act: Questions and Answers" and is available from the U. S. Equal Employment Opportunity Commission (1801 L Street NW, Washington, D.C. 20507).

THE TECHNOLOGY-RELATED ASSISTANCE FOR INDIVIDUALS WITH DISABILITIES ACT AMENDMENTS OF 1994 (TECH ACT)

Public Law 103-218 (1988) "is a federal competitive grants program which provides monies for states to establish a statewide, consumer-responsive service delivery system designed to effect systems change regarding assistive technology" (Ourand & Gray, 1997, p. 345). The original act delineated a broad definition of assistive technology that encompasses all devices regardless of the level of technology.

The programs under the Tech Act do not necessarily provide direct funding for AAC services and devices. Rather, "most states use Tech Act grants to fund broad programs to disseminate information and provide referrals to increase access to assistive technology" (Ourand & Gray, 1997, p. 345). Some states also conduct financial and/or equipment loan programs.

SECTION THREE
Disorders

CHAPTER SIX
Aphasia

DEFINITION/DESCRIPTION

Aphasia is defined by Robert T. Wertz as "an impairment due to acquired damage of the central nervous system of the ability to comprehend and formulate language." (Helm-Estabrooks & Holland, 1998, p. 12). Furthermore, it is a multimodality disorder, and it is important to note that the language deficits are not due to a dementia, a motor dysfunction, or a sensory loss.

Most patients with neurogenic language disorders initially will be seen in the acute care setting. Thus, the assessment may be limited to a bedside screening until the patient has the stamina for a more comprehensive battery of standardized tests. Typically, the clinician starts with a bedside screening and formal assessment of the patient's attention, his memory, and his orientation because the speech-language pathologist needs an estimate of the patient's ability and stamina for further assessment and intervention (Golper, 1998).

Patients with suspected language disorders may present with a variety of disorders including traumatic brain injury, stroke, right hemisphere deficits, confusion, and dementia. The role of the speech-language pathologist is "determining candidacy for treatment, selecting appropriate treatment avenues, implementing treatment services for neurogenic language disorders, and counseling family members" (Golper, 1998, p. 3).

Etiology of Stroke

Strokes can be caused by an ischemic or hemorrhagic event, brain trauma, intracranial tumors, bacterial infections, viral infections, brain abscesses, or cerebral toxemia.

Ischemic strokes are caused by a blockage of blood flow, typically by a thrombosis or an embolism. A thrombosis is a blockage that develops in an artery and impedes the flow of blood to the brain. An embolism is also a clot, but it forms in one location, travels through the bloodstream, and becomes lodged in another location, thereby impeding the blood flow to the brain (Hegde, 1998, p. 61). Approximately two-thirds of all ischemic strokes are caused by a thrombosis (Hegde, 1998, p. 60).

Hemorrhagic strokes are due to the rupturing of cerebral blood vessels, resulting in the unimpeded flow of blood into the brain tissues. Weakened blood vessels can be caused by trauma to the blood vessel, high and/or fluctuating blood pressure, weakened arterial walls, or malformations of the vessels. Hemorrhages can be intracerebral or extracerebral (see Table 6–1). An intracerebral hemorrhage in the basal ganglia may cause a subcortical aphasia,

TABLE 6-1 Comparison of intracerebral hemorrhage and extracerebral hemorrhage

Intracerebral Hemorrhage	*Extracerebral Hemorrhage*
Hemorrhage caused by ruptures within the brain or brainstem	Hemorrhage caused by ruptures within the meninges
In most cases, ruptures as caused by high blood pressure (hypertension)	Three types and their causes:
More common in small arteries deep within the brain structures, especially around the thalamus and basal ganglia	*Subarachnoid:* The most common of the extracerebral hemorrhages on the surface of the brain, brainstem, or cerebellum; ruptures beneath the arachnoid; frequently caused by aneurysms
	Subdural: Rupture is beneath the dura mater; often caused by traumatic head injury
	Epidural (Extradural): Ruptures above the dura mater, between the dura and the skull; often caused by traumatic head injury

Adapted from *A Coursebook on Aphasia and Other Neurogenic Language Disorders* (2nd ed.) (p. 61), by M. N. Hegde, 1998, San Diego, CA: Singular Publishing Group. Copyright 1998 by Singular Publishing Group. Adapted with permission.

and is typically associated with a high mortality rate and more permanent brain damage. These types of strokes typically have a sudden onset as the hemorrhaging blood forms a clot and destroys the surrounding brain cells.

An aneurysm is a "balloon-like swelling of a weak and thin portion of an artery that eventually ruptures" (Hegde, 1998, p. 62). The base of the brain is a common site of extracerebral aneurysms, and they can involve the Circle of Willis, the vertebral arteries, and the basilar artery. Other major sites for aneurysms are the anterior and cerebral arteries (Hegde, 1998). Hemorrhages and aneurysms are parenchymal lesions since the blood escapes into the brain tissue.

Patterns for recovery from ischemic and hemorrhagic strokes vary as outlined in Table 6–2.

Bacterial meningitis affects the cerebrospinal fluid and the meninges. This disease moves rapidly and can be fatal if not treated with antibiotics soon after its onset. Viral infections include AIDS, rabies, mumps, measles, and herpes simplex encephalitis. The herpes simplex virus frequently causes aphasia. Brain abscesses are caused by bacteria, fungi, or parasites that migrate into the brain from the middle ear, the mastoid cells, or the sinuses. Finally, cerebral toxemia as a sequela to drug use, heavy metals (e.g., lead), and drug interactions can result in stroke (Hegde, 1998).

TABLE 6-2 Different patterns of recovery from typical ischemic and hemorrhagic strokes

Ischemic	*Hemorrhagic*
Greater and sooner recovery	Little recovery in the first 4–8 weeks
Noticeable recovery in the first few weeks	More rapid recovery after 4–8 weeks
Maximum recovery in 3 months	A slowing down of recovery, stabilizing with greater residual deficits

Adapted from *A Coursebook on Aphasia and Other Neurogenic Language Disorders* (2nd ed.) (p. 62), by M. N. Hegde, 1998, San Diego, CA: Singular Publishing Group. Copyright 1998 by Singular Publishing Group. Adapted with permission.

Timing of Strokes

With regard to the time course, which is sometimes called the clinical presentation, strokes fall within one of four categories: (1) a transient ischemic attack (TIA), (2) a reversible ischemic neurological deficit (RIND), (3) a stroke in evolution, or (4) a completed stroke. (Vinson, 1999, p. 298)

A TIA is a rapidly resolving disruption of blood flow to the brain. Symptoms include "headache, dizziness, blurred or double vision, confusion, slurred speech, swallowing difficulty, and weakness or numbness on one side of the body" (Shipley & McAfee, 1998, p. 52). However, the symptoms dissipate when circulation of blood to brain is restored, and the patient is left with no residual effects. RINDs typically last longer than TIAs, and they may leave the patient with some mild residual deficits, which may last for days or weeks. However, over the course of time, minimal, partial, or no residual neurological deficits may remain (Aronson, 1991).

A stroke in evolution "is a classic, full stroke from which the person can expect residual problems, including physical weakness and language deficits or aphasia. In a full stroke, the symptoms persist longer than 24 hours and an associated progressive deterioration occurs in the patient's neurological status" (Vinson, 1999, p. 228). The amount of residual damage that remains will depend on whether the lesion is diffuse or focal, and on the severity of the attack.

The completed stroke is one in which the deterioration stops, and the patient's condition stabilizes. Although neurological deficits remain, they typically do not worsen after the patient is medically stable. During this period, one type of aphasia may evolve into another, but the symptoms do not worsen with regard to the time course, or the area of the lesion.

ASSESSMENT

Aronson (1991) developed a series of prerequisite questions that should be addressed by the team evaluating an individual with a neurological deficit. The team should include, at a minimum, the neurologist, the speech-language pathologist, and the neurosurgeon. The questions are listed in Table 6–3.

TABLE 6–3 Prerequisite questions to guide the evaluation of patients with neurological deficits
1. What is malfunctioning?
2. How is it malfunctioning?
3. Is a lesion causing the malfunction?
4. Where is the lesion?
5. What is the lesion?
6. What can be done to reduce or eliminate the lesion?
7. What can be done to reduce or eliminate the malfunction?

Adapted from *Neurology for the Medical Speech-Language Pathologist*, by A. E. Aronson, 1991, Workshop presented in Tampa, FL. Adapted with permission.

Questions three through six primarily address the issue of the lesion, so these questions are the purview of the neurologist and/or neurosurgeon. The other three questions focus on the functioning aspects of the disorder, so the speech-language pathologist can be a contributor in the answering of these questions. Question one is related to the patient's complaints. Question two is based on the clinician's observations, and question seven is answered according to the clinician's plans for rehabilitation.

Components of Assessment

Depending on the site of the lesion(s), the patient with aphasia will show different symptoms. Therefore, the first step beyond the history in assessing aphasia or other neurological disorders is typically a neuroimaging study to determine the site and nature of the lesion. This is done by the neurologist, but the speech-language pathologist needs to be familiar with the types of neuroimaging studies, and with the results of the studies.

The Neurological Exam

The next step is to complete a neurological exam. A list of the cranial nerves is in Table 6–4.

Much of the neurological exam can be obtained while the clinician and physician are taking the patient's history, because a good neurological examination relies heavily on clinical observation skills. Initially, the patient's behavior should be analyzed. Does the patient interact appropriately? What kind of mood and affect does the patient generate? Is the patient clean and neat? What thought processes does the patient exhibit? Does the patient appear to be anxious or confused? (Helm-Estabrooks & Albert, 1991).

In addition to behavior, the patient's gait and posture should be observed, looking for signs of asymmetry, unsteadiness, or weakness. The patient's mental status similarly should be evaluated during the history-gathering process. For example, is the patient alert and attentive to the examiner's questions and comments? What is the memory status of the patient?

TABLE 6-4	The cranial nerves	
I	Olfactory	Sensory
II	Optic	Sensory
III	Oculomotor	Motor
IV	Trochlear	Motor
V	*Trigeminal*	*Sensory and Motor*
VI	Abducens	Motor
VII	*Facial*	*Sensory and Motor*
VIII	Acoustic	Sensory
IX	*Glossopharyngeal*	*Sensory and Motor*
X	*Vagus*	*Sensory and Motor*
XI	*Spinal Accessory*	*Motor*
XII	*Hypoglossal*	*Motor*

Nerves in italic type are most frequently involved in speech.

Memory can be addressed informally by teaching the patient a list of four unrelated items, then asking him to recall the list after a five minute interlude of other questions and conversation. Recall of immediate events ("Tell me what happened to you") and recall of major events from the past ("Are you married? How many children do you have?") similarly are important aspects of memory to assess (Helm-Estabrooks & Albert, 1991). Knowledge of recent nonpersonal events should be explored, depending on the patient's areas of interest. For example, if the patient likes baseball, questions such as, "Who won the World Series this year?" would be a way to explore memory.

The cranial nerve examination is done by the neurologist, although the speech-language pathologist can contribute to this portion of the examination. While assessing the cranial nerves, the astute physician and clinician will also evaluate the patient's motor skills, the status of his sensory system, and the presence or absence of reflexes. General tests for the assessment of cranial nerves involved in speech are outlined in Table 6–5.

TABLE 6–5 General tests for the assessment of cranial nerves involved in speech (nerves V, VII, IX, X, XI, XII)

Nerve	*Tests*
Trigeminal (V)	Check sensation with cotton wisps, pinpricks, warm and cold objects
	Ask if patient can sneeze
	Check ability to chew
	Palpate masseters and temporal muscles with jaw clamped tightly
	Look for wasting of masseter on affected side and deviation of the mandible to one side when lowering jaw against resistance
Facial (VII)	Check ability to smile
	Check ability to whistle
	Check results of electromyographic studies
	Offer taste tests (sweet with sugar, sour with citric acid, bitter with quinine, salty with salt)
	Look for facial symmetry at rest
	Look for facial symmetry during voluntary facial movement
Glossopharyngeal (IX)	Elicit pharyngeal gag (stroking of affected side does not produce gagging if nerve is injured)
	Ask patient to say "ah" (look for presence of constriction of pharyngeal wall)
	Administer taste tests on the posterior one-third of the tongue
Vagus (X)	Perform a laryngoscopic examination to check motor status of the larynx and pharynx
	Check sensory status of the larynx and pharynx (gag reflex)
Accessory (XI)	Check ability of patient to shrug shoulders and rotate head against resistance
	Complete objective examination for muscle atrophy and shoulder drop
	Evaluate electromyography (EMG) results
Hypoglossal (XII)	Test tongue strength by having patient push tongue tip against the cheek against clinician's finger resistance
	Check for deviation of the tongue upon protrusion
	Notice atrophy or tremors of the tongue
	Evaluate EMG stimulation of tongue muscles

Oftentimes, the clinician may have difficulty differentiating between aphasia and various motor speech disorders. For example, both can be characterized by trial-and-error, groping articulatory movements. Thus, one must use other diagnostic criteria to make the differential diagnosis. Table 6–6 sums up aspects the clinician can use.

In addition, motor speech disorders can occur with aphasia. Table 6–7 shows differential diagnosis of aphasia without dysarthria and dysarthria without aphasia.

TABLE 6-6 **Differential diagnosis of aphasias and motor speech disorders**

Aphasia Without Apraxia of Speech	Apraxia of Speech without Aphasia
Neurogenic language problem	Neurogenic speech problem
Trial-and-error, groping articulatory movements are not significant	Trial-and-error, groping articulatory movements are significant
Misarticulations less variable, more consistent	Misarticulations more variable, more inconsistent
Some impairment of auditory comprehension	Generally, no impairment in auditory comprehension
Prosodic problems not dominant	Prosodic problems dominant
Difficulty in initiating utterances is less obvious	Difficulty in initiating utterances is more obvious
Omission of function words	No significant tendency to omit function words
Word-finding problems	No word-finding problems, although articulatory groping can make it look like such problems
Limb or oral apraxia not dominant	Limb or oral apraxia or both may be dominant

Adapted from *A Coursebook on Aphasia and Other Neurogenic Language Disorders* (2nd ed.) (p. 191), by M. N. Hegde, 1998, San Diego, CA: Singular Publishing Group. Copyright 1998 by Singular Publishing Group. Adapted with permission.

TABLE 6-7 **Differential diagnosis of aphasia and dysarthria**

Aphasia Without Dysarthria	Dysarthria Without Aphasia
Neurogenic language problem	Neurogenic speech problem
The language problems are not due to muscle weakness	The speech problems are due to muscle weakness
No consistent misarticulations	Consistent misarticulations
Intelligibility clearly related to the rate of speech	Intelligibility of speech not clearly related to the rate of speech
No respiratory problems associated with speech production	Respiratory problems associated with speech production
Phonatory problems not significant	Phonatory problems may be significant
Resonance disorders not significant	Resonance disorders significant
Prosodic disorders not dominant	Prosodic disorders may be dominant
Abnormal voice quality not significant	Abnormal voice quality may be significant
Abnormal stress not significant	Abnormal stress may be significant

Adapted from *A Coursebook on Aphasia and Other Neurogenic Language Disorders* (2nd ed.) (p. 192), by M. N. Hegde, 1998, San Diego, CA: Singular Publishing Group. Copyright 1998 by Singular Publishing Group. Adapted with permission.

Aphasia must also be differentiated from dementia and right hemisphere disorders, as outlined in Tables 6–8 and 6–9.

Table 6-8 Comparison of aphasia and dementia

Aphasia	*Dementia*
Sudden onset	Slow onset
Damage in left hemisphere	Bilateral brain damage
Focal brain lesions	Diffuse brain damage
Mood is usually appropriate, though depressed or frustrated at times	May be moody, withdrawn, agitated
Nonverbal cognitive functions are mostly intact	Mild to severely impaired mostly cognition
Most memory functions are typically intact	Memory is impaired to various degrees, often severely
Generally relevant, socially appropriate, and organized	Often irrelevant, socially inappropriate, and disorganized
Semantic, syntactic, and phonologic performance simultaneously impaired	Progression of deterioration from semantic to syntactic to phonologic performance
Fluent or nonfluent	Fluent until dementia worsens

Adapted from *A Coursebook on Aphasia and Other Neurogenic Language Disorders* (2nd ed.) (p. 187), by M. N. Hegde, 1998, San Diego, CA: Singular Publishing Group. Copyright 1998 by Singular Publishing Group. Adapted with permission.

TABLE 6-9 Comparison of aphasia to right hemisphere problems

Aphasia	*Right Hemisphere Problems*
More severe problems in naming, fluency, auditory comprehension, reading, and writing	Only mild problems
No left-sided neglect	Left-sided neglect
No denial of illness	Denial of illness and lack of insight into their problems
Speech is generally relevant	Speech is often irrelevant, excessive, and rambling
Generally normal affect	Often lack of affect
Recognizes familiar faces	May not recognize familiar faces
May simplify drawings	Rotation and left-sided neglect
Some prosodic deficit	More pronounced prosody defect
Appropriate humor	Inappropriate humor
May retell the essence of a story	May retell only nonessential, isolated details (no integration)
May understand implied meanings of statements	Understands only literal meanings
Pragmatic impairments less striking	Pragmatic impairments more striking (eye contact, topic maintenance, etc.)
Although limited in language skills, communication can often be good	Although possessing good language, communication can be very poor
Pure linguistic deficits are dominant	Pure linguistic deficits are not dominant

Adapted from *A Coursebook on Aphasia and Other Neurogenic Language Disorders* (2nd ed.) (p. 190), by M. N. Hegde, 1998, San Diego, CA: Singular Publishing Group. Copyright 1998 by Singular Publishing Group. Adapted with permission.

Language Testing

Naming

Anomia is a hallmark symptom of aphasia. That is to say, without anomia the diagnosis of aphasia cannot be made. When assessing anomia, the clinician needs to consider the semantic category, word frequency, and the nature of the task. Confrontational naming (showing the patient an item and asking for the name) and free recall (i.e., listing items in a specified category, usually under a time limit) should both be tested when assessing naming abilities.

Fluency

Word output of fewer than 50 words per minute is significant (normal amount of speech is 100–200 words per minute). The patient may have reduced fluency in nonfluent aphasia; he may have excessive speech in fluent aphasia. Also important is whether or not the patient has difficulty initiating speech. Difficulty initiating is characteristic of nonfluent aphasias.

Paraphasias

Verbal paraphasias can often be observed in patients with aphasia. A semantic paraphasia is the unintentional substitution of a word with similar semantic content for the target word. For example, the patient may call a spoon a fork. Neologistic paraphasias consist of made up words that bear little or no resemblance to the target word. For example a patient may call a fork a "stumple." Phonemic paraphasias occur when the patient unintentionally substitutes a sound in the target word, such as saying "tat" for "cat."

Auditory Comprehension

Auditory comprehension is good in Broca's, transcortical motor, conduction, and anomic aphasia. It should be tested initially using single word identification. "In this task, the clinician asks the patient to respond with single words to identify or describe an object, a picture, or an action. A second task is to have the patient follow simple commands. Finally, the patient should be asked a series of questions" (Vinson, 1999, p. 238). The questions should be designed to explore four different types of interactions:

1. Personal information (name, address, marital status, number of children, etc.);

2. Impersonal questions ("Is it raining outside?", "Who is President of the United States?");

3. Questions related to well-known stories such as *Sleeping Beauty* or *The Three Little Pigs*;

4. Questions related to obscure facts ("Who was the first man to walk on the moon?").

Repetition Skills

Repetition skills are remarkably preserved in the transcortical aphasias. In fact, the excellent repetition skills in transcortical motor and transcortical sensory aphasia can be considered their hallmark features. Repetition is also good in anomic aphasia.

Repetition skills should be assessed using tasks of increasing complexity. "The single words used in the initial testing of repetition skills should be selected from a wide variety of semantic categories. The words should progress from single to multisyllabic words and from simple to complex words with regard to their phonetic content" (Vinson, 1999, p. 238). In the initial testing, the clinician should ask the patient to repeat frequently used words, and progress to low frequency words. After having the patient repeat single words, the clinician should progress to short common phrases and sentences ("Sit down"), longer common phrases and sentences, ("Go to the store and buy some bread"), then short unfamiliar phrases and longer unfamiliar phrases and sentences.

Standardized Assessment Tools

There are many standardized assessment tools that the clinician can employ in the evaluation of language and communication skills in patients with aphasia. These are enumerated in Table 6–10.

TABLE 6–10 Standardized assessment tools	
ASHA Functional Assessment of Communication Skills for Adults (Frattali, Thompson, Holland, Whol, Ferketic)	Assesses functional communication skills in a variety of settings and environments
Assessment of Nonverbal Communication (Duffy & Duffy)	Assesses comprehension and expression of gestures through picture selection
Auditory Comprehension Test for Sentences (Shewan)	Assesses comprehension of spoken sentences
Boston Assessment of Severe Aphasia (Helm-Estabrooks et al.)	Assesses communication skills in patients with severe aphasia
Boston Diagnostic Aphasia Examination (Goodglass & Kaplan, 1983)	Profiles various aphasia syndromes
Boston Naming Test (Goodglass, Kaplan, & Weintraub)	Assesses naming skills using line drawings
Communicative Ability in Daily Living (Holland)	Assesses communication in daily life
Communicative Effectiveness Index (Lomas, Pickard, Bester, Elbard, Finlayson, & Zoghaib)	Assesses pragmatic communication skills using a questionnaire completed by a significant other
Examining for Aphasia (Eisenson)	Assesses receptive and expressive language skills
Functional Auditory Comprehension Task (LaPointe & Horner)	Assesses functional auditory comprehension of spoken language
Functional Communication Profile (Sarno)	Assesses communication in daily life
Minnesota Test of Differential Diagnosis of Aphasia—Revised (Schuell & Sefer)	Profiles various aphasia syndromes
Multilingual Aphasia Examination—3rd edition (Benton, Hamsher, & Sivan)	Assesses oral expression, spelling, verbal understanding, articulation, reading, and writing in English, German, Spanish, and French
Porch Index of Communicative Ability (Porch)	Quantifies a prediction for recovery
Reading Comprehension Battery for Aphasia (LaPointe & Horner)	Assesses reading comprehension of words, sentences, and paragraphs
Revised Token Test (McNeil & Prescott)	Assesses auditory processing
Western Aphasia Battery (Kertesz, 1982)	Profiles various aphasia syndromes

Adapted from *Pocketguide to Assessment in Speech-Language Pathology,* by M. H. Hegde, 1996, San Diego, CA: Singular Publishing Group. Copyright 1996a by Singular Publishing Group; and *Language Disorders Across the Lifespan,* by B. Vinson, 1999, San Diego, CA: Singular Publishing Group. Copyright 1999 by Singular Publishing Group. Adapted with permission.

Aphasia Syndromes

Subcortical Aphasias

The subcortical aphasia syndromes include (1) anterior capsular or putaminal aphasia; (2) posterior capsular or putaminal aphasia; (3) global capsular or putaminal aphasia; and (4) thalamic aphasia. The subcortical aphasia syndromes are evaluated in the same way as the cortical aphasias, concentrating on the four primary tasks of naming, repetition, auditory comprehension, and fluency. However, verbal agility, nonverbal agility, and the presence of hemiparesis or hemiplegia must also be assessed. Most subcortical aphasia are believed to be caused by "lesions in or surrounding the left basal ganglia or the left thalamus" (Hegde, 1994, p. 148).

Fluent Cortical Aphasias

Fluent and nonfluent aphasia are compared in Table 6–11, and a chart delineating the characteristics of three fluent aphasias (Wernicke's, conduction, and transcortical sensory) is in Table 6–12.

Wernicke's Aphasia

In Wernicke's aphasia, the lesion causes damage to Wernicke's area and neighboring temporal and parietal regions. This area centers on the posterior third of the superior temporal gyrus (Helm-Estabrooks & Albert, 1991). When the lesion is in Wernicke's area and the inferior parietal area, fluent speech and phonemic paraphasias predominate. When the lesion is in the occipital area and the more posterior angular gyrus, the patient uses verbal paraphasias, whereas lesions that are even more posterior lead to the use of neologisms.

In Wernicke's aphasia, the "spontaneous speech is fluent with normal phrase length, prosody, intonation, and inflection, although little meaning is conveyed (content or important words are absent)" (Guilmette, 1997, p. 41).

Conduction Aphasia

Conduction aphasia is characterized by extremely poor ability to repeat. This is because the lesion in conduction aphasia lies in the arcuate fasciculus (the white matter pathways), or

TABLE 6–11 A comparison of fluent and nonfluent aphasias	
Fluent Aphasias	*Nonfluent Aphasias*
Voice onset time not impaired	Voice onset time often impaired
Phonemic substitutions used that differ by more than one feature	Phonemic substitutions usually differ from the target by a single feature
Many substitutions and additions of sounds	Use of intrusive vowels and prolongations
Transposition and sequencing errors	Prevalence of substitutions
Errors tend to be more toward the end of words	Errors tend to be at the beginning of words
Errors on vowels and consonants	Errors primarily on consonants
	Timing errors and transition errors in speech

Adapted from *Language Disorders Across the Lifespan,* by B. Vinson, 1999, San Diego, CA: Singular Publishing Group. Copyright 1999 by Singular Publishing Group. Adapted with permission.

TABLE 6–12	**A comparison of the three primary fluent aphasias**		
Diagnostic Entity	*Wernicke's Aphasia*	*Conduction Aphasia*	*Transcortical Sensory Aphasia*
Spontaneous speech	Fluent, but pauses for word retrieval; press of speech; lacks content; jargon; monologue-like	Fluent, but frequent use of inappropriate words; good intonation	Fluent; discourse incoherent and circumlocutory; lacks content; uses stereotypical phrases
Articulation	Good	Good	Good
Auditory comprehension	Poor to severely impaired	Good	Poor
Reading comprehension	Poor	Good	Poor
Naming	Poor; neologisms	Very poor	Very poor; produces long, unrelated sentences
Writing	Mechanically good but lacks content	Poor to dictation but good volitionally	Poor
Grammaticism	Word strings empty of content but syntactically correct;	No problem	Word strings empty of content but syntactically correct
Error awareness	Little to none	Yes	Little to none
Echolalia	Doubtful	No	Present
Paraphasias	Semantic	Phonemic	Semantic or neologistic
Repetitions	Poor due to decreased auditory comprehension	Very poor	Good
Visual disturbances	Possibly	Variable	Frequently
Reading aloud	Poor	Poor	Good
Paralysis or paresis	No	Rare	Rare; mild if occurs

From Aronson (1991); Benson (1979); Davis (1993); Gonzalez-Rothi (1990); Helm-Estabrooks & Albert (1991); Rubens (1976).

the association tracts that connect Broca's and Wernicke's areas. Although it is classified as a fluent aphasia, the more anterior the lesion, the less fluent the speech.

Transcortical Sensory Aphasia

Transcortical sensory aphasia is caused by damage in the parietal-temporal junction area posterior to Wernicke's area. Transcortical sensory aphasia bears a very close resemblance to Wernicke's aphasia with the exception of repetition. Patients with transcortical sensory aphasia maintain excellent repetition skills.

> It is not unusual for global aphasia to resolve into transcortical sensory aphasia. In such cases, the patient initially may experience no comprehension and little or no verbal output. This is followed by a period of jargon replete with numerous neologisms. As the neologistic paraphasias decrease, words and meaningful phrases begin to appear, although they typically have little or no relationship to the clinician's questions or remarks. As the words and phrases appear, the ability to repeat begins to emerge (Vinson, 1999, p. 243).

According to Benson (1979), the most common etiological factor in transcortical sensory aphasia is vascular disease, with occlusive problems being most causative. Typically, there is an occlusion of the left internal carotid artery leading to infarction in the parietal-temporal junction area. Tumors in the same area can also produce transcortical sensory aphasia.

Nonfluent Aphasias

The most striking features of the nonfluent aphasias are the effort and difficulty the patient has in generating spoken language. A chart comparing the nonfluent aphasias (Broca's, transcortical motor aphasia, and global) is in Table 6–13.

Broca's Aphasia

Broca's aphasia is a nonfluent, expressive aphasia with the lesion being in the third frontal convolution immediately anterior to the precentral gyrus. The lesion typically "involves the left lateral frontal, prerolandic, suprasylvian region (Broca's area) extending necessarily into the periventricular white matter deep to Broca's area. This lesion is in the territory of the

TABLE 6-13 A comparison of the three primary nonfluent aphasias

Diagnostic Entity	Broca's Aphasia	Global Aphasia	Transcortical Motor Aphasia
Spontaneous speech	Nonfluent; apraxic labored; telegraphic	Nonfluent and infrequent; stereotypic utterances	Nonfluent; decreased verbal output; paucity of speech; difficulty initiating speech
Articulation	Poor	Poor (scarce)	Poor
Auditory comprehension	Good	Very poor	Good
Reading comprehension	Usually good	Poor	Good
Naming	Poor	Poor	Poor
Writing	Mechanically poor; content like speech	Poor	Poor; letters are large and clumsily produced
Grammaticism	Agrammatism	Not applicable	Possibly agrammatic; reduced complexity
Error awareness	Yes	Probably not	Probably
Echolalia	Rare	Not likely	Maybe (not a true echolalia because will correct errors in the original statement)
Paraphasias	No	No	No
Repetitions	Mechanically poor	Poor	Excellent
Visual disturbances	No	Possibly	Rare
Reading aloud	Poor	Very poor	Poor
Paralysis or paresis	Yes	Possibly	Probably; often right hemiparesis

From Aronson (1991); Benson (1979); Davis (1993); Gonzalez-Rothi (1990); Helm-Estabrooks & Albert (1991); Rubens (1976).

superior division of the middle cerebral artery and often extends posteriorly to include the parietal lobe" (Helm-Estabrooks & Albert, 1991, p. 21).

The spontaneous speech is "nonfluent, agrammatical, (and) produced as single words or short phrases, telegraphic, with absent prosody, intonation, and inflection" (Guilmette, 1997, p. 40). The patient with Broca's aphasia understands what is said to him, and is frequently frustrated by his own awareness of his errors.

Transcortical Motor Aphasia

Transcortical motor aphasia is similar to Broca's aphasia "with the exceptions of repetition which is intact, and reading which is also generally well preserved" (Guilmette, 1997, p. 42). Also, the speech of an individual with transcortical motor aphasia will more closely resemble stuttering than does the speech of a patient with Broca's aphasia.

The lesion is located in the border zones of the perisylvian area, typically in the region of the brain that is superior or anterior to Broca's area (Benson, 1979). Patients with transcortical motor aphasia, and with Broca's aphasia often exhibit dysarthria, which is a generalized weakness of the oral musculature (see the chapter on Dysarthria).

Global Aphasia

The most devastating and pervasive of all the aphasia syndromes, global aphasia is characterized by damage in the entire perisylvian region (along the sylvian fissure). Many of the lesions extend deep into the white matter below the cortex. Patients with global aphasia have difficulty with all aspects of language, both expressive and receptive.

TREATMENT

In general, treatment of aphasia is aimed at reducing "the effects of the residual deficits on the personal, emotional, social, family, and occupational aspects of the client's life" (Hegde, 1996b, p. 5). Treatment may be designed to rebuild language and/or to rebuild communication (Wertz, 1998). Frequently this is done by teaching compensation methods. "Ultimately, patients with aphasia must compensate for their language problems through a dynamic process of problem-solving that requires them to assess communicative situations, generate plans for conveying target messages and then put these plans into effect" (Helm-Estabrooks & Holland, 1998, p. 70). Thus, the clinician must carefully determine the levels of competence in all areas of cognition as a foundation for the implementation of treatment of aphasia in those patients for whom cognition is not spared. As expressed in Helm-Estabrooks & Holland (1998), Von Mourik, Vershaeve, Boon, and Harskamp (1992) espoused the belief that "patients with impairment of basic cognitive skills should be treated nonverbally to create a sufficient basis for language-oriented treatment and communication strategies" (p. 70).

In planning one's approach to therapy, the clinician should first determine if the patient is a candidate for therapy. If the patient has complicating medical conditions that could interfere with remediation, it is advisable to wait until the patient is medically stable before beginning treatment. Also, one should remember that immediately post-onset, there may be swelling of the brain. There may be some spontaneous recovery as the swelling reduces and the injured cells begin to function. Thus, it may be advisable to wait and see what is going to occur in the spontaneous recovery period before undertaking an extensive rehabilitation program.

It is also important that the clinician take into account the functionality of the approach chosen. It may be preferable to target communication in natural settings rather than strictly focusing on language in a clinical setting. Family support and involvement in this approach is absolutely critical. In fact, current emphasis of managed care administrators on the need for proof that clinically based treatment methods have a functional impact may dictate a change in historical treatment methodology (Lyon, 1998). The "use of communication in daily life has become the reimbursable criterion of today's health care system" (Lyon, 1998, p. 206).

> "Total communication" is a clinically based technique for augmenting spoken transactional aspects of communication in people with severe aphasia. This therapy depends on the implementation of a patient-specific blend of gestural, written, drawn, and visual linguistic/nonlinguistic aids. Much of this therapy is targeted at a patient and carried out within a clinical setting. Its prime purpose is to provide a transactional base from which interactants might share a joint "topic" or "referent". That is, by learning a combined use of speech, gesture, print, and drawing, the person with aphasia is able to share a level of content otherwise not possible through speech alone. (Lyon, 1998, p. 208–209)

In this type of therapy, the first step is to establish a means in which the conversation partners can comfortably participate in communicative turn-taking (Lyon, 1998).

Addressing Underlying Processes

Luria believed that effective therapy for aphasia relied on leading the cortex into reorganizing itself using cross-modal stimulation. Based on this approach, new pathways for receiving and acting on stimuli are developed, with consequent improvement in language and memory being expected.

Schuell espoused the theory that training reauditorization was the key to improving auditory comprehension. Through reauditorization, internal sound organization would improve, leading to the improvement in auditory comprehension.

Deblocking is another technique that addresses the underlying basic cognitive processes. "Deblocking is a system of reorganizing the cortex by using an intact function to facilitate the use of other modalities" (Kerns, 1997). Hemispheric specialization, in which the right hemisphere is taught to assume some of the responsibilities previously held by the left hemisphere, is an example of deblocking. Melodic Intonation Therapy (MIT) and visual imaging are both examples of deblocking. The research on which MIT is based was originally done in 1945 by Backus who suggested that words and phrases be presented to the patient in a rhythmical, unison manner. Albert, Sparks, and Helm (1973) assigned simple pitch patterns to phrases and sentences to facilitate speech in nonfluent patients. The conceptual thinking that led to the development of MIT is that "functions associated with the intact right hemisphere may be exploited for purposes of rehabilitating speech in left-brain damaged individuals" (Helm-Estabrooks & Albert, 1991, p. 207).

Visual Action Therapy (VAT) is another example of hemispheric specialization and reorganizing the representational system. VAT was developed by Helm and Benson in 1978 after using visual communication as a treatment methodology for patients with global aphasia. The VAT approach uses hand and arm gestures to represent objects and actions. No verbalizations are required since communication is via a gestural system.

Promoting Auditory Comprehension

Berndt, Mitchum, and Haendiges (1996) wrote that patients who have difficulty interpreting structural cues from sentences may depend on other factors in order to interpret sentences that they hear. "For example, a patient might assume that the first mentioned noun is always the agent of the action. This strategy would fail for sentences that do not follow agent-first word order, such as those in the passive voice" (Berndt & Mitchum, 1998, p. 92). The use of semantically reversible and semantically nonreversible sentences to describe pictures is one approach to improving sentence comprehension. For instance, the clinician could show a picture denoting a girl kicking a boy in one segment and a distractor picture of a boy kicking a girl in another segment, then ask the patient to indicate which picture denotes "The girl is kicking the boy." This is an example of a semantically reversible sentence. A semantically nonreversible sentence could be assessed using a picture of a girl kicking a ball, and a foil of a girl throwing a ball. Upon hearing the sentence, "The girl is kicking the ball," the patient should point to the appropriate picture (Berndt & Mitchum, 1998).

Initially, auditory comprehension tasks should focus on frequently used words, using nouns instead of verbs, adjectives, and adverbs. When verbs are introduced, they should be those which can be easily visualized. It is advisable to use short, syntactically simple sentences. Hegde recommends the following progression of activities in the remediation of auditory comprehension:

1. Single words (body parts, objects, pictures of objects, clothing items, food items, action pictures);

2. Spoken sentences (move from simple to complex, more redundant to less redundant, familiar information to unfamiliar information);

3. Spoken questions (concrete yes/no, abstract yes/no, simple open-ended, complex open-ended);

4. Spoken directions (point to single objects or pictures, point to objects in sequence, manipulate stimuli in sequence, manipulate objects according to directions);

5. Comprehension of discourse (turn-taking, topic maintenance) (Hegde, 1996b, pp. 6–7).

Promoting Naming

Generally speaking, therapy should begin with high frequency words and names of objects that can be manipulated. It is helpful to use objects rather than pictures in the initial stages of therapy. When progression is made to pictures, realistic drawings should be used. The clinician can offer phonemic cues, and provide extra time to respond. When presenting stimuli, it is often helpful to provide visual and auditory information.

Naming can be of two types: general naming and confrontational naming. In confrontational naming, the clinician presents a stimulus, and the patient is expected to name the picture or object. In general naming, the clinician can use cuing hierarchies and different types of cues to facilitate the naming. For example, the clinician may model the response for the patient to imitate. Sentence completion is another type of cue in which the clinician provides a semantic cue in a sentence format, and the patient completes the missing word (i.e., "You listen with your _____ "). Phonetic cues in which the clinician provides the first sound in the target word can also be used. If the patient cannot get the word with a phonetic cue, the clinician can provide the majority of the syllable to prompt the correct response. The clinician can also give silent phonetic cues such as posturing to produce the /p/ silently as a prompt for the word "pen." Functional descriptions can also be offered. It may also be helpful, along with a functional description, to demonstrate the use of the item, or point to the item that is the target response. The patient can also be asked to demonstrate the use of the object prior to naming it. For some patients, it may be helpful to have objects or pictures with their name printed alongside the item. For patients in whom spelling and writing are intact, the clinician may want to have them write the word prior to saying it (Hegde, 1996b).

Promoting Functional Communication

In promoting functional communication, the intended goal should be communication, regardless of linguistic accuracy. During the stages of therapy when naming and auditory comprehension are being stressed, it is helpful to use words that relate to the natural environment of the patient. For example, if the patient is an avid baseball fan, some of the vocabulary targeted in treatment should relate to the game of baseball. Other targets should include words needed for "personal experiences, bodily needs, emotions, and thoughts" (Hegde, 1996b, p. 11). The clinician should gradually shape the communicative efforts into phrases and sentences. If the patient can only utter a few syllables, add other syllables to create words. Once words are produced, add additional words to create phrases, and, eventually, sentences. Use prompts as needed, moving through the treatment hierarchy of physical assistance, modeling, visual cues, and verbal cues, but remove the prompts as quickly as possible so the patient does not become dependent upon them.

The clinician should lead the patient into conversational speech, starting with engaging him in meaningful conversation, such as discussions of, for example, personal experiences, family events, professional experiences, vacations, and entertainment. The clinician can also promote conversational speech by telling the patient a story and having him retell it. The story telling can also be an opportunity to work on conversational turn-taking and topic maintenance.

Maintenance programs will revolve around getting the involvement of the family and friends. The patient should be taught to self-monitor, and to generate his own cues to assist in word recall and other strategies addressed in direct therapy. The emotional support of the family will be particularly critical during the generalization and maintenance stages of therapy.

Specific Treatment Programs

Gestural Reorganization

Developed by Rosenbek, LaPointe, and Wertz (1989), this is a method of "teaching verbal expression by first pairing them with gestures and then fading the gestures" (Hegde, 1996b, p. 17). The clinician first selects the target phrases or sentences, then chooses gestures that mean the same as the targets. The gestures and procedures are then explained to the patient. The gestures are taught through modeling and imitation, then by having the patient match the gestures to pictures. The gestures are then modeled along with the verbal expression. After the patient can imitate the gestures and verbal expression, either the gesture or the speech is modeled. The gestures are faded, and the verbal expressions are reinforced.

Melodic Intonation Therapy (MIT)

MIT was developed by Albert, Sparks, and Helm (1973) for use with patients who have severe nonfluent aphasia. The technique uses continuous voicing, musical intonation, and rhythmic tapping to facilitate verbal expression. The program consists of three levels based on the following general principles:

1. Target high frequency words, phrases, and sentences;

2. For each target utterance, use environmental cues or pictures;

3. Maintain constant voicing of each word, phrase, or sentence;

4. Keep the pitch and stress variations of normal speech constant;

5. For each intoned syllable, tap the patient's left hand one time;

6. The clinician signals with his/her own hand when to listen and when to speak.

If the patient fails at one step, the clinician should return to the previous step in the exercise (Hegde, 1996b). A complete outline of the three levels can be found in Helm-Estabrooks, Nicholas, and Morgan (1989).

Promoting Aphasics' Communication Effectiveness (PACE)

PACE was developed by Davis and Wilcox, and was designed to promote face-to-face conversation. The program emphasizes the "exchange of new information, functional communication (as opposed to linguistic precision) with turn taking, free choice for the client to communicate in any modality, and natural feedback" (Hegde, 1996b, p. 21). In the PACE program, the clinician places a large number of cards containing pictures of objects, actions, and stories on the table face down. The clinician and the patient take turns drawing a card and making comments about the stimulus item. The comments may be made using any modality (speech, writing, pointing, gesturing, or any combination of expressive modes). Following the utterance of the patient, the clinician should clarify the message as necessary (Hegde, 1996b).

Auditory Stimulation Approach for Aphasia

The auditory stimulation approach for aphasia was developed by Schuell on the premise that reauditorization would facilitate the use of language in patients who have aphasia. The approach focuses on intensive auditory stimulation or auditory bombardment. In this method, auditory stimulation is combined with visual stimulation to facilitate the use of words, phrases, and sentences. As in other techniques, the clinician should begin with easy, familiar tasks, gradually increasing the complexity of the stimuli. In the auditory stimulation program, the clinician proceeds through the following steps:

1. Pointing to objects;

2. Following directions;

3. Answering yes-no questions;

4. Responding to alternate items;

5. Repeating words, phrases, and sentences;

6. Answering different kinds of questions;

7. Forming simple sentences;

8. Retelling stories;

9. Describing pictures and events;

10. Engaging in conversation;

11. Copying and writing words (Hegde, 1996b).

In this approach, the clinician does not correct responses made by the patient. Instead, he/she repeats the stimulation.

Visual Action Therapy (VAT)

Visual Action Therapy was developed by Helm-Estabrooks, et al. In this technique, neither the clinician nor the patient talks. All communication is done through the use of visual and gestural communication. VAT has been used with some success in patients with global aphasia. Prerequisite criteria for using this approach require that the client be able to match an object with a tracing of that object. The clinician chooses "seven real objects, shaded line drawings of the objects, and seven action pictures involving the objects" (Hegde, 1996b, p. 25). The program progresses through three levels, with the first level using pictures and objects, the second level using action pictures of the objects, and the third level using only drawings. More complete information on the steps in each level can be obtained from Helm-Estabrooks and Albert (1991) or Hegde (1996b).

CHAPTER SEVEN
Apraxia

DEFINITION/DESCRIPTION

Apraxia is defined by Wertz (in Helm-Estabrooks & Holland, 1998) as "a neurogenic speech disorder resulting from sensorimotor impairment of the capacity to program and execute, in coordinated and normally timed sequences, the positioning of the speech musculature for the volitional production of speech sounds with loss or impairment of phonologic rules not being adequate to explain the observed pattern of deviant speech" (Helm-Estabrooks & Holland, 1998, p. 12). Furthermore, the disorder is not due to weakened musculature.

McNeil, Robin, and Schmidt (1997, p. 311) posit that apraxia is only present when "assurance could be given that the patient had the intent, the underlying *linguistic representation*, and the fundamental *motor abilities* to produce speech, but could not do so *volitionally*."

Wertz, LaPointe, and Rosenbek (1984, p. 81) did a detailed review of the characteristics of apraxia, but found the following four features to be the most salient clinical characteristics of apraxia of speech:

> (1) Effortful, trial and error, groping articulatory movements and attempts at self correction. (2) Dysprosody unrelieved by extended periods of normal rhythm, stress, and intonation. (3) Articulatory inconsistency on repeated productions of the same utterance. (4) Obvious difficulty initiating utterances.

Wertz et al., (1984) further suggested that patients who demonstrate these four behaviors in imitative and spontaneous speech should be diagnosed as apraxic. However, it should be noted that "only the dysprosody, in the context of these three (and other) behaviors is likely to separate it from phonemic paraphasia" (McNeil et al., 1997, p. 328).

Acquired apraxia of speech may occur as the result of a stroke, traumatic brain injury, or a tumor. It is typically defined as involving "disruption in the planning and programming of voluntary, complex motor activity for speech production" (Caruso & Strand, 1999b, p. 14). The deficits do not carry over to vegetative functioning. If the individual has difficulty with voluntary movement of the lips, tongue, or jaw, it is referred to as oral apraxia. It may also occur with verbal (speech) apraxia.

The pathology of apraxia of speech is in the left hemisphere. It is not unusual for apraxia of speech to coexist with a nonfluent aphasia. Vascular pathology typically involves the left middle cerebral artery. According to Hegde (1996), the dominant symptoms of apraxia of speech include "speech programming difficulties with inconsistent errors of articulation, groping and struggling, notable difficulties in volitional speech production, and prosodic problems" (p. 67).

Guilmette (1997) defines apraxia as "an inability to carry out purposeful or skilled movements to command by an individual who has normal motor functions (e.g., strength, tone, coordination, reflexes) and who has generally adequate auditory comprehension and intellectual skills" (Guilmette, p. 44). He goes on to identify three types of apraxia:

Ideomotor: a disruption in the selection, sequencing, and spatial orientation of movements in response to a verbal command, especially involving a tool or object;

Ideational: an inability to carry out a sequence of acts in their proper order . . . although each individual activity can be performed normally;

Buccofacial: the inability to perform learned skilled movements of the face, lips, tongue, cheeks, larynx and pharynx on command; occurs in greater than 90% of patients with Broca's aphasia; usually results from frontal or Corpus Callosum lesions (Guilmette, 1997, p. 45).

McNeill et al., (1997) present a table delineating the differences between apraxia of speech and dysarthria. The information in this table (Table 7–1) is based on the work of Wertz, LaPointe, and Rosenbek in 1984.

In apraxia of speech, the most frequent misarticulations are omissions and substitutions. Also, the number of misarticulations typically increases when the complexity of the speech task increases. Both consonants and vowels are affected, although more errors are noted on consonants than on vowels. Also, sounds in the initial position are affected more than

TABLE 7–I Traditional differentiating characteristics of AOS and dysarthria

Feature	AOS	Dysarthria
Lesion location	Unilateral/anterior	Bilateral if cortical, usually subcortical
Psychophysioloigcal level/ mechanism	Motor programming	Movement execution
Observed deviant speech behavior	Speech initiation, selection, & sequencing; phoneme substitution; abnormal prosody; infrequent metathetic errors	Sound-level distortions
Speech processes involved	Essentially normal: 1. Resonance 2. Respiration 3. Phonation	Frequent disturbance of: 1. Resonance 2. Respiration 3. Phonation
Physiological manifestations	Free from paralysis, paresis, ataxia, involuntary movements	Presence of paralysis, paresis, ataxia, involuntary movements
Influence on nonphonologic (phonetic) factors	Affected by word length; error inconsistency	Less affected by word length; errors are more consistent
Oral Nonverbal Apraxia	Frequently present	Absent

From "Apraxia of Speech: Definition, Differentiation, and Treatment," by M. R. McNeil, D. A. Rubin, & R. A. Schmidt, 1997, in *Clinical Management of Sensorimotor Speech Disorders* by M. R. McNeil (Ed.), New York: Thieme Medical Publishers. Copyright 1997 by Thieme Medical Publishers. Reprinted with permission.

sounds in the medial or final positions. It is important to note that the errors are inconsistent. The patient may produce a syllable, word, or phrase correctly one time, then incorrectly another time. Reactive and automatic speech tasks typically are freer of errors than regular speech efforts. Metathetic errors also occur (Shipley & McAfee, 1992).

Developmental apraxia of speech (DAOS) refers to the "inability or difficulty with the ability to perform purposeful voluntary movements for speech, in the absence of a paralysis or weakness of the speech musculature" (Caruso & Strand, 1999b, pp. 14–16). Developmental apraxia of speech typically occurs at a time when children are acquiring language, implying that there is a motor-linguistic processing deficit in apraxia. Crary (1993) writes that the motor-linguistic deficit is present in adults and children, but is more pronounced in children since they are still learning language.

ASSESSMENT

Shipley and McAfee designed checklists for limb, oral, and verbal apraxia. These checklists are included in Appendix 7–A.

Hegde (1996) recommends testing for coexisting aphasia using standard tests for aphasia (see chapter on Aphasia). Other problems associated with aphasia (auditory comprehension, reading, and writing) should also be assessed. Wertz, LaPointe, and Rosenbek developed the *Motor Speech Evaluation* (1991), which can be used to assess speech production in adults.

The patient's speech should be recorded and transcribed phonetically. One should also make note of groping behaviors, dysfluencies such as repetitions, facial grimacing, delayed reactions, and self-corrections. Diadochokinesis should be assessed by having the patient say each CV combination in p t k individually for several repetitions as evenly as possible. Then, the patient should be instructed to say "p t k" as long and evenly as possible.

Imitated production of selected words should then be elicited. A list of some of these words is in the Appendix 7–A checklist. Other suggested words are in Appendix 7–B. Repetition of words and phrases, as well as sentences, should be evoked. Sample sentences could include:

> The valuable watch is missing.
>
> In the summer they sell vegetables.
>
> The shipwreck washed up on the shore.
>
> Please put the groceries in the refrigerator.
>
> Please tell the gardener to fertilize the plants.
>
> I do not understand the reasons for repeating it. (Hegde, 1996, p. 63)

Automatic speech, such as counting from one to twenty should also be assessed. Spontaneous speech can be assessed by having the patient describe a picture such as the "Cookie Thief" picture from the *Boston Diagnostic Aphasia Examination* (Goodglass & Kaplan, 1983). Oral reading can be assessed using standard passages such as the "Rainbow Passage" or the "Grandfather Passage."

In addition to the *Motor Speech Evaluation,* published tests for apraxia include the *Screening Test for Developmental Apraxia of Speech* (Blakeley, 1980), the *Apraxia Battery for Adults* (Dabul, 1986), *The Test of Oral and Limb Apraxia* (Helm-Estabrooks, 1992) and the *Comprehensive Apraxia Test* (DiSimoni, 1989).

With regard to differential diagnosis, one should evaluate the muscle forces produced during nonspeech tasks. If there is weakness present, the diagnosis should be dysarthria, not apraxia of speech.

> If disorders of postural control are evidenced, the diagnosis of oral-nonverbal apraxia or dysarthria (depending on its precise nature) are the likely diagnoses. In fact, it is usually part of the criteria for the diagnosis of AOS that individual articulator strength (usually measured as maximum muscle force) as well as articulatory positioning (usually measured as accurate articulatory placement and speed of movement) be judged within normal limits. (McNeil, Robin, & Schmidt, 1997, p. 320)

In 1979, Dabul proposed "a list of 15 speech and nonspeech behaviors that characterize AOS, any five or more of which were sufficient for its diagnosis." These 15 characteristics are listed in Table 7–2. However, it should be noted that in 1991, Pierce found that only three of the 15 behaviors were unique to speakers with AOS. The other 12 were also characteristic of phonemic paraphasia. These three behaviors were "difficulty initiating speech, intrusion of a schwa, and abnormal prosody" (McNeil et al., 1997, p. 326).

With regard to developmental apraxia of speech, Crary (1993) suggests that evaluation should consist of observation and documentation of "motor and motor speech functions, articulation/phonological performance, language performance, and potential interactions among these aspects of communication" (p. 171). Regarding pre-evaluation clinical observations, Crary (1993) suggests several observations that are summarized in Table 7–3.

TABLE 7-2 Dabul's speech and nonspeech behaviors that characterize AOS
anticipatory phonemic errors
perseverative phonemic errors
phonemic transposition errors
phonemic voicing substitutions
phonemic vowel substitutions
visible and audible searching behavior
numerous and varied off-target attempts at the word
highly inconsistent errors
increase in errors with increase in phonemic sequence
fewer errors in automatic speech than volitional speech
marked difficulty initiating speech
intrusion of a schwa between syllables or in consonant clusters
abnormal prosodic features
awareness of errors and inability to correct them
receptive-expressive gap

Adapted from "Apraxia of Speech: Definition, Differentiation, and Treatment," by M. R. McNeil, D. A. Rubin, & R. A. Schmidt, 1997, in *Clinical Management of Sensorimotor Speech Disorders* by M. R. McNeil (Ed.), New York: Thieme Medical Publishers. Copyright 1997 by Thieme Medical Publishers. Adapted with permission.

Table 7–3 Suggestions for pre-evaluation clinical observations of children with developmental motor speech disorders

Nonspeech Motor Functions

General Sensorimotor Organization
Posture and gait
Movement patterns
Gross and fine sensorimotor coordination

Oral Sensorimotor Organization
Overt paresis—asymmetry in the mechanism
Mouth posture
Drooling, mastication, swallowing, etc.

Speech Motor Functions

Nonspeech Indicators
Struggle, strain during speech
Visible groping of the oral articulators

Speech Indicators
Fluency of speech
Prosodic deviations
Hyper-Hyponasality
Voice deviations

Articulation/Phonological Performance

Amount of Verbal Output
Quiet, reluctant to speak
Highly interactive
Overall intelligibility

Type of Errors
Indication of "dominant" error type

Language Performance

Comprehension
Understand basic questions, instructions
Answers, interacts appropriately

Expression
Gestures and/or verbal output
Type of utterances (single words, sentences, etc.)

Other Observations

Attention
Focus, shift, sustain
Easily distracted/self-distracted

Reaction to Speech
Shy, withdrawn, crying
Aggressive
Other

From *Developmental Motor Speech Disorders,* by M. A. Crary, 1993, San Diego, CA: Singular Publishing Group. Copyright 1993, by Singular Publishing Group. Reprinted with permission.

The actual evaluation should address five aspects: motor, motor-speech, articulation/phonology, language, and other. Whether the evaluation can be completed in one session is dependent on the clinical environment and the child's ability to attend to and complete the tasks at hand. Based on the pre-evaluation observations, the clinician can alter the sequence of the assessment tasks, which are outlined in Table 7–4. It may be advisable, particularly in young and/or frustrated children, to begin with the more simple tasks, then intermingle the speech and nonspeech tasks (Crary, 1993).

TABLE 7-4 Basic components of the evaluation of developmental motor speech disorders

Motor

    Oral Structural-Functional Examination
        Anatomy and asymmetry
        Basic movement characteristics (range, speed, etc.)
        Reflexes
        Lingual/labial-mandibular dependency

    Volitional Oral Movements (Praxis)
        Traditional praxis examination
        Volitional oral movement task (single-sequential)

    Volitional Limb Movements (Praxis)
        Test of limb apraxia
        Fist-Edge-Palm task
        Communicative gestures

Motor Speech

    Basic Performance Patterns
        Prosody, fluency
        Nasality, voice deviations
        Maximum performance tests

    Speech Diadochokinesis
        Alternate motion rate
        Sequential motion rate
        Bite block effects

Articulation/Phonological Assessment

    Standardized Articulation Tests
        Objective severity assessment
        Normative comparison
        Typically sound based

    Phonological Analysis
        Patterns of errors
        Choice of elicitation technique

    Performance Load Effects
        Performance at increasing levels of complexity

    Other Phonological Functions
        Parallels with written language deficits
        Internal phonological processing

Language Assessment

    Comprehension
        Semantic, syntactic comprehension
        Effect of increased length of input

    Expression
        Standardized tests
        Interactive conversation and/or extended description
        Bottom up interference

Extended Evaluations

    Attention, perceptual, memory functions, etc.

    Intelligence, educational evaluation

    Medical evaluation

    Extended sensorimotor evaluation

From *Developmental Motor Speech Disorders,* by M. A. Crary, 1993, San Diego, CA: Singular Publishing Group. Copyright 1993 by Singular Publishing Group. Reprinted with permission.

TREATMENT

If one accepts the assumption that apraxia of speech is defined as a motor control problem, it will be imperative that the clinician apply "principles of motor control and learning to the therapeutic process" (McNeil et al., 1997, p. 329). The approach and timing of treatment for apraxia of speech in adults also depends, in part, on the presence of other conditions such as aphasia and/or dysarthria. If aphasia is present, the clinician may want to consider deferring treatment until the client is producing some language.

Once treatment begins, clinicians should structure the session to move from easy to more difficult tasks. The speech tasks should be carefully sequenced as follows:

> automatic speech before spontaneous speech;
>
> frequently occurring sounds before less frequently occurring sounds;
>
> stimulable sounds before nonstimulable sounds;
>
> sounds in word-initial positions before those in other positions;
>
> visible before nonvisible sounds;
>
> oral-nasal distinctions before voicing distinctions;
>
> voicing distinctions before manner distinctions;
>
> manner distinctions before place distinctions;
>
> bilabial and lingua-alveolar sounds before others;
>
> singletons before clusters;
>
> high-frequency words before low-frequency words;
>
> meaningful words;
>
> single-syllable words before multisyllable words;
>
> single words before phrases or sentences (Hegde, 1996b, pp. 27–28).

Procedurally, the clinician should provide models for the client to imitate, particularly during the early stages of treatment. The rate should initially be reduced, but, as articulatory proficiency increases, speech rate can be increased. Shaping should be used to facilitate the production of normal prosody. As always, immediate feedback is the best type of reinforcement. It is a good idea to promote the use of total communication (i.e., speech, gestures, writing, and AAC devices if so indicated) to facilitate communication in all settings. Monitoring frustration, depression, and motivation levels is critical. Offering counseling and support for the client and his family should be part of the treatment regimen.

Other therapy suggestions include working on large muscle group training prior to fine movements. Providing compensations, particularly in the early stages of therapy may be helpful for some patients (Guilmette, 1997, p. 46).

Some traditional approaches to therapy for apraxia of speech are delineated in McNeil et al. (1997). They include the following:

1. Phonetic derivation, which is the "shaping of speech sounds based on their nonspeech postures and/or actions" (p. 330). This approach may be problematic if oral apraxia is also

present. However, the clinician is able to control the complexity of the tasks by using nonspeech movements.

2. Progressive approximation involves the shaping of speech segments from other speech segments.

3. Phonetic placement is a technique in which the "clinician focuses on the position of the articulators during speech production and the coordination between speech production subsystems" (p. 330).

4. The key word technique builds upon words that the client can produce consistently. The key words are produced "under conditions whereby the patient exhibits greater degrees of control and lesser degrees of automaticity in the responses. Once the patient shows fairly good control of the key words, practice is expanded to include new words that contain the same phonemes as the key words" (p. 330).

5. Phonemic contrasts or minimal pairs is a technique in which the client imitates words that have minimal contrasts in terms of voicing, manner, and place.

6. Targeting the temporal schemata of speech and sequencing of segments into longer utterances forms the basis for a technique based on the premise that there is a rhythmic or temporal basis underlying the control of motor behaviors, including speech. Kent and Adams (1989) proposed that apraxia may be considered as a breakdown in the "normal temporal coherence of speech production" (McNeil et al., 1997, p. 331). Melodic Intonation Therapy (MIT) is an example of this technique. In MIT, the patient varies the pitch of the utterance, and uses a lengthened tempo in which the natural rhythm and stress of speech are exaggerated.

7. PROMPT is an acronym standing for Prompts for Restructuring Oral Musculature Phonetic Targets. This technique was originally developed for use with children, but later adapted for adults. It uses a highly structured system of finger placements on the face and neck to represent the different oral positions of the articulators during speech (Pierce, 1991). The finger placements are a cuing system that alerts the client "about such aspects of production as muscular tension, duration of production, and continuance" (McNeil et al., 1997, p. 331). Treatment efficacy data supporting the PROMPT technique is available.

8. Many other methods are incorporated into an Eight Step Task Continuum (Rosenbek, Lemme, Ahern, Harris, & Wertz, 1973). In the first step of this technique, the clinician instructs the client to watch and listen to him/her as they simultaneously produce a speech target. The final step involves role playing with the clinician, family members, and friends. "The intermittent stages move the patient systematically from simultaneous imitation to role-play by delayed imitation, removal of visual cues, the addition of successive productions and so on" (McNeil et al., 1997, p. 331–332).

More recent techniques have focused on learning motor movements through practice and experience. Inherent in practice and learning are the critical components of attention and memory. Acquisition of sounds is achieved through practice, and once the sounds are learned, they are retained. McNeil et al. (1997) discuss the importance of prepractice with the client. Prepractice encompasses the following activities:

1. Verbal pretraining: Some aspects of this portion of the training will be nonverbal. The point of this activity is to expose the client to the various stimuli that will be used in the training portion of the therapy.

2. During the second stage of prepractice, the clinician provides graphic representations of how specific movements and sounds are produced. The clinician can use models, videos, and/or drawings, but verbal input should be kept to a minimum.

3. The establishment of a "prepractice reference of correctness" should be the final aspect of the prepractice portion of therapy. This will help the client to practice away from the therapy session because he will have a level of reference for what is an acceptable response.

Also during prepractice, the client should be involved in helping to set goals to be attained in the practice portion of the therapy.

Both quantity of practice and quality of practice are critical concerns during the practice portion. The clinician should be striving to increase the efficiency with which the client makes the motor movements, be they verbal or nonverbal. Another critical concern is the type of feedback which is given to the client. McNeil et al. (1997, p. 335) differentiate between knowledge of results (KR) and knowledge of performance (KP). "KR refers to feedback about the outcome of a movement pattern with reference to the environmental goal. KR is *not* feedback about the parameters of the movement pattern itself, which is termed KP. KR refers to information provided by the clinician, to the patient, about the success of the movement." The timing of the feedback is of crucial importance. McNeil and his colleagues recommend approximately three seconds between the response and the feedback. They also have found that summary feedback after a series of trials (up to 15 for easy tasks; limited to 5 trials for difficult tasks) is more effective than immediate feedback after each trial. Extensive information about KR and KP is provided in McNeil et al. (1997).

Techniques for treating children with developmental apraxia of speech (DAOS) are summarized by Haynes in Table 7–5.

TABLE 7-5 Techniques for treating children with DAOS summarized by Haynes (1985)

Concentrated drill (both imitative and on command) of isolated movements of tongue and lips

Imitation of sustained vowels and consonants, followed by imitation of CV and VC combinations

Imitation of syllables and words

Avoid auditory discrimination drills (unless deficits in auditory discrimination have been determined)

Use slow rate and facilitate self-monitoring

Introduce a core vocabulary

Use carrier phrases to provide the basis for increased meaningful sentences

Use rhythm, intonation, and stress, paired with limb movement to facilitate speech motor sequencing

Use intensive, frequent, and systematic drill

Develop and heighten presensory perceptual awareness

From *Clinical Management of Motor Speech Disorders in Children* (p. 117), by A. J. Caruso and E. A. Strand, 1999, New York: Thieme Medical Publishers. Copyright 1999 by Thieme Medical Publishers. Reprinted with permission.

In summary, there are five principles which underlie the treatment of apraxia of speech based on motor training:

1. Intensive treatment is required;

2. A large number (20 is suggested) of repetitions are needed;

3. Move from nonspeech tasks to speech tasks as soon as feasible;

4. Progress systematically through hierarchies based on task difficulty; and

5. Emphasize prosody simultaneously with articulation.

APPENDIX 7-A CHECKLISTS FOR LIMB, ORAL, AND VERBAL APRAXIA

Name: _____ Age: _____

Date: _____

Examiner: _____

Instructions: Select several items from each section and ask the client to complete the task or repeat the utterance. Many items are provided to offer a wide range of tasks; you do not need to complete each item. Score each presented item as correct (+ or) or incorrect (– or). Transcribe errors phonetically on the right hand side. Also note accompanying behaviors such as delays with initiation, struggling, groping, or facial grimacing. The diagnosis of apraxia is made by evaluating the nature and accuracy of movement, as well as the type and severity of error patterns present.

Limb Apraxia   **Comments**

_____ wave hello or good bye   _____

_____ make a fist   _____

_____ make the "thumbs up" sign   _____

_____ make the "okay" sign   _____

_____ pretend you're zipping your coat   _____

_____ pretend you're combing your hair   _____

_____ pretend you're petting a dog   _____

_____ pretend you're turning a doorknob   _____

_____ pretend you're hitting a baseball
        (or golf ball)   _____

_____ pretend you're tying a shoe   _____

_____ pretend you're using scissors to cut a
        piece of paper   _____

_____ pretend you're knocking on a door   _____

_____ pretend you're writing   _____

_____ pretend you're going to make a fire   _____

_____ pretend you're going to make coffee   _____

_____ pretend you're going to drive a car

out of a driveway _____

Oral Apraxia   **Comments**

_____ smile   _____

_____ open your mouth   _____

_____ blow   _____

_____ whistle   _____

_____ puff out your cheeks   _____

_____ chatter your teeth as if you are cold   _____

_____ pucker your lips   _____

_____ bite your lower lip   _____

_____ smack your lips   _____

_____ lick your lips   _____

_____ stick out your tongue   _____

_____ touch your nose with the tip of your
       tongue   _____

_____ move your tongue in and out   _____

_____ wiggle your tongue side to side   _____

_____ click your tongue   _____

_____ cough   _____

_____ alternately pucker and smile   _____

Verbal Apraxia   **Comments or Transcription**

_____ love - loving - lovingly   _____

_____ jab - jabber - jabbering   _____

_____ zip - zipper - zippering   _____

_____ soft - soften - softening   _____

_____ hope - hopeful - hopefully   _____

_____ hard - harden - hardening   _____

_____ thick - thicken - thickening   _____

_____ please - pleasing - pleasingly   _____

_____ sit - city - citizen - citizenship   _____

_____ cat - catnip - catapult - catastrophe   _____

_____ strength - strengthen - strengthening   _____

_____ door - doorknob - doorkeeper - dormitory   _____

_____ tornado   _____

_____ radiator   _____

_____ artillery   _____

_____ linoleum   _____

_____ inevitable   _____

_____ delegation   _____

_____ probability   _____

_____ cauliflower   _____

_____ declaration   _____

_____ refrigeration   _____

_____ unequivocally   _____

_____ thermometer   _____

_____ parliamentarian   _____

_____ catastrophically   _____

_____ disenfranchised   _____

_____ statistical analysis   _____

_____ alternative opinion   _____

_____ regulatory authority   _____

_____ ruthlessly malicious   _____

_____ barometric pressure   _____

_____ indescribably delicious   _____

_____ Mississippi River   _____

_____ Tallahassee, Florida   _____

_____ Kalamazoo, Michigan   _____

_____ Boston, Massachusetts   _____

_____ Sacramento, California   _____

_____ Madison Square Garden   _____

_____ Minneapolis, Minnesota   _____

_____ Chattanooga, Tennessee   _____

_____ Encyclopedia Britannica

_____ Saskatoon, Saskatchewan

_____ Philadelphia, Pennsylvania

_____ Oakland - Alameda Coliseum

_____ Vancouver, British Columbia

_____ Nuclear Regulatory Commission

_____

_____

_____

_____

_____

_____

APPENDIX 7–B: SUGGESTED WORDS FOR IMITATION WHEN ASSESSING APRAXIA OF SPEECH

several	parliamentarian	please	coke
tornado	statistical analysis	pleasing	gag
artillery	Encyclopedia Britannica	pleasingly	fife
linoleum	Boston, Massachusetts	jab	sis
snowman	Minneapolis, Minnesota	jabber	zoos
television	San Francisco, California	jabbering	church
catastrophe	Nuclear Regulatory Commission	mom	churn
gingerbread	thick	judge	lull
probability	thicken	peep	shush
thermometer	thickening	bib	roar
refrigeration	love	nine	
responsibility	loving	tote	
unequivocally	lovingly	dad	

Source: Hegde, M. N. (1996). *Diagnosis in Speech-Language Pathology.* San Diego, CA: Singular Publishing Group. Reprinted with permission.

CHAPTER EIGHT
Articulation and Phonological Disorders

DEFINITION/DESCRIPTION

An "articulation disorder" implies that the individual has a motor speech disorder which negatively affects his ability to enunciate specific sounds. The term "phonological disorder" implies that there is a language component to the disorder. That is to say, language is required to learn speech. Both terms are used to describe individuals who have difficulty pronouncing sounds in the absence of physical problems such as an unrepaired cleft lip and/or palate, cranial nerve damage, problems with respiratory control, and laryngeal anomalies, although articulation and/or phonological problems can co-exist with any of these disorders (Bleile, 1995).

Diacritic markers are those used to modify symbols to describe phonetic detail. Bleile (1995) compiled a listing of the most frequently used symbols and diacritics, which is delineated in Table 8–1. American English consonants are displayed according to manner and place of production in Table 8–2, and the vowels and dipthongs are listed in Table 8–3.

TABLE 8-I Most frequently used symbols and diacritics		
A. Place of Production		
[Φ] [β]**	Bilabial fricatives (two lips approximate each other)	Φ
[͟]	Labiodental oral and nasal stops (upper teeth to lower lip)	p b m
[͡]	Dentolabial plosives and nasal (lower teeth to upper lip)	p b m
[͟]	Interdentalized (also called lisped) (tongue tip/blade between teeth)	t θ l
[͜]	Bidental (teeth approximated)	h u
[͜]	Bidental percussive (teeth brought percussively together)	t d
[ɲ]	Palatal nasal (nasal stop made at palatal region)	
[x] [ɣ]	Velar fricatives (fricatives produced in the velar region)	x ɣ
[fŋ]	Velopharyngeal fricative (fricative made in velopharyngeal region)	fŋ
[ʔ]	Glottal stop (stop produced at vocal folds)	ʔ
		continued

TABLE 8-1 continued

B. Manner of Production

[↔]	Labial spreading (lips spread)	s̷↔ t↔
[_]	Unrounded (lips at rest, unpursed)	w̲
[ˣ]	Denasal (little air through nose)	m̽ n̽
[ˣ]	Nasal escape (air through nose)	p̽ s̽
[‿]	Bladed (produced with tongue blade)	s̺ z̺
[r̮]	[w]-coloring ([r] with a [w]-like quality)	r̮
[ɾ]	Flap (quick stop-like consonant as in "butter")	ɾ
[|s]	Lateralized [s] and [z], respectively (air over the sides of tongue)	[|s] [|z]
[„]	Stronger production (produced with greater force than is typical)	f„
[ᵓ]	Weaker production (produced with less force than is typical)	ᵓ
[↑]	Whistled (high pitched sound)	s̝↑
[t̥]	Wet sound (produced with excess saliva)	t̥

C. Airstream

[↓]	Ingressive (air moves inward)	p↓
[(X)]	Silent or 'mouthing' (no sound produced)	(s)

D. Vocal Fold Activity

[ˌ] [ˌ]	Pre- and post-voicing of sounds (voicing begins earlier or ends later than expected)	ˌb zˌ
[₍ₒ₎]	Partial devoicing (normally voiced sound is partially devoiced)	z₍ₒ₎
[₍ᵥ₎]	Partial voicing (normally voiceless sound is partially voiced)	f₍ᵥ₎
[ʰ]	Pre-aspiration (sound begins with aspiration)	ʰp
[°]	Unaspirated (normally aspirated voiceless stops produced without aspiration	p° t° k°

E. Syllables and Stress

[ˌ]	Syllabic (consonant standing as a syllable)	l̩
[.]	Syllable boundary (separation between syllables)	bi.twin
[']	Primary stress (syllable with main stress)	bitwín

**Whenever two symbols are presented, the first is unvoiced and the second is voiced.

From *Manual of Articulation and Phonological Disorders* (pp. 37–39), by K. M. Bleile, 1995, San Diego, CA: Singular Publishing Group. Copyright 1995 by Singular Publishing Group. Reprinted with permission.

Table 8-2 American English consonants according to manner and place of production

Manner of Production	Place of Production							
	Bilabial	Labiodental	Interdental	Alveolar	Postalveolar	Palatal	Velar	Glottal
Stop								
Oral	p b			t d			k g	
Nasal	m			n			ŋ	
Fricative		f v	θ ð	s z	ʃ ʒ			
Affricate					tʃ dʒ			
Liquid								
Central				r				
Lateral				l				
Glide	w					j		h

From *Manual of Articulation and Phonological Disorders* (p.13), by K. M. Bleile, 1995, San Diego, CA: Singular Publishing Group. Copyright 1995 by Singular Publishing Group. Reprinted with permission.

Table 8-3 American English vowels and diphthongs

Height	Place				
	Front		Central	Back	
	+ Sprd[a]			- Rnd[b]	+ Rnd
Close	i				u
		I		ʊ	
Close mid	eI				oʊ
			ə		
Open mid	ε			ʌ	ɔ
		æ			
Open		a			ɑ

[a] = Sprd = lips spread
[b] = − Rnd = lips unrounded
   + Rnd = lips unrounded

Notes:
[ɔI] = tongue begins as for [ɔ] and moves toward [I]
[aI] = tongue begins as for [a] and moves toward [I]
[aʊ] = tongue begins as for [a] and moves toward [ʊ]
[ə^] = tongue shape has both [ə]-like and [r]-like qualities

From *Manual of Articulation and Phonological Disorders* (p. 14), by K. M. Bleile, 1995, San Diego, CA: Singular Publishing Group. Copyright 1995 by Singular Publishing Group. Reprinted with permission.

Terms related to the phonological aspects of language are outlined in Table 8–4.

TABLE 8-4 Phonological processes

Process	Description
Syllable reduction	Reducing the number of syllables in the verbal production of a word or utterance
Multisyllabicity	Difficulty producing words of 4 or more syllables
Postvocalic singleton deletion	The omission of a single consonant that terminates a consonant word or syllable
Prevocalic singleton consonant deletion	The absence of single consonants that initiate words
Intervocalic singleton consonant deletion	The omission of word-medial consonants
Consonant sequence reduction	The omission of one or more sound segments from two or more contiguous consonants
Consonant sequence deletion	The omission of more than one segment in a cluster
Coalescence	The replacement of two adjacent consonants by one that retains features from both of the original sounds
Migration	The moving of a sound to another position in the utterance
Epenthesis	The insertion of an additional sound in a word
Glottal replacement	The use of a glottal stop to replace a standard consonant
Substitutions	The demonstration that the position of the sound in a syllable or a sequence is within their capabilities, but some key characteristic of the class of which that sound is a member may not yet have been acquired. Thus, the sound is replaced with another sound with similar features.
Fronting	The substitution of alveolars for velars
Backing	The reverse direction of place-shift, in which anterior sounds are replaced by back phonemes
Palatization	Adding a palatal component to a nonpalatal phoneme
Depalatization	The deletion of the palatal component from a palatal phoneme target
"th" shifts	The replacing of /θ, ð / by anterior strident phonemes /f, v, s, z/
Stopping	Substituting stops for "nonstop" phonemes, with fricatives being the phoneme class most often affected. May also occur for sonorants.
Gliding	The substitution of a glide for a sound in another class
Vowelization	Substituting a vowel for a liquid
Affrication	The substitution of an affricate for a nonaffricate sound
Deaffrication	The replacement of a target affricate with a continuant phoneme
Postvocalic devoicing	Replacement of a voiced postvocalic obstruent with a voiceless phone
Prevocalic voicing	The replacement of a voiceless prevocalic consonant with a voiced sound
Prevocalic devoicing	The replacement of a voiced prevocalic obstruent with a voiceless phone
Postvocalic voicing	The replacement of a voiceless postvocalic consonant with a voiced sound; the rarest of voicing changes
Neutralization	A deviation involving vowels wherein all or many vowels are reduced to one or two; a major problem for children with profound hearing impairment
Assimilation	Altering a phoneme so that it takes on a characteristic of another sound in the word or phrase, presumably due to the influence of that other sound

TABLE 8-4 continued	
Process	*Description*
Metathesis	The reversal of the position of two sounds
Reduplication	Repeating a sound or syllable in a word in place of all the others
Tongue protrusion	The forward positioning of the tongue tip during productions of consonants
Lateralization	Emission of a sound to the side(s) rather than centrally; primarily affects the sibilants
Nasalization	Nasal emission during the production of typically nonnasal sounds; primarily affects the vowels, and occasionally nonnasal consonants
Denasalization	Speech that is produced strictly in the oral cavity
Pharyngealization/ velarization	The production of consonants with an inappropriate constriction in the velopharyngeal area

Adapted from *Targeting Intelligible Speech: A Phonological Approach to Remediation* (2nd ed.), by B. W. Hodson and E. P. Paden, 1991, Austin, TX: Pro-Ed. Copyright 1991 by Pro-Ed. Used with permission.

DSM DIAGNOSTIC CRITERIA FOR 315.39 PHONOLOGICAL DISORDER

A. Failure to use developmentally expected speech sounds that are appropriate for age and dialect (e.g., errors in sound production, use, representation, or organization, such as, but not limited to, substitutions of one sound for another [use of /t/ for target /k/ sound] or omissions of sounds such as final consonants).

B. The difficulties in speech sound production interfere with academic or occupational achievement or with social communication.

C. If mental retardation, a speech-motor or sensory deficit, or environmental deprivation is present, the speech difficulties are in excess of those usually associated with these problems.

Coding Note: If a speech-motor or sensory deficit or a neurological condition is present, code the condition on Axis III.

ASSESSMENT

A screening is a simple method of determining if a child's speech is within normal limits or not. Typically, it should not take more than five minutes to screen a child's speech. If the child fails a screening, or exhibits signs of an articulation or phonological disorder, a complete assessment should be done. Actual screening of the articulation should be preceded by a quick review of the client's oral-facial structures. Signs of asymmetry and malocclusion should be noted. The palate should be observed to determine if there is a submucous or repaired cleft. The position and size of the tongue should also be noted. If the child is an infant between 9–12 months of age, the parent should be encouraged to elicit vocalizations from the child. The clinician should note whether the child uses reduplicated babbling ("ba ba") and/or non-reduplicated babbling ("ba da"). If the child does not engage in either type of babbling, he should be referred for a complete speech and language evaluation. (Bleile, 1995)

For toddlers (18–24 months), the clinician should inquire as to how many and what words the child is using. If the child is not using words, he, too, should be referred for a complete speech and language evaluation.

For all other ages, a short speech sample should be elicited in order to assess the individual's articulatory skills. (Bleile, 1995)

In addition to the above mentioned nonstandardized methods of screening, there are numerous published screening instruments. A list of some of these follows:

A Screening Deep Test of Articulation: designed to screen children in K–3rd grade (McDonald, 1968a)

Speech and Language Screening Test: intended for use with children 2–6 years of age (Fluharty, N., 1978)

Predictive Screening Test for Articulation (Van Riper & Erickson, 1973)

Templin-Darley Test of Articulation: intended for use with children aged 3–8 years. (Templin, M. & Darley, F., 1969)

Articulation Subtest of the Preschool Language Scale: intended for use with children aged 1–7 years. (Zimmerman, I., Steiner, V., & Pond, R. 1992)

Quick Screen of Phonology: intended for use with children aged 3–7 years old (Bankson, N., & Bernthal, J. 1990)

Screening portion of the *Test of Minimal Articulation Competence* (Secord, W., 1981).

Complete Assessment

A complete articulation or phonological examination includes an oral-facial examination, analysis of a speech sample, and the use of nonstandardized or standardized assessment tools to analyze the client's speech production at the single word and connected speech levels.

Oral-Facial Examination

The oral-facial examination should include the areas outlined in Table 8–5.

The Speech Sample

A speech/language sample should contain a minimum of 50 to 100 utterances (Bleile, 1995). Bleile (1995) recommends that children in stages 2 and 3 (age 12–60 months) be encouraged to produce two or three productions of the same words since they are frequently

TABLE 8-5 Oral-facial examination

Structure	Assessment
Tongue	Position at rest
	Elevation of tip to alveolar ridge
	Lateral movement within oral cavity
	Lateral movement protruded
	Protrusion/retraction (symmetry in movement and at rest)
	Color (dark spots—cancer; grayish—muscular paralysis or paresis)
	Lingual frenum (Does it allow adequate movement of tongue?)
Velum	Symmetry at rest and with elevation
	Gag reflex (presence, absence, strength)
Tonsils	Enlarged, normal, or absent
Hard Palate	Height of arch
	Color (white borders indicative of possible submucous cleft; dark or translucent indicative of a fistula or cleft
Teeth	Caries
	Gum Disease
	Alignment
	Malocclusions
	Absence
Mandible	Symmetry at rest and in movement
Maxilla	Symmetry at rest and in movement
Lips	Position at rest
	Pucker
	Retract corners
	Symmetry at rest and in movement
	Cleft
Face	Bilateral symmetry at rest and in movement
	General muscle tone
Intraoral	Pressure
	Puff cheeks and hold
Reflexes	Gag
	Bite (clonic/tonic)
Diadochokinetic rate	

From "Assessment in Speech-Language Pathology," by K G. Shipley and J. G. McAfee, 1998, in *Assessment in Speech-Language Pathology: A Resource Manual* (2nd ed.), 1998, San Diego, CA: Singular Publishing Group. Copyright 1998 by Singular Publishing Group. Used with permission.

variable in their speech productions. How one transcribes a sample may depend, in part, on the child's age. Again using Bleile's stages, transcription of the speech of a Stage 1 child (birth–12 months) may consist of transcribing the entire vocalization, or using a checklist to mark off the sounds produced. For children at Stage 2 (12–24 months) and Stage 3 (2–5 years), the whole word should be transcribed. For individuals who are over 5 years of age, the clinician can transcribe individual sounds, or use a checklist format to mark off the sounds as correctly or incorrectly produced (Bleile, 1995).

There are a variety of methods that can be used to collect a speech sample. Bleile outlines these as illustrated in Table 8–6.

With younger children, speech samples can be elicited using, among others, books, toys, family photos, picture cards, category games, Bingo, tossing games, toy boxes, and I Spy. For older children and adolescents, questions such as "Tell me how to make a ham sandwich" or simple problem-solving questions can be used. Adults can be asked what their typical day is like, what route they used to get to the clinic, etc. (Bleile, 1995).

Shipley and McAfee (1998) suggest these facilitating techniques when gathering a speech sample:

- Strive for a long sample.

- Vary the subject matter of the sample.

- Seek out multiple environments (e.g., clinic, playground, home, work place, etc.)

- Alter the contexts (e.g., conversation, narratives, responses to pictures, etc.)

- Request other people to record samples for you (e.g., spouse, parent, teacher, etc.)

Clinicians should also avoid yes-no questions, and short-answer questions. The use of "how" and "tell me about . . ." statements help to elicit complete thoughts and sentences so that intelligibility in connected speech can be assessed.

When transcribing a speech sample or a standardized test, Bleile (1995) recommends the use of square brackets to reflect the child's pronunciation. However, if one wants to indicate the phonological status of an enunciation, slashes should be used.

TABLE 8-6   Methods used to collect a speech sample

Elicitation techniques	Definition
Spontaneous speech	Naturally occurring speech
Elicited speech	
Naming	Single words typically elicited through naming objects or pictures. (For example, the clinician shows the child an object or picture and says, "What is this?")
Sentence completion	Single words typically elicited through the client finishing the clinician's sentence. (For example, the clinician shows the client an object or picture and says, "This is a ____.")
Delayed imitation	Single words typically elicited through placing a short phrase between the clinician's model and the client's response. (For example, the clinician makes a statement such as, "This is a cat. Now you say it.")
Imitation	Single words typically elicited through the client's immediate imitation of the clinician's model. (For example, the clinician says, "Say these words after I do.")

From *Manual of Articulation and Phonological Disorders* (p. 57), by K. M. Bleile, 1995, San Diego, CA: Singular Publishing Group. Copyright 1995 by Singular Publishing Group. Used with permission.

Standardized Assessment Instruments

The decision as to whether to use nonstandardized or standardized tests may depend, in part, on the client's age as outlined in Table 8–7.

A list of various published instruments is as follows:

Arizona Articulation Proficiency Scale (Fudala, B., & Reynolds, W., 1986)

The Assessment of Phonological Processes—Revised (Hodson, B., 1986)

The Assessment of Phonological Processes—Spanish (Hodson, B., 1986)

Bankson-Bernthal Test of Phonology (Bankson, N., & Bernthal, J., 1990)

Clinical Probes of Articulation Consistency (Secord, W., 1981)

A Deep Test of Articulation (McDonald, E., 1964)

Fisher-Logemann Test of Articulation Competence (Fisher, H., & Logemann, J., 1971)

Goldman-Fristoe Test of Articulation (Goldman, R., & Fristoe, M., 1986)

Khan-Lewis Phonological Analysis (Khan, L., & Lewis, N., 1986)

The McIntosh Interactive System for Phonological Analysis (Masterson, J., & Pagan, F., 1994)

Natural Process Analysis (Shriberg, L., & Kwiatkowski, J., 1980)

Phonological Assessment of Child Speech (Grunwell, P., 1986)

Phonological Process Analysis (Weiner, F., 1979)

Photo Articulation Test (Pendergast, K., Dickey, S., Selmar, T., & Soder, A., 1969)

Spanish Articulation Measures (Mattes, 1993)

Structured Photographic Articulation Test featuring Dudsberry (Kresheck, J. D., & Werner, E. O., 1989)

Smit-Hand Articulation and Phonology Evaluation (Smit, A. B., & Hand, L., 1997)

The Templin-Darley Tests of Articulation (Templin, M., & Darley, F., 1969)

Test of Minimal Articulation Competence (Secord, W., 1981)

Test of Phonological Awareness (Torgesen, J., & Bryant, B., 1994)

Weiss Comprehensive Articulaton Test (Weiss, C., 1980)

Articulation and phonology can be analyzed using five forms of analysis as outlined by Bleile in Table 8–8.

TABLE 8–7	Use of non-standardized procedures and standardized instruments at four developmental levels	
Developmental Level	*Assessment Strategy*	
Stage 1	**Primarily nonstandardized assessments supplemented by standardized instruments**	
Stage 2	**Primarily nonstandardized assessments supplemented by standardized instruments**	
Stage 3	**Combination of nonstandardized procedures and standardized instruments**	
Stage 4	**Primarily standardized assessment instruments supplemented by nonstandardized assessment procedures**	

From *Manual of Articulation and Phonological Disorders* (p. 48), by K. M. Bleile, 1995, San Diego, CA: Singular Publishing Group. Copyright 1995 by Singular Publishing Group. Used with permission.

TABLE 8-8 Clinical purposes of five forms of analysis

Type of Analysis	Clinical Purposes
Severity	A primary means used to establish the need for clinical services
Intelligibility	A possible means to establish the need for clinical services, also a possible means to help select treatment targets
Age norms	A primary means to help select treatment targets, also used to establish the need for clinical services
Better abilities	A primary means to help select treatment targets
Related analysis	A primary means to identify client characteristics important to the articulation and phonological analysis (adjusted age, developmental age, dialect, acquisition strategies)

From *Manual of Articulation and Phonological Disorders* (p. 127), by K. M. Bleile, 1995, San Diego, CA: Singular Publishing Group. Copyright 1995 by Singular Publishing Group. Used with permission.

TREATMENT

Again referring to the stages of development, Bleile outlines the primary purposes of care at four stages in articulation and phonological development as indicated in Table 8–9.

Short-term goals for clients at four different stages in articulation and phonological development are delineated in Table 8–10.

Two significant contributions to the treatment of articulation and phonological disorders are centered around the use of distinctive features and error patterns. Both were developed to "speed remediation through generalization of treatment results from a treated sound to untreated sounds" (Bleile, 1995, p. 194). Bleile defines each approach as expressed in Table 8–11.

TABLE 8-9 Primary purposes of care at four stages in articulation and phonological development

Stages	Age Range in Typically Developing Children	Primary Purpose of Care
Stage 1	0–12 months	Facilitate practice of vocal skills that serve as the basis for later speech development
Stage 2	12–24 months	Facilitate the acquisition of sounds and syllables in specific words
Stage 3	2–5 years	Facilitate the elimination of errors affecting classes of sounds
Stage 4	5 years and older	Facilitate the elimination of errors affecting late-acquired consonants, consonant clusters, and unstressed syllables in more difficult multisyllabic words

From *Manual of Articulation and Phonological Disorders* (p. 3), by K. M. Bleile, 1995, San Diego, CA: Singular Publishing Group. Copyright 1995 by Singular Publishing Group. Used with permission.

TABLE 8-10	Short-term goals for clients at four different stages in articulation and phonological development
Stages	*Short-term Goal*
Stage 1	Increase opportunities to vocalize
	Facilitate acquisition of developmentally advanced vocalizations
Stages 2 & 3	Reduction in homonyms
	Reduction of variability
	Maximization of established speech ability
	Elimination of errors affecting sound classes
Stage 4	Facilitation of late-acquired consonants, consonant clusters, and unstressed syllables in more difficult multisyllabic words

From *Manual of Articulation and Phonological Disorders* (p. 189), by K. M. Bleile, 1995, San Diego, CA: Singular Publishing Group. Copyright 1995 by Singular Publishing Group. Used with permission.

TABLE 8-11	Distinctive features vs. error pattern approaches to treatment
Approach	*Description*
Distinctive Features	Organizes sounds into classes based on shared acoustic and articulatory features; the hoped-for result of treatment is that generalization will occur from the treated sounds to other sounds that share similar features
Error Patterns	Organizes sounds according to the errors they typically undergo; the hoped-for result of treating one sound is that the results will generalize to other sounds that undergo the same error

Adapted from *Manual of Articulation and Phonological Disorders* (p. 194), by K. M. Bleile, 1995, San Diego, CA: Singular Publishing Group. Copyright 1995 by Singular Publishing Group. Used with permission.

Selection of Treatment Targets

Typically, treatment targets are selected based on stimulability, emerging sounds, key words, and phonetic placement and shaping. Stimulability refers to the client's ability to imitate a treatment target, which indicates that the child is developmentally and physically ready to produce the sound. The purpose of treatment is to generalize the use of the sound into spontaneous speech (Bleile, 1995).

Emerging sounds are those that "are produced correctly on 10 to 49% of all occasions in one or more phonetic environments" (Bleile, 1995, p. 198). The goal is to increase the frequency with which the individual produces the correct sound. A key word is one in which the client is able to successfully produce the selected target. Treatment in this case is based on generalizing the production of the sounds in the key word to other words.

Finally, phonetic placement, which is the "physical placement of a client's articulators into position to produce a sound" (Bleile, 1995, p. 199), and shaping, which "involves developing a new sound from a sound already in the client's phonetic inventory" (Bleile, 1995, p. 199) comprise prominent teaching techniques. In both cases, the goal is to generalize the success in the treatment to spontaneous speech.

Questions also arise regarding which position to work on when learning sounds. Bleile also addresses this issue as outlined in Table 8–12.

TABLE 8-12 "Best bets" for environments within which to establish treatment targets	
Treatment Targets	*Environments*
All treatment targets	Establish in CV, CVCV, or VC syllables
All treatment targets	Establish in stressed syllables
Consonants	Except for the instances noted below, establish consonants in the beginning of words
Voiced	Establish either between vowels or in the beginning of words and syllables
Voiceless	Establish at the end of syllables and words
Velar stops	Establish at the end of words or at the beginning of words before a back vowel
Alveolar stops	Establish at the beginning of words before front vowels
Voiced fricatives	Establish between vowels

From *Child Phonology: A Book of Exercises for Students* (p. 78), by K. Bleile, 1991, San Diego, CA: Singular Publishing Group. Copyright 1991 by Singular Publishing Group. Used with permission.

The Cycles Approach

According to Hodson and Paden (1991), phonology "refers to the speech sound *system* of a language and includes the study of how speech sounds are classified and organized and how they are used contrastively in a given language" (pp. 3–4). The cycles approach to phonological therapy was designed by Hodson and Paden over a period of 15 years, and was published in 1983. It is primarily designed for use with children who have multiple misarticulations and a high degree of unintelligibility. The approach incorporates auditory stimulation and production practice, with each cycle lasting between five to sixteen weeks.

Phonological assessment prior to beginning therapy is essential. Hodson and Paden (1991) propose that the key requirements "of phonological assessment for *clinical* purposes are that the results provide (a) information about the *severity* of the disorder, (b) a direction for *remediation*, and (c) baseline data for *accountability* purposes" (p. 14).

Table 8–13 lists phonological deviations that are observed in children's utterances.

The first step in the cycles approach to phonological remediation is to assess the child's phonological status using tests such as *The Assessment of Phonological Processes—Revised* (Hodson, 1986) or the *Khan-Lewis Adaptation of the Goldman-Fristoe Test of Articulation*. Both of these tests assess phonology at the single word level, so additional analysis via a conversational speech sample is recommended.

Next, the clinician analyzes the results of the phonological processes assessment and develops a hierarchy of the phonological processes on which the child is stimulable in a minimum of 40% of the contexts. It is recommended that the clinician first treat the most stimulable process so that the child has a sense of accomplishment early on in the therapy. It is also suggested that only one phonological process be addressed in a session, and that each phoneme within the process be treated for approximately 60 minutes per cycle before another phoneme is introduced.

Each session begins with auditory bombardment in which the client listens to the clinician produce 12 words containing the target sound, and sentences containing the target words.

TABLE 8-13 Phonological deviations observed in children's utterances

Omissions of Sound Segments	Palatalization	Metathesis
Syllables	Depalatalization	Reduplication
Reduction	"th" shifts	Idiosyncratic rules
Weak syllable deletion	Manner Changes	*Nonphonemic Alterations*
Multisyllabicity problems	Stopping	Tongue protrusions
Singleton consonants	Gliding	Lateralization
Postvocalic	Vowelization	Nasalization
Prevocalic	Affrication	Denasalization
Intervocalic	Deaffrication	Pharyngealization/
Consonant sequences	Voicing Changes	velarization
Reduction	Postvocalic devoicing	*Suprasegmental*
Deletion	Prevocalic voicing	*Modifications*
Other Syllable Structure	Prevocalic devoicing	*Sound Class Deficiencies*
Alterations	Postvocalic voicing	Obstruents
Coalescence	*Vowel Alterations*	Stridents
Migration	Dialectal	Posterior obstruents
Epenthesis	Allophonic	Anterior nonstrident
Schwa insertion	Neutralization	obstruents
Diminutive	*Context-Related Alterations*	Sonorants
Cluster creation	Assimilations	Liquids
Glottal Replacement	Labial	Nasals
Substitutions	Velar	Glides
Place changes	Nasal	
Fronting	Alveolar	
Backing	Palatal	
	Liquid	

From *Targeting Intelligible Speech: A Phonological Approach to Remediation* (2nd ed) (p. 37), by B. W. Hodson and E. P. Paden, 1991, Austin, TX: Pro-Ed. Copyright 1991 by Pro-Ed. Reprinted with permission.

The client should wear an auditory trainer during bombardment. During auditory bombardment, the client sits silently and listens attentively; he does not produce the target words.

Following auditory bombardment, the clinician asks the client to say one of five target words, then to draw, color, or paste a picture of the target word on a 5 × 8 index card. The clinician then writes the word on the card. There should be five words per sound. After the child utters the target word, the clinician can model the target word, using auditory, visual, and tactile cues if necessary. Once this practice is complete, the clinician should test for stimulability of the target sounds planned for the next treatment session. Then, auditory bombardment is repeated. A sample lesson plan is in Appendix 8–A.

During the time intervening between sessions, the family members and other significant persons should be asked to read the same list of words used in auditory bombardment to the client, and to have the client repeat the words on the picture cards (Hodson & Paden, 1986).

The Distinctive Features Approach

The distinctive features approach consists of analyzing a child's speech sample to determine if there is any consistency of distinctive features in the client's misarticulations. Once the distinctive features are identified, remediation is begun. In therapy, a few sounds containing the targeted distinctive feature are taught, with the hope that they will generalize to other sounds. Typically, this approach is used with children who have numerous misarticulations that can be grouped together based on distinctive feature analysis. Used to address primarily omissions and substitutions, the approach is typically not employed in the remediation of distortions, or if the client only has a few errors that warrant intervention.

The sounds of the client's speech are analyzed based on a conversational speech sample, paying particular attention to omissions and substitutions. Then, the clinician should select the target features that have the highest rate of occurrence. Phonemes that contain those identified features should then be chosen and used in remediation. In remediation, a traditional approach is characteristically employed, teaching the sounds in isolation first, followed by practice in syllables, words, phrases, and sentences. The clinician models the sounds in each of these contexts, and fades the modeling as the client's imitations become consistently accurate. At this point, the clinician should probe sounds that have the same distinctive features as the target sounds to determine if generalization of the treated sounds to the untreated sounds occurs. If there is no generalization, the clinician should target additional sounds with the same distinctive features (Hegde, 1996).

APPENDIX 8-A: REMEDIATION PLAN: PHONOLOGICAL CYCLES APPROACH

Client _____ Clinician _____

Birthdate/Age _____ Supervisor _____

Disorder(s) _____ Semester _____

Date _____ Targets: _____ _____
                                      Pattern   Phoneme(s)

1. Review of preceding session's production-practice words.

2. Auditory bombardment (with slight amplification) of this week's target to facilitate development of auditory image.

3. Potential word list for production practice of words selected carefully for facilitative phonetic environments. (Actual selection depends on child's abilities.)

_____   _____   _____

_____   _____   _____

Child draws/colors pictures of most stimulable words on 5 by 8 inch index cards.

4a. Production-practice activities to help child develop new kinesthetic image to match with auditory image.

    1. _____

    2. _____

    3. _____

    4. _____

    5. _____

    6. _____

    7. _____

    8. _____

4b. [Break (3–4 minutes) about halfway through session: cookie, walk, free conversation, group activity, etc.]

4c. Probing to ascertain next session's target phoneme(s).

5. Repeat of amplified auditory bombardment (same list as in #2 above).

6. Home program (parents to read this week's auditory bombardment word list and child to name picture cards of production-practice words once a day.)

Daily Log Comments:

DEFINITION/DESCRIPTION

Attention deficit disorder (ADD) is best defined in terms of what it is and what it is not. ADD is not just a behavior management problem. It is not a learning disability, nor is it an auditory processing disorder, although these disorders can co-occur with ADD. Most importantly, it is not a label to be randomly applied to any child who has trouble sitting still or paying attention (Vinson, 1999).

ADD is an inability to maintain focused, selected attention. It is thought to be related to disruptions in transmission and metabolism along subcortical pathways connecting the midbrain to the prefrontal cortex. These are the areas of the brain that play roles in directing attention, self-regulation, and planning (Vinson, 1999).

Children with attention deficit hyperactivity disorder (ADHD) have more conduct and behavioral problems than do children with ADD. They also are more impulsive and reported to be less anxious than children with ADD. Children with ADD tend to be more shy and withdrawn than do children with ADHD. Learning differences also exist between the two groups, with children with ADD showing a higher co-morbidity of learning disabilities and more underachievement, particularly in mathematics. They are also slower on rapid naming tasks than are the children with ADHD (Edelbrock, Costello, & Kessler, 1984; Lahey, Schaughency, Strauss, & Frame, 1984; Lahey, Schaughency, Hynd, Carlson, & Nieves, 1987; Hynd, et al., 1991; Cantwell & Baker, 1992).

Fragile Control Systems in Children with ADD/ADHD

Children with ADD/ADHD have difficulty controlling their attention. There are seven types of control systems that merit recognition as problematic for individuals with ADD/ADHD (Heyer, n.d.).

Focal Control

Focal control refers to the ability to focus on what is important among a myriad of stimuli. For example, a child with ADD/ADHD may assign equal importance to the traffic outside the school and to what the teacher is saying. Obviously, this will have an impact on a child's academic progress.

Mental Effort Control

Mental effort control is the energy and concentration needed to maintain focal control. Individuals with ADD/ADHD may complain of mental fatigue caused by the effort it takes to maintain focal control. One adult that was referred for learning disability testing had legs that were in constant motion throughout the testing. When asked if she could keep her legs still, she indicated that she could, but the effort it took to do so took away from her ability to concentrate on the assessment tasks.

Associative Control

The ability to state issues that are relevant to a designated topic without the use of tangential remarks is known as associative control. Heyer (n.d.) points out that associative control is what "enables people to maintain a conversation by stating issues that are relevant to the conversation" (Vinson, 1999, p. 147). Children with ADD/ADHD frequently give answers that are somewhat tangential to the question. They may also respond to questions with answers that are related to the question, but not a direct answer. For example, when asked what his name was, a child responded, "The same as my father's."

Appetite Control

Appetite control does not refer to eating, but rather to the ability to delay gratification. "Delayed gratification refers to the ability to continue providing the correct and expected behaviors even when a delay exists between the response and the provision of reinforcement" (Vinson, 1999, p. 148). Delaying gratification is problematic for children with ADD/ADHD. Frequently, they are considered to be non-compliant because they have difficulty following the rules and meeting the expectations of others when reinforcement is not immediate. Reinforcement for good behaviors needs to be immediate and meaningful in order to be effective.

Behavior Control

The disorganization of the central nervous system results in an inability to control impulsivity. Impulsivity refers to a neurological inability to sustain inhibition. Thus, the child acts "reflexively" in many situations. The child with ADD/ADHD cannot predict the consequences of his own behavior. Usually, the acts are not intentionally malicious or purposefully disruptive. Behavior management techniques are often ineffective since the child has other symptoms, such as poor internal control systems, poor quality control, and impulsivity.

Affective Control

Affective control is the ability to control emotions, particularly with regard to laughing and crying. This, too, is problematic for children with ADD/ADHD. Frequently, they are teased by classmates for their inappropriate emotional reactions.

Quality Control

Related to ADD, quality control refers to the ability to explain and account for one's own actions. Many individuals with ADD/ADHD cannot verify their own actions. If asked why they did a specified behavior, they typically will respond with, "I don't know" (Heyer, n.d.).

DSM CRITERIA FOR ATTENTION DEFICIT/ HYPERACTIVITY DISORDER

The DSM-IV (American Psychiatric Association, 1994) suggests that ADD has two dimensions: (1) hyperactivity with impulsivity, and (2) inattention. The DSM-IV describes three subtypes of ADD and ADHD:

1. ADHD with inattention, in which a child must have six of the nine inattention symptoms listed in Table 9–1. This classification does not include the specified number of hyperactivity or impulsivity symptoms;

2. ADHD with hyperactivity and impulsivity, in which the child must have four of the six hyperactivity or impulsivity symptoms, but not the specified number of inattention symptoms;

3. ADHD combined type, in which the child meets the criteria for hyperactivity or impulsivity and inattention (Morgan, Hynd, Riccio, & Hall, 1996).

The complete diagnostic criteria are listed in Table 9–1.

TABLE 9–1   DSM criteria for Attention Deficit/Hyperactivity Disorder

A. Either (1) or (2):

1. six (or more) of the following symptoms of *inattention* have persisted for at least 6 months to a degree that is maladaptive and inconsistent with developmental level:

   Inattention
   a. often fails to give close attention to details or makes careless mistakes in schoolwork, work, or other activities
   b. often has difficulty sustaining attention in tasks or play activities
   c. often does not seem to listen when spoken to directly
   d. often does not follow through on instructions and fails to finish schoolwork, chores, or duties in the work place (not due to oppositional behavior or failure to understand directions)
   e. often has difficulty organizing tasks and activities
   f. often avoids, dislikes, or is reluctant to engage in tasks that require sustained mental effort (such as schoolwork or homework)
   g. often loses things necessary for tasks or activities (e.g., toys, school assignments, pencils, books, or tools)
   h. is often easily distracted by extraneous stimuli
   i. is often forgetful in daily activities

2. six (or more) of the following symptoms of *hyperactivity-impulsivity* have persisted for at least 6 months to a degree that is maladaptive and inconsistent with developmental level:

   Hyperactivity
   a. often fidgets with hands or feet or squirms in seat
   b. often leaves seat in classroom or in other situations in which remaining seated is expected
   c. often runs about or climbs excessively in situations in which it is inappropriate (in adolescents or adults, may be limited to subjective feelings of restlessness)
   d. often has difficulty playing or engaging in leisure activities quietly
   e. is often "on the go" or often acts as if "driven by a motor"
   f. often talks excessively

continued

TABLE 9–1 continued

Impulsivity
  g. often blurts out answers before questions have been completed
  h. often has difficulty awaiting turn
  i. often interrupts or intrudes on others (e.g., butts into conversations or games)

B. Some hyperactive-impulsive or inattentive symptoms that caused impairment were present before age 7 years.

C. Some impairment from the symptoms is present in two or more settings (e.g., at school [or work] and at home).

D. There must be clear evidence of clinically significant impairment in social, academic, or occupational functioning.

E. The symptoms do not occur exclusively during the course of a Pervasive Developmental Disorder, Schizophrenia, or other Psychotic Disorder and are not accounted for by another mental disorder (e.g., Mood Disorder, Anxiety Disorder, Dissociative Disorder, or a Personality Disorder).

Code based on type:

314.01 Attention-Deficit/Hyperactivity Disorder, Combined Type: if both Criteria A1 and A2 are met for the past 6 months

314.00 Attention-Deficit/Hyperactivity Disorder, Predominantly Inattentive Type: if Criterion A1 is met but Criterion A2 is not met for the past 6 months

314.01 Attention-Deficit/Hyperactivity Disorder, Predominantly Hyperactive-Impulsive Type: if Criterion A2 is met but Criterion A1 is not met for the past 6 months

Coding note: For individuals (especially adolescents and adults) who currently have symptoms that no longer meet full criteria, "In Partial Remission" should be specified. (p. 83–85)

From *Diagnostic and Statistical Manual of Mental Disorders* (4th ed.) (pp. 83–85), by American Psychiatric Association, 1994, Washington, DC: American Psychiatric Association. Copyright 1994 by the American Psychiatric Association. Reprinted with permission.

ASSESSMENT

Children are frequently referred to a speech-language pathologist for testing of potential learning disabilities caused by failure to succeed in school. Many of these children do not have a language-based learning disability, but they may show signs of ADD or ADHD. If a language-based learning disability is ruled out, the child should be referred to a psychiatrist or a psychologist with expertise in the areas of ADD/ADHD. Typically, there are three reasons for the evaluation of a child with a suspected language-based learning disability:

1. To determine if the child has a language-based learning disability, and to analyze the child's learning style;

2. To provide a baseline against which progress can be measured;

3. To determine the child's eligibility for school-based services.

Eight Diagnostic Categories

There are eight diagnostic categories that merit attention in the assessment of ADD/ADHD. A description of these follows.

Cognition

Assess what the child knows through multi-modality testing to determine the best avenues for receiving and giving back information. The tests/subtests should be analyzed in terms of input modalities (auditory, visual, tactile, gustatory, olfactory) and response modalities (oral, written, or gestural).

Processing

Assessment of processing determines how the child handles information that is presented orally and visually. "Children can have normal vision and hearing but have a breakdown in the neurological connections that permit them to process and understand the information that is presented" (Vinson, 1999, p. 153). Once the clinician has determined what modalities are most effective for the child to use when processing information, teaching strategies can be developed to accommodate the child's best learning modalities.

Achievement

Achievement is particularly important when a child has completed two or more years of school. Achievement testing assesses what the child has learned. Achievement tests are often done in the classrooms annually, although a school psychologist may also assess a child's academic achievement when his academic performance is suspect.

Language

This testing should focus on a variety of skills as outlined in Table 9–2. Language testing should include testing of metacognitive skills (the ability to reflect on the process of thinking), metapragmatic skills, (the conscious and intentional awareness of ways in which to use language effectively in different contexts), and metanarrative skills (the ability to analyze and comprehend a story).

Problem solving skills should be assessed, including the meta-skills listed above because "the child needs to know how to analyze language and develop sequenced plans of action to solve problems" (Vinson, 1999, p. 154).

TABLE 9–2 Areas of focus in language testing for children suspected of having ADD or ADHD

1. Problem-solving skills
2. Auditory skills
3. Visual skills
4. Sequencing
5. Pragmatic skills
6. Extracting detail
7. Story schema
8. Associative responses
9. Topic maintenance
10. Topic switching

Many children with ADD/ADHD have pragmatic deficits that interfere with social development. Typically, these children do not respond to nonverbal cues, and they ignore social rules. These behaviors lead to an impeding of their social skills, which can result in lowered self-esteem because of lack of friends. Testing of pragmatics should address topic maintenance and topic switching in addition to other pragmatic factors.

The assessment of the child's ability to participate in a story-telling scheme can yield important information with regard to the diagnosing of language problems that may be contributing to academic problems. Attention should be paid to how well the child extracts crucial information from the story. This may be hindered by problems with focal control. Efforts need to be made to help the child "stay on track" instead of using tangential comments. Finally, the child's ability to hypothesize about what is going to happen as the story progresses should be assessed.

Attention

It is important to determine the child's abilities to control his attention. This is especially critical with regard to focal and associative control since these two control systems have a powerful impact on the child's ability to succeed academically.

Behavior

Determine a reinforcement system that has meaning for the child, and discuss its implementation with all those involved with the child (all teachers and family members). The use of behavior management with children with ADD/ADHD can be a challenge. As stated previously, reinforcement needs to be immediate and meaningful in order for behavior management strategies to work.

Medical

Some children who have a hyperactive component may benefit from the use of psychostimulants. A physician with expertise in ADD/ADHD should evaluate the child and determine an appropriate dosage schedule, if so warranted. It should be noted that the use of medications is designed to help the child control his attention, not to control unruly behavior. Drugs create a window of opportunity in which the client with ADHD has an opportunity to do his best work socially, academically, and vocationally.

Social and Environmental Interaction

Multidisciplinary and parental reports on the child's social interactions, self-esteem, and general mood and affect are critical components of the assessment process. It is important to monitor the self-esteem of children with ADD/ADHD. Many children with ADD/ADHD suffer from depression related to their social and academic performances. The social and environmental interactions of the client need to be monitored so that intervention can take place as needed to bolster the client's self-esteem.

TREATMENT

Four Areas of Management of ADD and ADHD

Academic

Teachers and homework helpers should work together to individualize the interactions with the child, and to facilitate working through the modalities that are most effectively utilized by the child. Structuring the environment to encourage the completion of all work should be done, for example, breaking up long assignments into several shorter assignments. Memory deficits should also be addressed as outlined in Table 9–3.

Of the types of memory components, sustained attention, divided attention, and vigilance are the most problematic for children with ADD/ADHD (Heyer, n.d.).

Behavior

Behavior management must be consistent across all settings, and administered without excessive delay since children with ADHD often have difficulty with delayed gratification.

Medical

Medical management is sometimes necessary as a way to make the system amenable to learning. Medications can create a window of opportunity during which the child is better able to control and focus his attention on what is needed to learn. Ritalin and Adderall are the most commonly prescribed medications.

Social

Children with ADD/ADHD need to be taught how to handle their emotions appropriately. Behavior therapy should be implemented, including role play, to assist the children in developing their social skills.

Additional suggestions for the management of ADD/ADHD are found in Table 9–4.

TABLE 9–3 Memory deficits in children with ADD or ADHD	
Selective attention	Focusing on what is important amid myriad stimuli
Focused attention	Having a specific activity that must be done, usually under a time constraint
Sustained attention	Similar to, but a little less restrictive than, focused attention
Divided attention	Determining how much attention can be given to each activity
Vigilance	Completing the whole task without falling behind; needed to develop a memory bank

Adapted from *Programming for Children with Attention Deficit Disorders*, by J. L. Heyer, n.d., West Lafayette, IN: Purdue Research Foundation. Copyright by Purdue Research Foundation. Adapted with permission.

TABLE 9-4 Treatment strategies to use with children who have ADD or ADHD

Provide a consistent routine across all environments

Break assignments down into smaller groups (e.g., 5 mathematics problems at one time instead of 15)

Simple, single instructions or directions

Prepare for changes

Strengthen the strengths as much as address the weaknesses

Maximize function and circumvent or minimize the weaknesses

CHAPTER TEN
Augmentative and Alternative Communication

DEFINITION/DESCRIPTION

It is estimated by the American Speech-Language-Hearing Association (1991) that there are over 2 million individuals in the United States who cannot rely on speech as their primary means of communication. These individuals include children who are non-speaking from the developmental period to those who acquire speech deficits in late adulthood. The deficits may be cognitive and/or physical. For these individuals, there is a need to rely on other systems of communication, such as gestures, sign language, picture or word boards, alphabet boards, and systems with synthesized or digitized speech. All these systems are collectively known as augmentative or alternative communication systems (AAC). The use of AAC has reached a new level of acceptance as a first approach to therapy for individuals with severe speech deficits. Historically, AAC was resorted to only as a "last ditch" effort when attempts to learn more traditional communication systems (i.e., speech) had failed.

There literally has been an explosion in the availability of AAC systems. A database known as Abledata was developed by the Trace Center to catalogue over 16,000 references from 2,200 manufacturers of AAC devices. Abledata is available on a CD-ROM, and it is accessible through the Internet (Glennen, 1997a). The field has grown to the point that ASHA has developed a set of roles and responsibilities for professionals working in the area of AAC. These roles are delineated in Table 10–1.

In addition to the growth of the AAC within the fields of speech-language pathology and special education, there has been legislation that has increased awareness and availability of AAC to individuals with handicapping conditions. In 1988, the Technology Related Assistance for Individuals with Disabilities Act (Tech Act, P.L. 100-407) was passed. This legislation was quickly followed by the Americans with Disabilities Act (ADA, P.L. 101-336) and the Individuals with Disabilities Education Act (IDEA, P.L. 101-476) in 1990. Together, "these statutes emphasize the importance of disseminating information about assistive technology including AAC, use of AAC as a civil right, and use of AAC as an educational tool" (Glennen, 1997a, p. 12).

The Tech Act was designed to provide states with the means to increase consumer access to AAC devices and services, and to develop projects focused on systems change. It includes "the provision of assistive technology evaluation services; funding equipment; fitting, customization, and repair of equipment; coordinating interventions; training the AAC consumer or family; and training other professionals" (Swengel & Marquette, 1997, p. 22). IDEA stated that students who needed assistive technology should have it provided as part of their educational plan. However, there was no increase in funding made available to the schools to provide assistive technology, so many students are still denied the most

TABLE 10-1   Roles of speech-language pathologists working in the area of AAC as defined by ASHA.

1. Identification of persons who are appropriate candidates for augmentative communication intervention.

2. Determination of specific augmentative communication components and the strategies to maximize functional communication.

3. Development of an intervention plan to achieve maximal functional communication between individuals who use augmentative components and their partners.

4. Implementation of intervention plan to achieve maximal functional communication.

5. Evaluation of the functional communication outcomes of the intervention plan.

6. Ability to evaluate evolving aids, techniques, symbols and strategies in augmentative communication and to determine their utilization.

7. Advocacy for increased attention to the communication and funding needs of severely speech and language impaired persons with community, regional, government and education agencies.

8. Provision of inservice education for medical and allied health personnel, other health and education professionals, and consumers on the communication needs and augmentative communication potential of severely handicapped persons.

9. Coordination of augmentative communication services. (This role is implicit in all of the previously listed roles.)

From "Competencies for Speech-Language Pathologists Providing Services in Augmentative Communication" in *Asha*, March 1989, pp. 107–110. Copyright 1989 by ASHA. Reprinted with permission.

appropriate devices. The Rehabilitation Act of 1973 addressed the vocational needs of individuals with handicapping conditions, and reprioritized assistive technology services. (Glennen, 1997a; Swengel & Marquette, 1997).

The provision of intervention in the field of AAC includes several components. First, the professional has a responsibility to increase awareness of available assistive technology. This includes educating public service groups about AAC in the hope that they will support funding for AAC research and the provision of AAC devices. The second responsibility is to provide consumer services. These include assessment, helping the consumer obtain funding, technical assistance, and training in the use of the device (See Appendix 10–A for funding sources). However, support for the consumer goes beyond these services. Individuals with handicaps often are involved with multiple agencies. The speech-language pathologist may be a key person in coordinating the services provided by the various agencies serving the consumer. This may include the provision of transitional services if the consumer is transitioning from home to school, one classroom to another, one school to a different school, school to the work force, or one living situation to another. Ongoing technical assistance and AAC system maintenance are also critical components of the services needed by AAC users (PennTech, 1994). In addition, AAC services are provided in a variety of settings as outlined in Table 10–2.

The use of AAC has advanced tremendously in light of recent advances in microcomputer technology. AAC devices can be part of an environmental control system in which the user can control any number of devices and appliances in the home or work place. Some have synthesized speech, and others have digitized speech output. A variety of scanning options are now available. Systems can be independent, or part of a larger computer network.

TABLE 10–2 AAC service delivery settings

1. **Home**
   a. **Individual Home**
   b. **Group Home**
   c. **Residential/Extended Care Facility**

2. **Community**
   a. **Child Day Care**
   b. **Adult Day Care**
   c. **Respite Care**
   d. **Community Resources**

3. **Educational**
   a. **Self-Contained Classroom**
   b. **Inclusive Classroom**
   c. **Combination**

4. **Transitional and Vocational**
   a. **Vocational Training Setting**
   b. **Employment Setting**

5. **Medical**
   a. **Intensive and Acute Care Facilities**
   b. **Inpatient and Outpatient Rehabilitation Facilities**

From "Service Delivery in AAC" by K. E. Swengel and J. S. Marquette, 1997, in *Handbook of Augmentative and Alternative Communication* (p. 42), by S. L. Glennen and D. C. DeCoste (Eds.), San Diego, CA: Singular Publishing Group. Copyright 1997, by Singular Publishing Group. Reprinted with permission.

Because of the advances and variations in the types of AAC devices now available, it behooves us to review some of the current terminology related to AAC devices.

AAC strategies can be categorized as aided or unaided. Unaided communication strategies are those which are based entirely on the communicator's body. For example, vocalizations, gestures, sign language, eye gazing, and head nodding are all unaided communication because they do not require the use of any external devices. In contrast, aided communication strategies are those that require the use of a device or tool that complements the user's body. Most communicators use aided and unaided communication.

Technological communication systems can be listed as lite technology or high technology. Lite technology primarily consists of nonelectronic aids such as homemade picture boards, eye gaze boards, and alphabet boards. Electronic devices that are not computer-based are also considered to be lite technology. Examples include a Clock Communicator, switch-activated tape recorders, and Light Pointers used with simple communication boards (Glennen, 1997b). High technology systems are those that consist of microcomputer components. They often have voice output, and have the ability to store and retrieve messages.

High-technology systems are further divided into dedicated and non-dedicated systems. Dedicated systems are those that are developed exclusively for the purpose of communication. Examples include a Lite Talker and a Dynavox. Non-dedicated systems are AAC devices that are supplemental to devices, such as a laptop or desktop computer. In other words, a non-dedicated system is used for purposes other than communication. Some dedicated systems can be attached to a microcomputer for use as an alternate keyboard, but their primary purpose and use remains communication (Glennen, 1997b).

ASSESSMENT

As with many communication disorders, the assessment of individuals for the use of AAC is a team effort. The team should involve the client's family members, physicians, occupational therapists, physical therapists, psychologists, social workers, educators, and speech-language pathologists. All of these individuals can be involved in determining the client's communication needs. The occupational therapist and the physical therapist can assess the client's sensory and motor systems. Educators and psychologists can participate in assessment of cognitive skills, and the speech-language pathologist is actively involved in the assessment of language and cognitive skills. All members of the team should participate in deciding the most appropriate AAC system for the client based on their individual assessments. Social workers can be of benefit in helping to secure funding for AAC devices, which can run into thousands of dollars.

A sample history form that relates directly to the use of AAC is found in Appendix 10–B. Of course, a complete medical and educational history, an oral-facial exam, and assessment of speech, cognitive and language skills should be done in addition to the information gained from the sample history form. When deciding on an AAC device, one must keep in mind the physical load and the cognitive load required by the device.

Much can be learned by observing the client in a variety of settings to assess the communication environments of the individual, and to determine what his communication needs are. The next question that needs to be addressed is, "What methods of expressive communication is the client currently using?" For example, does the client use gestures, head nods, sign language, Morse code, speech, vocalizations, or pointing to pictures or objects? It is also important to address the issue of the purposes for which the client communicates. The following is a list of some purposes for communication: requesting objects; requesting actions; requesting information; making a statement; offering yes/no responses; asking and answering WH questions; making acknowledgments. It should also be noted whether the client uses echolalia or perseveration, or if the client is nonresponsive (Glennen, 1997c).

Beukelman and Mirenda (1992) also addressed the issue of access barriers. The determination of access barriers requires an assessment of the client's physical abilities, perceptual skills, cognitive abilities, experience with AAC and other technologies, and the client's own personal views and opinions about the use of an AAC device. This last issue, personal views and opinions, is particularly important because if the client does not view AAC positively, he is unlikely to use any device that is determined to be appropriate to his needs.

Assessing Sensory-Motor Skills

Clients who need to use an AAC system to communicate frequently have sensory and physical deficits in addition to the communication deficit. Some of these deficits are described in the chapter on Pediatric Feeding Problems. It is critical that the client's sensory and motor capabilities be thoroughly assessed before recommending any type of AAC system. Specifically, the diagnosticians should be concerned about the client's positioning and movement abilities, motor dexterity, vision and hearing status, and the client's ability to visually track and scan. All of these skills are of concern when recommending an AAC system (Shipley & McAfee, 1998).

With regard to positioning, the first concern is whether the client is ambulatory or confined to a wheelchair. This can impact the type of system decided chosen. For example, if the client is ambulatory and will be carrying his device, the weight of the device becomes more important, so the clinician needs to assess the client's ability to maintain his balance when carrying a similar load. The client's ability to achieve an appropriate posture, and then to remain positioned, should also be assessed. Does the client need assistance in achieving a posture that would optimize his communication abilities? Does he need positioners (i.e., wedges, pillows, foam rolls) and restraints to maintain the optimal posture? In what position is the client best able to use his sensory and motor strengths to communicate?

The client's ability to visually track and scan should be assessed. "Visual tracking refers to the ability to watch an object or person move through more than one visual plane, and visual scanning refers to the ability to look for and locate an object among several other objects" (Shipley & McAfee, 1998, p. 378). The client should be assessed when tracking vertically, horizontally, and diagonally in two directions. His ability to scan words, pictures, symbols, and/or objects should be assessed. A checklist for assessing visual scanning and tracking is found in Appendix 10–C.

The client's sensory and motor skills should be carefully assessed, addressing some of the following issues. If the client has sensory defensiveness in his hands and/or fingers, he may not be willing to use his hands to select an item on a communication board. If arm and hand movement are impaired, can the client use a pointer attached to his head or leg or foot? Is head control adequate for following an eye gaze? Can the client focus on one word, picture, symbol, or object to depict his choice? Can the access method be modified in terms of time needed to activate a selection, scanning speed, and negation of a selection? What switches are available to use with the device? Of all the different access methods, which one (or ones) is most appropriate for the client to use on a consistent basis?

Assessment of Cognition and Language

Before assessing cognition and language, the clinician must determine what mode of response will be used in the assessment. Can the client point to pictures for receptive language testing? If not, can he use a head stick, an eye gaze, or a light pointer to respond?

Visual tracking abilities should also be determined to be sure the client is able to visually focus on all the selection options in the testing. It may be necessary to make some modifications, such as using wider spaces between the choices to accommodate an eye gaze or poor pointing skills.

The clinician should also explore the client's ability to follow simple commands that will be part of the assessment process. This can be done by asking the client to "Touch this picture" instead of giving the actual test item. "The goal is to determine whether standardized test procedures need adaptation, and the range and accuracy of responding with the direct selection method of choice" (Glennen, 1997c, p. 170).

If necessary, the clinician can resort to the asking of yes/no questions if the client is unable to use, reliably and consistently, any direct selection methods.

Regardless of the system of response chosen for the testing, it behooves the clinician and client to practice the response system several times to be sure it can be used consistently and reliably. It should also be determined how fatiguing the system is to be sure the client can use the system for the duration of the testing (Glennen, 1997c).

It is critical that the assessment team determine the client's "ability to comprehend language, to process information, and to learn educational material" (Glennen, 1997c, p. 170). This may be better done by observation and interaction with the client than by formal testing. However, in some settings, formal testing may be required. In Table 10–3, there is a list of standardized assessment tools that use multiple choice and pointing to visual stimuli as the format for responding.

Tests that can be answered using a yes/no format can also be used if direct selection techniques are too fatiguing or difficult for the client.

Assessment of the client's symbolic language skills should also be assessed. There is much debate as to whether or not it is necessary to go back and develop all the prerequisite skills

TABLE 10–3 Standardized assessment procedures using multiple choice and pointing to visual stimuli as testing formats

Test Name	Skills Assessed
CELF Preschool (selected subtests) (Wiig, Secord, & Semel, 1992)	Receptive vocabulary Comprehension of syntax Comprehension of directions
Clinical Evaluations of Language Functions—3 (selected subtests) (Widd & Semel, 1995)	Comprehension of directions Comprehension of syntax
Peabody Picture Vocabulary Test—III (Dunn and Dunn, 1998)	Receptive vocabulary
Preschool Language Scale III. Auditory Comprehension Scale (Zimmerman, Steiner, & Evatt-Pond, 1991)	Receptive vocabulary Comprehension of syntax Sequencing events
Receptive One Word Picture Vocabulary Test (Gardner, 1985)	Receptive vocabulary
Test of Auditory Comprehension of Language—Revised (Carrow-Woolfolk, 1985)	Receptive vocabulary Comprehension of syntax
Test of Early Reading Ability—2 (selected items) (Reid, Hresko, & Hammill, 1989)	Letter identification Sign/symbol identification Sight word reading Reading sentences
Test of Nonverbal Intelligence—2 (Brown, Sherbenou, & Johnson, 1982)	Visual spatial skills Visual spatial sequencing
Motor Free Visual Perception Test (Colarusso & Hammill, 1972)	Visual perception
Peabody Individual Achievement Test—Revised (Most subtests) (Markwardt, 1989)	Reading comprehension Reading recognition Spelling Mathematics
Woodcock-Johnson Tests of Cognitive Ability—Revised (selected subtests) (Woodcock & Bonner-Johnson, 1989)	Visual Processing Speed Visual Matching Spatial Relations

Adapted from "Augmentative and Alternative Communication Assessment Strategies," by S. L. Glennen, 1997, in *Handbook of Augmentative and Alternative Communication* (p. 171), San Diego, CA: Singular Publishing Group. Copyright 1997 by Singular Publishing Group. Adapted with permission.

for symbolic communication. Regardless of one's viewpoint on that debate, it is important to know where the client is at the current time with regard to his symbolic abilities. Successful use of an aided communication system requires that the client be able to understand that pictures, words, or symbols represent a thought to be communicated. In order to achieve more advanced levels of communication, the client must learn to combine and sequence pictures, symbols, or words, and to categorize them for easier access.

Initial assessment of the client's symbolic abilities should focus on the client's understanding of the functions of objects, and using objects as symbols. Additionally, the client needs to understand that looking at, touching, or pointing to an object can be a communicative act. For example, touching a cup may indicate that the client wants a drink. If the client understands this communicative act, a photograph or realistic drawing of the object should be placed within reach of the client, and the object moved out of reach (but still within sight). The client's ability to understand the cause and effect of touching the picture to obtain the item is then assessed. If the client is able to touch the picture to obtain the item, an array of 3–4 pictures should be introduced. Once the client's understanding of the pictures is determined, the pictures should be shuffled around to be sure the client is responding to the picture itself, and not to the location of the picture. When it is verified that the client understands the relationship between the picture and the object, the client should be assessed to determine if he understands the relationship between the picture and the spoken word.

Glennen (1997c) points out that clients who do not succeed at these tasks are still potential candidates for AAC devices. The client who does not understand the relationship between a picture and an object may benefit from cause-and-effect training, such as turning on a tape recorder to hear music. For the individual who understands that the picture represents an object, but does not understand that pointing to the picture constitutes a communicative act, training can take place to shape the behavior of pointing to a picture to communicate a desire or thought.

Clients who succeed in the first portion of symbol assessment should move on to sequencing of picture symbols. The goal of this segment of the evaluation is to determine if the client can combine and sequence symbols to communicate a message. If necessary, modeling and prompting can be used to see if the client can be taught to sequence symbols to accomplish their communicative intent. If a client cannot learn to sequence pictures or symbols, it will be necessary to limit the AAC device to one in which the selection of a single symbol is all that is required to communicate a message.

Clients who are able to learn to sequence pictures/symbols/words to express a thought can potentially have hundreds of items on their communication board. Thus, it becomes necessary for the client to understand categorization and association of the items in order to organize the board for quick access. Table 10–4 provides an overview of semantic categorization strategies that can be used to encode vocabulary in picture-based AAC systems.

Once it is clear that the client can categorize and use simple combinatory strategies, his ability to deal with complex sequencing and memory should be assessed. Some of the symbol systems available (e.g., Minspeak and Blissymbolics) may require some "conceptual leaps" to sequence symbols to create a message. Some symbols are organized in such a way as to save space when a client is able to sequence abstract combinations. For example, instead of

TABLE 10–4	Semantic categorization strategies used to encode vocabulary in picture-based AAC systems
Semantic Categorization	**Strategy**
Symbol Name	Identification of a picture by name
Object Function	Associating an object with its functions
Category Name	Associates an object with its category referent
Part/Whole Concepts	Can identify a named part of a whole object
Similar Item Associations	Associates items that belong together in groups
Location Concepts	Can associate an object with its typical location
Size/Shape Concepts	Associates size and shape terms with objects
Color Concepts	Can identify colors
Other Descriptive Concepts	Associates other descriptive terms with a picture
Rhyming and Phonetic Concepts	Associates words that rhyme or sound alike
Grammatical Concepts	Can understand grammatical terms such as action, verb, object

Adapted from "Augmentative and Alternative Communication Assessment Strategies," by S. L. Glennen, 1997, in *Handbook of Augmentative and Alternative Communication* (p. 179), San Diego, CA: Singular Publishing Group. Copyright 1997 by Singular Publishing Group. Adapted with permission.

using up space to put the name of every fruit on a board, the clinician could put one symbol for fruit, and have the client combine that symbol with a color and/or shape symbol to indicate a specific fruit. Individuals with short and/or long-term memory problems may find it difficult to use sequencing due to the memory involved in recalling the sequences. Elder (1987) developed a three-step process to assess picture sequencing and memory.

The client selects two pictures from a set of four to represent the following:

1. A sentence that is concretely associated with the picture symbol set;

2. A single-word associated with the symbol set; and

3. A sentence that is abstractly associated with the symbol set (Glennen, 1997c, p. 180).

The client is asked to remember the selected sequence of symbols and to reproduce them 10–15 minutes later. This determines the client's ability to use his memory to recall sequences for communicative intent.

Finally, the client's ability to use written language as a communication mode should be assessed. What are the client's literacy skills? Can the client write his messages? Words take up considerably less space and limit some of the guess work in using AAC devices. The client's knowledge of letters, sound/symbol associations, reading sight words, and spelling simple words should be assessed to determine if reading is a potential AAC system for the client (Glennen, 1997c).

It should be remembered that "the purpose of evaluating receptive language, cognitive, and academic skills is not to determine who would benefit from AAC intervention. Instead, this information should be used to determine how best to implement AAC interventions with a particular individual" (Glennen, 1997c, p. 171).

Assessing Access Methods: Direct Selection

Direct selection means that the user has "access to all possible symbol choices at all times" (Glennen, 1997b, p. 63). The most common type of direct selection is to depress a key on a keyboard using the fingers or hands. However, direct selection on a keyboard can also be achieved via adaptive pointers, head sticks, and other body parts. This type of direct selection is found on dedicated and non-dedicated AAC devices. The client must have the motor control and strength to depress the keys sufficiently to convey the signal that the key has been selected and needs to be activated. Thus, the clinician should be familiar with how much strength is required to activate a key on the devices being considered for a client. Examples of dedicated devices that require mechanical key depression in order to be activated include the Walker Talker, the Liberator, the Light Writer SL30, the Delta Talker, the Alpha Talker, and the Canon Communicator (Glennen, 1997b).

> Other direct selection keyboards rely on touch membrane or touch screen surfaces. A touch membrane keyboard consists of two electrically conductive flat surfaces separated by nonconductive spacers. Touching the keyboard lightly presses the two surfaces together which sends an electronic signal to the AAC system. (Glennen, 1997b, p. 63)

This is the same principle as a touch screen on a computer. Examples of dedicated devices with a touch screen or touch membrane keyboard are the Mega Wolf, Finger Foniks, Voice Mate, DynaVox, Say It All, Voice Pal, Digivox, and Parrott. Non-dedicated devices that have a touch membrane are Intellikeys, the Discover: Board, and the TASH Mini Keyboard (Glennen, 1997b). Individuals who have low muscle tone and do not have the capability to depress and activate a key would benefit from the use of a touch screen or touch membrane keyboard.

Computers can be adapted to accommodate communication through direct selection. Examples of software available for this purpose, Speaking Dynamically, Intellitalk, Write Out Loud, and Talk About can be used with the Macintosh. EZ Keys, Handi Chat, and Talking Screen are compatible with IBM operating systems.

An advantage of direct selection methods is that they are relatively fast when compared to scanning methods. Foulds (1980) and Szeto, Allen, and Littrell (1993) have found that average speeds of 13–43 words per minute can be achieved when using direct selection. This rate can be increased when prediction and encoding systems are coupled with the direct selection technique. Another advantage is that many direct selection methods can be modified according to the client's needs. For example, the size of the keys can be altered on some devices. This can be done by defining the number of cells that a device will use, or by leaving an unprogrammed cell between two programmed cells. Keyguards can be placed over the keys to help stabilize the user's hand as he makes his selections. The sensitivity of the keys can sometimes be adjusted, as can the amount of time they must be depressed before activating a message.

The primary disadvantage of most direct selection devices is portability. Many devices that use direct selection weigh between 8–10 pounds, making them difficult to carry around, particularly when there may be a physical handicap complicating matters. However, as newer devices are produced, manufacturers are attempting to reduce the weight and size of the communicators.

Switch-Activated Direct Selection

Sometimes, switches are used in place of a keyboard to make a direct selection. Speak Easy, AlphaTalker, AIPS Wolf, Lync, Voice Mate, and Voice Pal are examples of switch activated AAC devices (Glennen, 1997b). Some devices can accommodate up to 12 switches at one time. They are advantageous for clients who cannot physically use a keyboard, usually because of the proximity of the keys to each other. Switches can be placed further apart for more gross motor activation than can be used with a keyboard. There are many switches available that can be used with different body parts and differing amounts of pressure, so that a switch can be found for just about anyone who may require one. There is a limit to how many messages can be accessed at any one time, so more advanced users may be frustrated by their use.

Eye Gaze Direct Selection

Eye gaze displays, or E-Tran boards, may be fixed or dynamic. Symbols, letters, objects, or pictures are affixed to a sheet of clear plastic. When using a fixed display, the display remains stationary, with the user and listener sitting on opposite sides of the board and looking through it. The listener follows the communicator's eye gaze as he fixes on one of the items. On a fixed display, the symbols (or letters, objects, or pictures) are typically displayed on the periphery of the E-Tran board.

According to Goosens (1989), all eye gaze systems are based on a three-point reference to make the selections on the AAC device:

1. the AAC communicator scans the options on the communication display;

2. he or she decides on the targeted symbol;

3. the AAC communicator establishes eye contact with the communicative partner to indicate that a selection has been made (Millikin, 1997, p. 140).

Although it follows the same basic three steps, the use of a dynamic eye gaze board is more difficult. When using a dynamic system, the listener watches the communicator's eyes and moves the board for the communicator. The communicator "locks his or her eye gaze on a target and continues to visually track the target while the listener moves the board. . . . When the user's and listener's eye gaze lock together through the E-Tran, the symbol that both are looking at is selected" (Glennen, 1997b, p. 68). A dynamic display permits the placing of more symbols on the board. Encoding systems can be used that allow the placement of hundreds of items on a board (Goosens & Crain, 1986). For example, there could be 10 blocks of 16 items per block. Using an encoding system, the communicator could indicate the row and column of the item after fixing on the block with the desired item.

Light and Optical Pointers

A relatively inexpensive option with regard to light and optical pointers is to purchase a Class II laser pointer from an office supply store and attach it to a body part on the user over which he has optimal control. The pointer emits a narrow beam of light (typically red) that can be used to focus on an item that expresses the desired communicative intent. Most of these light pointers have a long battery life, and some come with rechargeable battery packs. The beam is readily visible to anyone in the room, and care should be taken to ensure that the beam is not directed at someone's eye (although a reflexive blink should prevent damage from occurring).

Other optical pointers are not actually light beams, but rather combinations of reflective mirrors and an LED. In these devices, the mirror on the pointer reflects the beam from the LED that is beside each symbol. The mirror reflects the beam back to the LED, and the symbol is selected. Sonar and Infrared pointers are also available.

Typically, if head and neck control are adequate, the pointer is attached to the use's head using a hat, headband, or glasses. Preferably, it is mounted at midline. However, if head control is poor, it can be mounted on another body part such as the back of the hand, or on a knee. Whichever body part is used, fine motor control is needed in order to direct the beam to the desired location. The beam must be steady enough to activate the message. Also, there is no tactile feedback, so frequently there is a small "beep" to indicate that the item has been selected. Users who require tactile feedback would be better served by a head stick.

Assessing Access Methods: Indirect Selection

Scanning is the most prevalent type of indirect selection, and it can be used on dedicated and nondedicated devices. In scanning, selections are presented systematically to the user, and he chooses the desired selection by activating a switch or some other mechanism. Some AAC devices that can be adapted for scanning include the DeltaTalker, the Digivox, the DynaVox, the Alpha Talker, the Voice Pal Plus, the RealVoice, and the Macaw. Non-dedicated devices can be adapted for scanning access through the use of Talking Screen, Talk About, Scanning WSKE, KE:nx, Handi Chat, and Speaking Dynamically (Glennen, 1997b).

Single Switch Scanning Methods

Single switch scanning only requires one repetitive motor movement, making it much more feasible than direct scanning for people with severe motor deficits. For example, one hit on the switch will activate the scanning, and another hit will stop the scanning.

Scanning can be linear or circular. In linear scanning, the options are presented one at a time in a line-by-line pattern. When the desired selection is reached, the user hits a switch to stop the scanning. Circular scanning operates in a similar fashion except that the items are scanned in a circular pattern instead of a linear pattern. An example of an indirect selection circular scanner is a Clock Communicator in which a dial rotates clockwise and the user depresses a switch when the dial is on the item he wishes to communicate. The advantage of linear and circular scanning is that they are simple to use. The disadvantage is that they are very slow. Therefore, one may want to use this type of scanning only when there are a few choices of items from which to make a selection.

Indirect selection can be sped up through the use of row-column scanning. In row-column scanning, an entire row of symbols/pictures/words is highlighted at one time. When the row or column containing the desired item is lit, the user activates the switch, which stops the row or column scanning and then illuminates each item on that row or column until the user again depresses the switch indicating the item he wishes to select. A variation of row-column scanning is group-item scanning in which a group of items is scanned, and the user depresses the switch when the desired group is reached. Within the group, the user can then activate row-column scanning, or scanning of a smaller group of items. The items are then individually scanned. Row-column scanning is usually a two-step process, whereas group scanning is a three- or four-step process.

Another variation within single switch scanning is the choice between automatic scanning, directed scanning, and step scanning. In automatic scanning, the cursor moves across the choices while the user waits for the desired symbol to be marked. When that desired item is marked, the user depresses the switch to stop the movement of the cursor. In directed scanning, the user depresses the switch continuously until the cursor reaches the desired item. At that point, he releases the switch and the cursor stops on the designated item. In step scanning, the switch is activated each time the user wants the cursor to move.

The advantage of automatic scanning is that it is less labor intensive than direct scanning and step scanning. However, it requires a level of patience that young or immature users may not have. Direct scanning and step scanning are more physically demanding, but require less waiting time between hits (Glennen, 1997b).

Joystick and Multiple Switch Scanning

According to Glennen (1997b, p. 71), "joysticks are used to control the movement of the cursor on the AAC device. A joystick feeds vertical and horizontal movement coordinates to the AAC system to control the direction of the cursor." The speed and starting point of the cursor can usually be changed to meet the needs of the user. In order to use a joystick, the user must have good fine motor skills, since the smallest movement can result in a large jump by the cursor.

Multiple switch scanning requires a stronger physical and cognitive load to operate than does a joystick or single switch scanning. Multiple switch scanners have several different switches to control the movement of the cursor on the AAC device. For example, one switch may control vertical movement, one horizontal movement, and another control diagonal movement. There may be a fourth switch that is used to confirm the selection of the item.

As seen from the previous discussion, there are a variety of factors which should be considered when assessing a client to determine the suitability of using an AAC device, and determining which AAC system to use. Before any final decisions are made, the client should be observed using the system in his natural settings to determine if the system meets his communication needs in his daily communication efforts.

TREATMENT

Switch Selection

There are a variety of switches available for use in activating scanning on communication boards. The only requirement is that the individual can make replicated movements of a body part in a controlled manner. "Switches vary in terms of the body movement necessary to activate the switch, the mechanism that triggers switch activation, and the pressure or length of touch necessary to activate the switch. In addition switches also vary in terms of the kind of feedback given to the user" (Glennen, 1997b, p. 75). Some switches offer visual feedback by illuminating a light when the switch is pressed. Others offer auditory feedback such as a click or a tone when the switch is activated. Still others provide tactile feedback by making a physical movement. The kind of switch chosen for the AAC user depends largely on his muscle tone.

Individuals with low muscle tone need to use switches that require little physical movement. These switches are pressure sensitive; that is, they require little pressure to be activated. Pressure sensitive switches include TASH's MicroLight Switch and Zygo's Leaf Switch and Lever Switch. Touch membrane switches are also good for individuals with low muscle tone as they also require only light pressure to be activated. The TASH Plate Switch is an example of a switch with touch membranes (Glennen, 1997b). Finally, AdapTech has produced Taction Pads. Taction Pads "are flat pliable wires or stickers that can be wrapped around objects. Touching the pads on the objects activates the switch" (Glennen, 1997b, p. 76).

Some pressure switches are not as sensitive, and they are more appropriate for individuals with normal muscle tone or high muscle tone. These switches are activated by force and body movement, usually by pushing or pressing the switch. The advantage of switches that require higher pressures to be activated are that they are usually more durable. Thus, they will withstand the force that frequently accompanies the movements of individuals with high tone. Those switches that require less force are usually not as durable, but may be more appropriate for the individual with normal muscle tone. Also, the amount of surface area varies from switch to switch. Some switches for young and/or physically impaired children have large surface areas, whereas those for individuals with more control have smaller surface areas. Examples of switches that require higher force to activate and have a large surface area include Ablenet's Big Red Switch, TASH's Square Pad, and the Plate Switch from Toys for Special Children (Glennen, 1997b).

There are other switches that do not require touch for activation. These are generally designed for individuals with paralysis and/or spinal cord injuries. For example, there are mercury switches (often called Tip Switches). Mercury switches have to be tipped by a body part in order to result in activation. When they are held in balance, no activation occurs. The author once worked with a young man with spastic cerebral palsy who had the most control over his left knee. The mercury switch was attached to his left knee, and he used it to activate his electronic communicator as well as certain computer programs on a PC. The Blink Switch (Innocomp) can also be used for individuals with little or no controlled movement of the body parts. The Blink Switch relies on an infrared light beam which, when "broken," activates the switch. The beam is aimed toward the user's eye, and then reflects back to the light source. When the individual blinks, the beam is broken and the switch is activated.

Another switch that requires little or no movement is the sip-and-puff switches frequently used by individuals with high level spinal cord injuries. The sip-and-puff switch is activated or deactivated by breath inhalations and exhalations. The P-Switch (Prentke-Romich) "consists of a piezo-electric sensor that is strapped onto the user's body" (Glennen, 1997b, p. 76). The P-Switch can be activated by any movement or muscle tensing, and the sensitivity of the switch can be adjusted. It can be strapped onto the leg, around the arm, on the forehead, jaw, or cheek (Glennen, 1997b).

Training Access Skills

DeCoste (1997) writes that the client "must be able to reliably and effortlessly access an augmentative communication system (operational knowledge) to effectively utilize that system for communicative exchange (social and linguistic knowledge)" (p. 275).

DeCoste advocates MSIPT Assessment (see Appendix 10–D). A MSIPT assessment is composed of five major components: movement, control site, input method, position, and targeting. Movement evaluation consists of assessing the range of motion, the ease of movement, and the time required to contact and release the input method. Generally speaking, the clinician needs to identify movements that are controlled, done with relative ease, do not result in overflow motions, and occur without abnormal muscle tone and abnormal reflexes. Movements of the upper extremities and head are the most common and natural methods of access. If these are not possible, movements of the lower extremities, the chin, the mouth, and the shoulder should be evaluated (DeCoste, 1997).

The next area of concern is the control site which refers to the point of contact with the input device. Positioning adaptations done to improve contact with the switch should be noted so that they can be replicated at a later date for additional training and use. Also, the exact site of the contact should be noted. Do not simply indicate that the head is the point of contact; rather, indicate if it is the back of the head, the side of the head, the right cheek, the left temple, and so on.

Assessment of the input method is the next area of evaluation. This requires specifying the equipment that the client will use to communicate using his AAC device. Input methods would include all those access modes discussed previously, or any combination of those modes. According to DeCoste (1997, p. 263), the following factors should be considered when evaluating the input method: (1) the appropriate type of input method relative to the individual's movement skills; (2) the accuracy associated with the combined movement and input method; and (3) whether the individual is using direct selection or scanning.

"P" on MSIPT refers to the positioning of the input device. This decision will be dictated by the client's motor and visual skills, as well as the type of AAC switch and device. Assessment of the positioning of the input device will take place throughout the MSIPT process, since it is affected by the motor skills and the input site. It will probably be necessary to go through a trial-and-error process, trying several different positions to determine the optimal position for the input device.

Evaluating targeting methods is the final step of the MSIPT process. "Targeting refers to the ability of an individual to access a desired symbol using direct selection or scanning" (DeCoste, 1997, p. 271). It will require a combination of visual and motor skills, or auditory and motor skills, depending on the feedback of the input device. Targeting also taps into the memory and cognition abilities of the client. Initially, targeting is considered as part of the motor assessment and as a component of the selection of the input device. In the later stages of the assessment, targeting refers to the design of the overlay. Specifically, it will address the size of the symbols, the number of symbols, and the spacing between the symbols.

Even though MSIPT is a systematic approach to evaluation, it is discussed under treatment because it guides the treatment phase. Because of the extensive nature of the MSIPT system, the client may tire during the evaluation, or there may simply not be enough time to complete the assessment. The MSIPT system may take place over several sessions, and provide the basis for planning intervention. It may also be used to provide guidance in upgrading a client's AAC system. Regardless of how the MSIPT system is implemented, it is critical that the clinician develop a comprehensive and complete training and implementation plan.

Parallel training is the training of the skills needed for the next level of advancement, concurrently with the skills needed for the current level of functioning. Obviously, this requires a training and implementation plan to guide the therapeutic intervention. Parallel training eases the process of upgrading a system to the next level of complexity, when the client is ready to advance.

Another type of training is "layering." Layering is described by Goosens and Crain (1986) as a system of reducing the initial cognitive, communication, and linguistic loads when the client is first being trained in the use of an AAC device. In layering, the first aspect of training focuses on the motor and visual components. When the client has mastered the physical aspects of accessing the AAC device, the cognitive components are added to the task. Thus, after mastering the motor and visual skills, the client works on the memory and learning aspects of using the AAC device. When the cognitive component is mastered, the ultimate goal of communicative components can be added. The clinician is cautioned not to lose sight of the fact that the point of the AAC training is to communicate (DeCoste, 1997). If the training gets too bogged down in the motor, visual, and cognitive components, this goal may be lost. Once the motor and visual skills are mastered, the clinician may choose to start the client with a direct selection method of input to facilitate the bridging to communicative use of the AAC device. At the same time, the cognitive demands needed for scanning can be addressed in therapy, which would eventually provide the client with access to more symbols for communication.

Choice of Symbol Systems

Millikin (1997) writes that "symbolic communication involves the use of arbitrary symbols which represent ideas, affective states, objects, actions, people, relationships, and events" (p. 97). Symbols can be graphic, spoken, or manual; regardless of the mode the meaning must be clear to the communicator and the listener. This fact guides the selection of symbols used on an AAC device.

Unaided symbol systems include speech/vocalization, sign language (American Sign Language, Signs Supporting English, or Signing Exact English), gestures and body language, or Amer-Ind (based on a gestural system used among Native Americans). Implementation of these systems does not require any device beyond the user's body.

Aided symbol communication is composed of a variety of systems that can be used from the lowest tech boards to the highest tech systems available. The choice of which symbol system to use for a client is one of the most critical decisions the assessment and intervention team will make. Aided symbols can consist of an array of objects or an array of seemingly abstract symbols, which may have meaning to the listener only when orthographic representations (words) are printed alongside the symbol. Mirenda and Locke (1989) developed a hierarchy of symbols from the most iconic to the least iconic: objects; color photographs; black and white photographs; miniature objects; black and white line drawings; Blissymbols; and traditional orthography.

The more iconic a symbol, the easier it is learned. However, the communication potential of a single object is less than that of some more advanced symbols, such as those found in Rebus, PCS, PIC, Picsyms, and Blissymbols. In all symbol systems, the nouns are the most iconic. When considered across the three word classes of nouns, verbs, and modifiers, in general, Rebus symbols were the most translucent, followed by PCS. However, specific symbols in PIC and Picsyms were more translucent than some of the Rebus and PCS symbols (Mizuko, 1987). Therefore, one has to look at the entire symbol system before deciding which symbols to use. The reader is warned that there is no need to have only one symbol system represented on an AAC device. It may look nicer, but there is no need to compromise communicability with aesthetics. The author frequently will show a client four or five representations of a single word (for example, a Rebus symbol, a Blissymbol, a line drawing, a word, and a Picsym) and ask him to identify which one represents the targeted word. This results in a board that is a hodge-podge of symbols, but it is the most meaningful to the client.

Use of Real Objects

In some cases, it may be necessary to use real objects or miniature versions of the objects for an AAC system. This is particularly true when developing AAC systems for very young children, or for individuals with cognitive delays. The reader is reminded, however, that miniature objects are less iconic than photographs of real objects. Two types of real objects are tangible symbols and tactile symbols. As explained by Rowland and Schweigert (1989), tangible symbols are "permanent three-dimensional symbols that can be tactilely discriminated and physically manipulated by the AAC communicator" (Millikin, 1997, p. 111). It may be necessary to use an identical object as a symbol. For example, if the child has a red cup on his board as a symbol for drink, the child may need to be given his drink in a red cup, identical to the one on his board, in order for the child to make the association. It is important that the child get his drink from a cup other than the one on the board so that he can learn that the cup on his board is a symbol of the one actually used. Obviously, tangible symbols do not require the cognitive and memory demand of other more advanced symbol systems.

Tactile symbols may be used with clients who have visual and/or auditory impairments. The basic premise is that the client learns to associate certain textures with specific referents. It is possible for a system to contain tactile and tangible symbols. For the sake of space, it is advisable to move from three-dimensional objects to two-dimensional symbols. For example, using the cup example, once the child is able to make the symbolic association of the cup on his board to the cup from which he drinks, the cup can be cut in half and mounted on a board. Gradually, the size of the cup can be reduced. It is also possible to use cut out photographs of objects that the client can trace with his fingers to identify the object.

Use of Photographs and Line Drawings

Photographs of actual objects used by the client represent the lowest cognitive demand beyond the use of objects. However, their use should be paired with more abstract photographs (for example, a different cup than the actual one used), to encourage generalization to other symbols. Generally speaking, when a client is able to identify objects using dissimilar photographs, he is ready to use black and white line drawings (Mirenda, 1985).

Line drawings can be done by the clinician, or a local artist, or they can be purchased commercially. The commercial sets are usually inexpensive, and may come in a sticker format. The sizes vary from set to set, making them applicable for just about any size cell. The main warning regarding commercial symbol sets is that the clinician should be careful not to let the contents of the symbol set dictate what appears on the communication board (Millikin, 1997). Many of the commercial sets are iconic, making them easy to teach in the initial stages of developing an AAC system.

Photographs may be effective as symbols for objects and other nouns, but they are less effective when used for verbs and modifiers. Graphic drawings can be made that depict movement by the use of arrows, dots, and lines that are not possible on photographs. Bloomberg et al. (1990) found that modifiers were more translucent when they were paired with a known referent. Millikin (1997) uses the example of representing "hot" by showing a thermometer, a hot stove, or a picture of an individual sweating in the sun.

Drawings can be either ideographic or pictographic. Pictographs are pictures representing actual things, whereas ideographs represent concepts and ideas (Bishop et al., 1994; Bliss, 1965). Most AAC displays contain ideographic and pictographic symbols.

Frequently, the communication is telegraphic, with functor words being omitted and only content carrying words being included in the message. Thus, the message is often up to the interpretation of the listener. The exception is when a symbol on an electronic voice output device is programmed to express a complete sentence, thus making the message clearer to the listener.

Some symbol systems are unique to the device into which they are programmed. For example, the DynaVox uses DynaSyms, and many of the Prentke-Romich devices use Unity symbols. Usually, these symbols are accompanied by a written word making their interpretation easier for the listener. Also, as mentioned above, the symbol for one word can be programmed as a complete sentence. For example, the symbol for cold could be programmed to say, "I am cold."

Picture symbols can be easily recalled and generalized to other communicative expressions. Some pictographic systems include Rebus (Woodcock and Davis, 1969), Picture Communication Symbols (Johnson, 1981), Pictogram Idiogram Communication Symbols (PIC) (Maharaj, 1980), Blissymbolics (Bliss, 1965), Picsyms (Carlson, 1986), DynaSyms (Carlson, 1994), Minspeak (Baker, 1986), and Sigsymbols (Cregan & Lloyd, 1990).

Orthographic Symbol Systems

For those capable of using them, orthographic symbol systems are the system of choice because they are essentially limitless in what they can express. However, they are the most difficult to learn, and have the least transparency of all the systems. "Traditional orthography (TO) consists of written letters that are combined together to form words, sentences, and other forms of written language. Other orthographic symbol systems include Morse Code, Braille, and phonemic symbols" (Millikin, 1997, p. 127). Many AAC users combine orthography with pictographic symbol systems in order to maximize the words they can communicate to another individual.

Traditional orthography consists of the 26 letters of the Roman alphabet, numbers, and punctuation marks. The system is unlimited as to what can be generated. However, it is slow when compared to some pictographic systems. Some rate enhancement strategies are available that can increase the rate of communication (Millikin, 1997).

Morse Code uses a series of dots (dits) and dashes (dahs) to represent the letters of the alphabet and punctuation marks. It combines auditory and visual feedback, making it appropriate for those with relatively normal cognitive ability but impaired visual or auditory systems. Using a single or dual switch, many dedicated AAC devices and adapted computers can interpret the Morse code and transmit the information to a speech synthesizer. Morse code is a viable alternative for clients with limited switch access methods, or slow direct selection abilities (Millikin, 1997).

Braille is a symbol system with symbols to represent letters, numbers, punctuation marks, and music through a series of raised dots. Traditionally used by blind individuals, Braille holds promise as an orthographic AAC system as well. "Braille can be used to access computers with specialized hardware and software. If the computer is adapted with a speech synthesizer and printer, Braille can be used to produce both written and spoken language" (Millikin, 1997, p. 128).

Selecting and Organizing a Symbol System

As mentioned previously, the potential AAC user should be observed in a variety of environments to determine his communication needs and abilities. If the client has a good head nod response for yes/no, there is no need to put "yes" and "no" on the communication board. For clients who have a lot to say, space is a premium on AAC devices. After observing the client, a vocabulary list should be generated, and the clinician and client should then decide which symbol systems to use and how it will be organized on the client's AAC device.

Numerous possibilities exist for the organization of a symbol system. The clinician should refer back to the assessment information, and particularly the information gained through the MSIPT evaluation, to determine the best organization of the symbol system. Some users will need to be limited to one item per page, whereas others can handle over a hundred items per page.

Eye gaze systems were previously discussed. In addition to the systems already described, the clinician can wear a vest with symbols attached by Velcro. The display can be static or dynamic, depending on the needs of the communicator.

Booklet systems are also popular methods of displaying symbols. The booklets can have as many symbols on a page as the client can handle. If the client has difficulty turning pages, tabs, which are easier to grasp, can be added to the pages (as in notebook divider pages). Another option is to put foam spacers between the pages so the client can easily slide his fingers between the pages (Millikin, 1997). It is suggested that book pages be put into plastic sleeves to promote longevity of the pages. It is also suggested that copies be made of the pages in case the communication book is lost.

Communication books can be organized according to topic, place of communication, holidays, or other methods appropriate to the client's needs. For example, one client who ate at restaurants frequently had a menu page for each restaurant he visited. These were kept in a special section and provided precise ordering in the restaurant, without taking up space on the main pages of his communication booklet. Similarly, holidays can have a page dedicated to the particular holiday, with a holiday section being added to the book.

The main pages of the book, or the total display on a communication board, can be organized in a variety of ways. One way is syntactically, with question words and nouns that are frequently used as subjects (people) on the left side of the page, verbs in the next column(s), followed by modifiers and other nouns. This is more commonly known as the Fitzgerald Key, with the words being organized from left to right according to the position they would assume in a sentence (Millikin, 1997). Symbols depicting time, numbers, months, days, and money can be added to the right side of the display.

Some symbols will carry a complete message and will not need to be combined with other symbols. It is suggested that frequently used remarks, such as "My name is ____." be handled in this fashion. There should also be a cell to indicate that the message is complete, one to indicate that there was a mistake and that the user is starting over, and one empty cell to indicate that there is no symbol on the board to express the desired word (Millikin, 1997).

Frequently used symbols may be displayed in such a way that no matter where the user is in his book, he can see the symbols that he uses on a regular basis. These may be down the sides of the book, across the top of the book, along the bottom of the book, or on all sides. The location of these most frequently used symbols should be in the areas that provide the easiest access for the client.

In summary, AAC is an exciting aspect of our field that is relatively new when compared to other areas of study. There are tremendous advances being made in the electronic applications for AAC. The clinician should keep abreast of the latest developments in order to best use the information gathered during the assessment and intervention stages of interaction with the client.

APPENDIX 10-A: AAC FUNDING SOURCES

AAC FUNDING SOURCES	Age of Eligibility			
	0 to 3	3 to 21	16 to 65	65+
Federal Entitlement Programs				
Individuals with Disabilities Education Act (IDEA)				
IDEA, Part H, Early Intervention Grants	X			
IDEA, Part B, State Grant Programs	X	X		
Rehabilitation Act Amendments of 1992				
Basic State Grants, Title I			X	
Supported Employment, Title VI - C			X	
Independent Living, Title VII - A			X	X
Section 504	X	X	X	X
Section 508			X	
Health Insurance Programs				
Medical Assistance (Medicaid, MA)				
EPSDT—Children's Services	X	X		
Adult Services			X	X
Waiver Programs	X	X	X	X
Medicare Part B			X	X
Private Insurance	X	X	X	X
SSA Work Incentive Programs				
Plans for Achieving Self-Support (PASS)			X	X
Impairment Related Work Expenses (IRWEs)			X	X
Continued Medicaid Eligibility (Section 1619b)			X	X
Continuation of Medicare Coverage			X	
Medicare for People with Disabilities Who Work			X	
Internal Revenue Code (IRS)				
Medical and Dental Expense Deductions	X	X	X	X
Depreciation of Capital Equipment	X	X	X	X

AAC FUNDING SOURCES

	Age of Eligibility			
	0 to 3	3 to 21	16 to 65	65+
Section 44: Disabled Access Credit			x	x
Section 51: Targeted Jobs Tax Credit			x	x
State Sales Tax	x	x	x	x
Charitable Contributions	x	x	x	x
Impairment Related Work Expenses (IRWEs)			x	x
Alternative Funding Sources				
Technology Related Assistance Programs	x	x	x	x
Monetary Loan Programs	x	x	x	x
Equipment Loan Programs	x	x	x	x
Disability Organizations	x	x	x	x
Service Clubs	x	x	x	x
Private Funds or Foundations	x	x	x	x

APPENDIX 10-B: AUGMENTATIVE AND ALTERNATIVE COMMUNICATION INFORMATION AND NEEDS ASSESSMENT

Name: _____ Age: _____ Date: _____

Examiner: _____

Informants: Relationship to Client:

_____   _____

_____   _____

_____   _____

I.   **Current Methods of Communication.** For each modality ask the informant (1) whether the modality is used, and if it is, to describe the client's current use of the modality; (2) to indicate the size of the client's vocabulary using the modality; and (3) to indicate how well the client is understood when using the modality. Use the spaces provided to record notes.

Modality	Description	Vocabulary Size	Intelligibility
Speech			
Vocalizations			

Sign language

Gesture/pointing

Head nods

Eye gaze

Facial expression

AAC device

Other

II. **Past AAC Experience.** Ask the informant the following questions. Record notes in the spaces provided.

Has this individual ever used a picture or letter-based AAC device in the past? If yes describe the system.

Name of device: _____

Length of time used: _____

Number of symbols: _____ Size of symbols: _____

Symbol system used: _____

Organization of symbols: _____

Access method: _____

What were the strengths and limitations of the AAC system described above?

III. **Communication Environments.** Ask the informant to describe how the AAC will be used and with whom. Also determine barriers to using the AAC. Take notes in the spaces provided.

Environment	Description	Interaction Partner
Home		
School		
Work		
Community		
Other		

What barriers to AAC implementation exist in any of the environments listed above?

IV. Mobility and Access. Ask the informant to describe the client's mobility and access regarding use of an AAC system. Also determine specific mobility, seating, or positioning concerns.

Mobility	Description	Environment Used
Fully ambulatory		
Ambulatory with assistance		
Manual wheelchair		
Power wheelchair		
Other		

Are there any mobility, seating, or positioning concerns that will affect the implementation of an AAC system? If yes, describe.

Functional Access	Description	Access Limitations
Left arm/hand		
Right arm/hand		
Head		
Left leg/foot		
Right leg/foot		

Eye gaze

Other

V. **Other Technologies.** Ask the informant what other technologies will need to be integrated with an AAC system. Record notes in the spaces provided.

Technology	Description	Environment Used
Wheelchair		
Computer		
Environmental controls		

Switch toys

Other

VI. AAC Expectations. Ask the informant the following question. Record notes in the space provided. What goals could be achieved if the client had access to an AAC system?

APPENDIX 10–C: VISUAL SCANNING AND TRACKING CHECKLIST

Name: _____ Age: _____ Date: _____

Examiner: _____

Instructions: Make the following observations. Mark a check (√) if a statement describes the client. Record additional comments in the right-hand column.

Comments

Client is able to track from:

_____ left to right _____

_____ right to left _____

_____ up and down _____

_____ down and up _____

_____ diagonally up and down, left to right _____

_____ diagonally up and down, right to left _____

_____ diagonally down and up, left to right _____

_____ diagonally down and up, right to left _____

Client is able to:

_____ read words (indicate size of print) _____

_____ read phrases (indicate size of print) _____

_____ recognize pictures or objects _____

_____ recognize symbols _____

Client is able to:

_____ visually focus on stimuli _____

_____ scan stimuli for desired word/picture/symbol (circle
one and indicate number of stimulus items in field) _____

Comments

_____ identify desired stimulus quickly/slowly
(circle one and indicate seconds) _____

_____ identify desired stimulus consistently _____

_____ identify desired stimulus with cues (indicate type) _____

Client demonstrates:

_____ visual neglect (indicate areas) _____

_____ nystagmus (oscillating movements of the eyeball) _____

_____ strabismus (eyes turn in or out) _____

_____ poor ability to move eyes together _____

_____ difficulty seeing stimuli more than 12 inches
away from face _____

Note any identifiable patterns of scanning, including where the client begins visually searching (e.g., at midline, top left, top right, etc.)

APPENDIX 10-D: MSIPT ASSESSMENT

Client: _____ Date: _____ Evaluator: _____

Date:	MSIPT #1	MSIPT #2	MSIPT #3

Position of client

Positioning adaptations

Motivators

M: Movement

   Movement concerns

S: Control Site

   Site adaptations

I: Input method

   Direct selection features: (Keyboard size and configuration, keyguards/grids, pressure sensitivity)

   Scanning features: (Scan method, scan pattern, scan speed, reactivation time, auditory scan, auditory feedback)

P: Position of input method

   (Device/switch)

T: Targeting method

   (Target size, number of keys/cells, number of active keys/cells)

Speed of overall response

Accuracy of overall method

Reliability

Overall quality

Additional comments

Training and Implementation Plan:

CHAPTER ELEVEN
Autism

DEFINITION/DESCRIPTION

Autism is a pervasive developmental disorder of unknown etiology. It is proposed that it could have genetic factors, and/or a neurological basis. Studies at Duke University found a higher prevalence of manic depression in families of children with autism, leading them to hypothesize that autism may be an inherited psychiatric disorder (Trace, 1996). More recent studies at the University of North Carolina at Chapel Hill (and other affiliated centers) have found genetic markers on Chromosome 13 and Chromosome 7 that may play a causative role in autism. Other suspected/associated etiological factors include tuberous sclerosis, maternal rubella, fragile X syndrome, perinatal trauma, and seizure disorders (Hewitt, 1992, p. 265).

The reported incidence figures are 4–5 per 10,000 children. Even though it is more predominant in males, females tend to have more severe cases (Hegde, 1996). Approximately 75–80% of those with autism also have mental retardation.

The DSM-IV lists five subtypes of pervasive developmental disorder: autistic disorder, Rett's disorder, childhood disintegrative disorder, Asperger's disorder, and pervasive developmental disorder not otherwise specified (including atypical autism) (American Psychiatric Association, 1994). Schreibman (1988) suggested three subtypes of autism based on IQ levels: High (IQ of 70+; 20% of autistic population); Middle (IQ of 50–70; 20% of autistic population); Low (IQ below 50; 60% of autistic population).

Asperger's disorder "is essentially what used to be called high functioning autism. The two key differences between Asperger's disorder and autistic disorder are in the areas of language and cognitive development"(Nelson, 1998, p. 114). Typically, there is use of single words by age two years, and communicative phrases by age three, so no significant general delay in language exists. There is also no significant delay in cognition, self-help skills, or curiosity about the environment. "The children with Asperger's disorder do show the impairment in social interaction that is typically associated with autism, and the 'restricted, repetitive, and stereotyped patterns of behavior, interests, and activities'" (American Psychiatric Association, 1994, p. 77).

Table 11–1 lists characteristics associated with autism and related syndromes.

Historically, echolalia was considered to be a symptom of autism that served no meaningful purpose. More recent research by Prizant and Duchan (1981) hypothesizes that echolalia serves a variety of communicative purposes. The imitation may serve as a way to validate or

TABLE 11–1 Characteristics frequently observed in autism and related syndromes
Failure to develop normal responsivity to other persons
Social withdrawal in varying degrees
Typically fail to develop normal verbal and nonverbal communication
Failure to use objects functionally and/or appropriately
Abnormal fixations on inanimate objects
Abnormal sensory thresholds (over or underactive)
Cyclical behavioral extremes
Obsessive traits such as fixations on strange objects
Special abilities to calculate numbers or remember facts
Regression of social and language skills after an early period of normal development
Reluctance or difficulty in forming interpersonal relationships
Preference for being left alone
Use of echolalia (unsolicited imitative verbal behavior)
Monotone speech
Pronoun confusions (particularly I, you)
Articulatory skills exceeding vocabulary, syntax, and social language use (not the case with children who have SLI or MR)

Adapted from "Classification of Language Abnormalities by Etiology and Diagnosis," by B.Vinson, 1999, in *Language Disorders Across the Lifespan* (p. 45), San Diego, CA: Singular Publishing Group. Copyright 1999 by Singular Publishing Group. Adapted with permission.

acknowledge the speaker's input, even though the input may not have been processed by the child. Thus, "echolalia was no longer a disease symptom but a strategy for overcoming severe communication disability" (Hewitt, 1992, p. 264). Children with autism show much more echolalia than do children with specific language impairment or mental retardation. The imitation in children with autism is usually fully phrased and familiar words. This is opposed to the imitation of normal children, which centers on new and unfamiliar words.

Owens (1995) describes language impairment as consisting of the following characteristics:

1. Limited range of communication functions;

2. Perseverations;

3. Overuse of questions;

4. Word-retrieval deficits;

5. Morphological difficulties;

6. Less complex sentences;

7. Pragmatic and conversational deficits (lack of initiation, lack of topic maintenance, lack of turn-taking, poor conversational repair).

Ritvo and Freeman (1978) are referenced in Owens (1995) as delineating the definition of autism from the Autism Society of America. They state that the disorder has an onset prior to 30 months of age, with disturbances in the following areas:

> Developmental rates and the sequence of motor, social-adaptive and cognitive skills;

> Responses to sensory stimuli—hyper- and hyposensitivity in audition, vision, tactile stimulation, motor, olfactory and taste, including self-stimulatory behaviors;

> Speech and language, cognition, and nonverbal communication, including mutism, echolalia and difficulty with abstract terms;

> Capacity to appropriately relate to people, events, and objects, including lack of social behaviors, affection, and appropriate play (Owens, 1995, p. 44).

Owens (1995) goes on to say that the symptoms often become more pronounced around 18 months of age. These early symptoms include frequent tantrums, and extreme reactions to certain stimuli. The child may exhibit a lack of social play, and will have communication deficits. The child may also start to demonstrate ritualistic play and repetitive movements.

As delineated in Campbell (2000), Prelock has developed a list of red flags that may provide early detection of a child with autism. These red flags are listed in Table 11–2.

TABLE 11–2 Red flags for potential diagnosis of autism
Failure to develop anticipatory reach
Absence of pointing
Use of hand leading
Loss of language between 18–36 months
Failure to look at others
Lack of interest in other children
Inability to orient to name
Failure to show objects
Failure to demonstrate symbolic play
Lack of interest in or joint attention to games for pleasure or connection with another person

DSM CRITERIA FOR 299.00 AUTISTIC DISORDER

A. A total of six (or more) items from (1), (2), and (3), with at least two from (1), and one each from (2) and (3):

1. qualitative impairment in social interaction, as manifested by at least two of the following:

   a. marked impairment in the use of multiple nonverbal behaviors such as eye-to-eye gaze, facial expression, body postures, and gestures to regulate social interaction

   b. failure to develop peer relationships to developmental level

   c. a lack of spontaneous seeking to share enjoyment, interests, or achievements with other people (e.g., by a lack of showing, bringing, or pointing out objects of interest)

   d. lack of social or emotional reciprocity

2. qualitative impairment in communication as manifested by at least one of the following:

   a. delay in, or total lack of, the development of spoken language (not accompanied by an attempt to compensate through alternative modes of communication such as gesture or mime)

   b. in individuals with adequate speech, marked impairment in the ability to initiate or sustain a conversation with others

   c. stereotyped and repetitive use of language or idiosyncratic language

   d. lack of varied, spontaneous make-believe play or social initiative play appropriate to developmental level

3. restricted repetitive and stereotyped patterns of behavior, interests, and activities, as manifested by at least one of the following:

   a. encompassing preoccupation with one or more stereotyped and restricted patterns of interest that is abnormal either in intensity or focus

   b. apparently inflexible adherence to specific, nonfunctional routines or rituals

   c. stereotyped and repetitive motor mannerisms (e.g., hand or finger flapping or twisting, or complex whole-body movements)

   d. persistent preoccupation with parts of objects

B. Delays or abnormal functioning in at least one of the following areas, with onset prior to age 3 years: (1) social interaction, (2) language as used in social communication, or (3) symbolic or imaginative play.

C. The disturbance is not better accounted for by Rett's Disorder or Childhood Disintegrative Disorder (p. 70–71).

ASSESSMENT

Performance on assessments may be affected by a variety of factors including positioning of the child, temperature and lighting of the room, light and dark contrasts, placement of the materials, and visual and auditory distractions. The clinician may have to address issues of perseveration by reminding the child that all answers are not the same. Short-term memory deficits may result in the need to repeat directions and cues (Owens, 1995).

It is suggested that sensory profiles be assessed in children with autism. This should be done prior to any other testing in order to determine the sensory thresholds with regard to auditory, visual, and tactile stimulation. It is also helpful to observe the child with familiar persons and objects, but to introduce a stranger and new toys into the environment to gauge his reactions. The child should, preferably, be videotaped in two or three settings to get a more complete profile of the behaviors he typically displays. Also, as with all pediatric assessments, the parents/caregivers should be interviewed (Campbell, 2000).

Assessment of a child with suspected autism should follow the basic guidelines of any child being tested for receptive and/or expressive language deficits (see chapter on receptive and expressive language). Each assessment should address morphology, syntax, semantics, pragmatics, and cognition. A majority of children with autism are nonverbal; however, those that are verbal should also have their phonology/articulation assessed.

Children with autism usually have delayed morphology when compared to children without developmental disabilities. With regard to syntax, children with autism construct sentences with superficial form. However, they do not have a full understanding of the deep structures and generative principles associated with comprehending syntax.

Semantics is typical of language delay, with the children not using semantic cues to aid in the recall of information. They remember words without remembering their meaning or content.

Pragmatics is delayed and deviant. They have difficulty making the connection between content and form and content and use. They typically do not establish eye contact, nor do they participate in active turn taking, topic initiation, or topic maintenance.

Cognitively, there are wide variations, but, generally, there is a cognitive deficit. Argument exists as to whether the cognitive impairment is secondary to the language deficits generally displayed by children with autism, or whether it is a primary deficit (Nelson, 1998).

If the use of alternative and/or augmentative communication devices is being considered, prelinguistic issues related to communication need to be assessed. Specifically, means-end, causality, and communicative intent should be explored in assessing the potential uses of AAC, and deciding whether to use presymbolic or symbolic communication forms. The dysfunctional behaviors exhibited by some children with autism may, indeed, mask any existing communication behaviors. Thus, the child's behavior should be carefully analyzed to determine if he has such prelinguistic concepts as means-end, causality, cause-and-effect, and communicative intent. These are critical developmental steps that form a foundation from which communication skills (speech or nonverbal) can be built (Wetherby & Prizant, 1990).

TREATMENT

Treatment of language and speech disorders in children with autism should first address sensory stimulation. It was mentioned that, as part of the assessment, the child's sensory thresholds with regard to auditory, visual, and tactile stimulation should be tested. It would also be wise to assess the child's reaction to olfactory and gustatory stimulation since primary reinforcement is often used with these children. Other focuses of intervention should include social interaction, verbal and nonverbal communication, play, and behaviors (Campbell, 2000).

Incidental teaching may be an effective intervention strategy. Incidental teaching takes place as part of the caregiver's daily activities and the child's unstructured times. Whenever the child demonstrates interest in a person, an object, or an event, the caregiver responds accordingly. Thus, to effectively implement incidental teaching, the caregiver must "be aware of the learning potential within each situation and to structure events to enhance learning" (Owens, 1995, p. 462).

McCormick and Schiefelbusch (1990) propose that the language difficulties experienced by children with autism may be due to "overselectivity to both auditory and visual stimuli. The child who attends to only one irrelevant stimulus or only one aspect of a stimulus could not possibly learn the visual-auditory associations so necessary for language learning" (p. 169). Thus, when the child with autism is presented with a multimodal stimulus array, he may focus on only one stimulus, excluding all others from his attention. It also could be hypothesized that this inability to attend to multiple stimuli may affect social interactions because the child may be distracted by one aspect of the interaction to the exclusion of all other aspects (McCormick and Schiefelbusch, 1990).

There are a variety of approaches that can form the foundation of intervention with children with autism. Historically, a behavioral, stimulus-response approach has been used. "Behavioral approaches require intensive scheduling of one-on-one training sessions for teaching discrete behaviors with multiple massed trials with a heavy reliance on imitation" (Nelson, 1998, p. 117). However, since generalization is difficult to achieve in children with autism (Brown, Nietupski, & Hamre-Nietupski, 1976), one has to question the wisdom of doing the traditional stimulus-response training in therapy. "Low inference abilities may contribute to a lack of generalization across cues, modalities, persons, and settings for individuals with severe developmental disabilities. Teachers of students with autism cannot assume that a skill trained in one setting will spontaneously generalize to other settings" (Wertz, Dexter, & Moore, 1997, p. 419).

A more appropriate approach to therapy for children with autism may be grounded in a naturalistic language training. If the child has opportunities to learn within his natural context, the skills he learns are more likely to be generalized to other settings. The natural language teaching paradigm is espoused by Koegel, O'Dell, and Koegel (1987). This paradigm is based on basic parameters of normal language. These parameters are used in child-directed activities that are typical of the child's natural learning environment. When compared to the traditional behavioral stimulus-response training, there is more active learning and generalization.

Another naturalistic language training method is the TEACCH (*Treatment and Education of Autistic and Related Communication Handicapped Children*) program, which is a comprehensive program of intervention that focuses on therapy for communication, independence, and socialization. The three areas of focus are integrated throughout the child's day in his natural learning environments. Structured teaching methods are implemented in a child-directed model.

> One of the core goals of the TEACCH program is the training of functional communication. This is initiated by conducting an inventory of the child's communication demands across various program contexts (e.g., play time, circle time, work time, snack time). This inventory is then used to identify those situations that can be engineered for communication. It is here that the child's emerging communication skills are shaped into more conventional forms of expression using AAC setups as warranted. Much effort is given to developing the conditions from which natural consequences can be used to reinforce the communicative attempts offered by the child. (Wertz, Dexter, & Moore, 1997, p. 421)

The use of alternative and augmentative communication (AAC) devices is a much debated topic when discussing communication intervention for children with autism. AAC is not always successful as an intervention for children with autism. Possibly this is because they do not have a communication foundation from which to build a communication interaction system (Wertz, Dexter, & Moore, 1997).

Children with autism who are verbal usually have atypical speech. This speech is likely to include stereotypic expressions and extensive echolalia. Prizant (1983) theorized that children with autism process information in a gestalt fashion rather than an analytic one. Thus, they remember large blocks of auditory or visual information in a holistic manner, then reproduce the information using echolalic speech. The clinician must be careful not to let advanced echolalia mask a language deficit. Some children with autism repeat complex statements, some with quite a bit of delay between the original hearing of the utterance, and the actual repetition. However, these utterances serve little or no communicative value. Many of the utterances are self-stimulatory in nature (Wertz, Dexter, & Moore, 1997).

If a child's communication attempts are infrequent and predominantly preintentional, he may not be ready for a formal symbolic communication system (Prizant & Wetherby, 1988; Schuler & Prizant, 1987). Thus, according to Mirenda and Schuler (1988), the clinician should begin intervention by facilitating the existing nonsymbolic communication in an effort to prepare the child for later use of a symbolic system. The facilitation of eye contact and reaching behaviors with meaning as nonverbal communication systems may be more appropriate for establishing communication than would be an AAC system. Once some nonverbal communication systems can be used as a foundation for communication, introduction of AAC systems may be more beneficial (Wertz, Dexter, & Moore, 1997).

When AAC training begins, it needs to be "systematically linked to the ecological needs of school, community, and home" (Wertz, Dexter, & Moore, 1997, p. 414). The Picture Exchange Communication System (PECS) has been successfully implemented in developing symbolic communication skills in children with autism (Bondy & Frost, 1993). "The picture exchange technique teaches children to initiate a communicative act to receive a concrete outcome. Because children with autism are not highly reinforced by typical social rewards associated with the act of communication, the use of a picture exchange setup can provide for immediate and concrete reinforcement while teaching the social interaction necessary for communication. This type of communication training is excellent for those who are demonstrating emerging intentional communication" (Wertz, Dexter, and Moore, 1997, p. 415). Even if the child pays little attention to the picture, the child learns that if he gives the picture to another person, he will get something in return. The PECS format promotes communication as a social exchange, and it also teaches the child that he can use symbols to manipulate outcomes in his environment.

Another model for training nonverbal communication skills in children with autism is Aided Language Stimulation. Aided Language Stimulation is a receptive and expressive teaching strategy in which a facilitator points to an array of symbols on a communication display as he or she verbally interacts with the child (Goossens et al., 1992; Romski & Sevcik, 1992). The facilitator "attempts to simulate the natural modeling of verbal language skills typically provided for children who can speak. In doing so, the facilitator employs various semantic contingency techniques involving the recasting and expansion of the child's expressions as he or she points to various pictured symbols on a communication display" (Wertz, Dexter, & Moore, 1997, p. 416). In essence, the facilitator is shaping the use of more complex and correct communications.

Another use of AAC is with children who are hyperlexic. Most children who are hyperlexic use speech as their primary mode of communication, but they often have expressive difficulties due to pragmatic deficits. Since children with hyperlexia process information better through the visual channels, and they can decode written words, the use of an orthographic communication system to augment their speech efforts may help to improve their communication skills (Wertz, Dexter, & Moore, 1997).

Finally, there are several Computer Assisted technologies on the market that can be used with children with autism. Some examples are the Touch Window, IntelliKeys, and the Discover:Board. These devices provide an alternative or adaptive access to the keyboard, thereby simplifying the computer operation when accessing a variety of software. Programs can be adapted to the child's learning style, and provide a means of interaction between the facilitator and the child. "It appears that the use of computers is consistent with autistic cognitive styles and processing preferences as evidenced by the fact that many individuals with autism are remarkably interactive with educational and entertainment software (Wertz, Dexter, & Moore, 1997, p. 418).

CHAPTER TWELVE
Cleft Lip and Cleft Palate

DEFINITION/DESCRIPTION

In 1987, Surgeon General Koop called for the following goals in the treatment of craniofacial disorders: (1) parent-professional collaboration, (2) providing parents with accurate and complete information, (3) making emotional and financial support available, (4) being sensitive to cultural attributes, (5) encouraging parent-to-parent support programs, (6) including the developmental needs of babies, children, and adolescents, (7) ensuring comprehensive care that includes appropriate social, emotional, and cognitive elements, and (8) carrying out treatment in interdisciplinary settings (Crowe, 1997). In reaction the American Cleft Palate-Craniofacial Association (1993) developed a document entitled "Parameters for Evaluation and Treatment of Patients with Cleft Lip/Palate and Other Craniofacial Anomalies" that addressed ten principles:

1. Team management by
2. Teams with adequate numbers of patients;
3. Early initial evaluations;
4. Attention to family adjustment;
5. Provision of information to family and patients;
6. Encouraging their participation in treatment planning;
7. Executing treatment at convenient locations with complex diagnostic and surgical procedures restricted to major centers;
8. Sensitivity to family characteristics that affect team-patient dynamics;
9. Longitudinal assessment of patients and long-term outcomes evaluations that
10. Take into account both physical and psychosocial well-being (Crowe, 1997).

In addition to the client and the family, team members typically include prosthodontists, orthodontists, speech-language pathologists, audiologists, pedodontists, psychologists, pediatricians, neurosurgeons, oral-maxillofacial surgeons, otolaryngologists, plastic surgeons, ophthalmologists, genetic counselors, nurses, social workers, and educational personnel (Haynes & Pindzola, 1998; Bzoch, 1997a; Nackashi & Dixon-Wood, 1989).

A study by Weachter (1959) found that the major sources of worry to parents of children with craniofacial anomalies were the child's appearance, immediacy of surgery, feeding, speech, reactions of family members and friends, mental development, finances, and possibility of recurrence in future children. Other concerns included knowing the cause of the anomaly, what, if anything, they did wrong, the effects of hearing loss, and how their child would be accepted by peers (Crowe, 1997).

It should also be noted that cleft lip and/or palate are associated with over 350 syndromes. Over 50% of children with clefts of the palate only are likely to have developmental deficits or other associated malformations (McWilliams & Matthews, 1979). Approximately 76% of children who have velopharyngeal insufficiency but no palatal clefts have additional congenital anomalies.

Some of the associated anomalies are very mild, while others may be life threatening. Frequently, the associated anomalies include various syndromes, many of which are genetic. Therefore, it is critical to stress the need for genetic counseling and good pediatric care for individuals with cleft lip and/or palate, and other craniofacial anomalies and their families (Crowe, 1997).

Velo-Cardio-Facial Syndrome (VCFS)

VCFS is the most common cause of syndromic clefting. It is characterized by velopharyngeal insufficiency, facial dysmorphology, conotruncal heart defects, and vascular anomalies. Individuals with VCFS also present with learning disabilities, behavioral abnormalities, and neurologic deficits. Cranial nerve dysfunction in VCFS may account for VPI in children with normal palatal anatomy, and may compromise the outcome of pharyngoplasty. The presence of cranio-vertebral junction abnormalities may increase the risk for neurologic complications, and may warrant surgical management if the child is symptomatic. In addition, aberrant cervical vasculature may affect surgical decision-making. (Riski, 1999).

Assessment of VCFS includes orofacial examination, lateral cephalometric radiography, nasendoscopy, pressure flow, nasometry, MRA of cervical vasculature, and an MRI of the cranio-vertebral junction (Riski, 1999).

Therapy considerations include the developmental level and intellect of the patient, the degree of ability to be compliant with speech therapy activities, patency of the airway, stability of the cervical spine, and the severity of the cardiac disease. Surgical considerations include tissue deficiency, the anatomical configuration, innervation, the presence of scar tissue, and the presence of an obturator.

Clinical findings in velo-cardio-facial syndrome include good lateral wall movement with a short palate, poor lateral wall movement with adequate velar closure, or limited posterior and lateral wall and velar motion.

Velopharyngeal Function

The velopharyngeal (VP) mechanism consists of the pharynx and the soft palate (velum). The muscles of these two structures act together to close the connection between the oropharynx below and the nasopharynx above during swallowing, speech, and other activities. This closing of the connection between the oropharynx and the nasopharynx is called *velopharyngeal closure*. Individuals with cleft palate who are unable to achieve velopharyngeal closure are said to have *velopharyngeal insufficiency* (VPI) (Huang, 1999). Table 12–1 offers a summary of the anatomy of the important VP muscles. There are five muscles involved in velopharyngeal closure. The velar component of closure involves the palatopharyngeus, the levator veli palatini, and the musculus uvulae. The pharyngeal component of closure involves the superior constrictor and the palatopharyngeus muscles.

TABLE 12-1 The anatomy of the important VP muscles			
Muscle	*Attachments*	*Actions*	*Functions*
Palatoglossus	Hamulus (previously undescribed) to tongue	Tongue elevation	Increases oral impedance to airflow during certain speech sounds
Palatopharyngeus	Soft palate to (1) lateral & posterior walls, (2) larynx	(1) Stretches velum & orients it vertically, (2) Inward movement of pharyngeal walls	Acts synergistically with: (1) levator to maximize VP contact, (2) superior constrictor to constrict pharynx
Musculus uvulae	Tensor aponeurosis to base of uvula	(1) Increases dorsal midline velar bulk, (2) Velar extension	Maximizes midline VP contact
Levator veli palatini	Skull base & Eustachian tube to soft palate	(1) Velar elevation & retrodisplacement, (2) Dilatation of Eustachian tube	(1) Prime mover of velum in closure, (2) Clears tubal secretions & equalizes tympanic air pressure
Tensor veli palatini	Skull base & Eustachian tube to hard & soft palate (via aponeurosis)	Dilates Eustachian tube	Clears tubal secretions & equalizes tympanic air pressure
Superior constrictor	Hamulus & pherygomandibular ligament to pharyngeal ligament	Inward movement of pharyngeal walls	Acts synergistically with palatopharyngeus to constrict pharynx

From "Velopharyngeal Anatomy," by M. H. S. Huang, in *Proceedings of the 12th annual symposium on cleft lip and palate and related conditions*. October 8–10, 1999. Reprinted with permission.

ASSESSMENT

Appendix 12-A summarizes the following assessment information in a checklist format. Cases of velopharyngeal incompetence, whether they are associated with cleft lip and/or palate or not, are typically assessed in many of the same areas as are used in craniofacial anomalies. A listing of some of these areas is in Table 12–2.

Oral-Facial Examination

In addition to a complete oral-facial examination (See Table 8–5 in the Articulation and Phonology chapter), the clinician should pay attention to the following factors when assessing a child with cleft lip and/or palate:

1. The type of cleft should be described and classified. It should be noted whether the cleft is repaired or unrepaired.

2. The presence of other oral-facial anomalies should be documented.

3. Assessment to determine the presence of a submucosal cleft should be done. A submucosal cleft can be indicated when there is a bluish line due to thinning or translucency at the midline of the musculature of the hard palate, and/or a bifid uvula. Asymmetrical or reduced movement of the palate, and the presence of a palpable notch on the posterior edge of the hard palate are also indicators of a possible submucous cleft.

4. The presence of labial pits in the lower lip should be determined.

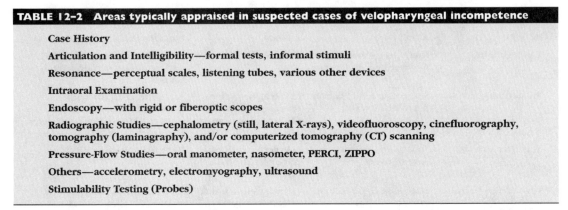

TABLE 12-2   Areas typically appraised in suspected cases of velopharyngeal incompetence

Case History

Articulation and Intelligibility—formal tests, informal stimuli

Resonance—perceptual scales, listening tubes, various other devices

Intraoral Examination

Endoscopy—with rigid or fiberoptic scopes

Radiographic Studies—cephalometry (still, lateral X-rays), videofluoroscopy, cinefluorography, tomography (laminagraphy), and/or computerized tomography (CT) scanning

Pressure-Flow Studies—oral manometer, nasometer, PERCI, ZIPPO

Others—accelerometry, electromyography, ultrasound

Stimulability Testing (Probes)

From *Diagnosis and Evaluation in Speech Pathology* (5th ed.) (p. 390), by W. O. Haynes and R. H. Pindzola, 1998, Boston, MA: Allyn & Bacon. Copyright 1998 by Allyn & Bacon. Reprinted with permission.

5. The presence of velar, palatal, labiodental, or alveolar fistulas should be determined.

6. The elevation pattern of the velum should be assessed, noting if the movement is symmetrical or asymmetrical, and the extent of the movement.

7. The perceived length of the velum, and the depth of the nasopharynx should be documented.

8. The shape of the alveolar ridge (collapsed, wide, notched, cleft) should be noted (Shipley & McAfee, 1998).

Oral Health in Children with Cleft Lip and Palate

Dahllof (1989) reported that decayed, missing, and filled teeth occurred at almost twice the rate in the cleft population as in the non-cleft population. Sandy, Williams et al. (1998) found that 40% of 5 year olds with unilateral cleft lip and palate had active caries. Paul and Brandt (1998) found that 20% of 3–18 year olds with cleft lip and/or palate had active dental caries (Shirley, 1999).

Caries can expose the pulp, a neurovascular bundle near the center of the tooth, resulting in infection and pain. However, removal of teeth that cannot be restored can have a negative effect on maxillary alveolar bone in the area of the cleft. Furthermore, untreated caries and subsequent infection can lead to a facial infection. Children are much more susceptible to rapid spread of infection because of the location of muscle attachments, density of the bone, and the relative size of the child. Congenital structural defects can also contribute to rapid spread of infection (Shirley, 1999).

Management of dental caries includes first determining the risk for developing caries. After determining the inherent risk, the patient and/or caregivers can be provided with preventative guidance that addresses diet, nutrition, and oral hygiene. Periodic evaluations are absolutely necessary. Both systemic and topical fluoride treatments should be provided. Finally, when possible, restorative treatment should also be provided. Also, presurgical management of cleft lip and palate should include orthodontics and orthopedics.

Voice

A frequent finding in individuals with cleft palate is poor vocal resonance. According to D'Antonio and Scherer (1995), as cited in Shipley and McAfee (1998), this may be directly related to the presence of the cleft, or indirectly the result of the development of laryngeal voice disorders due to the individual's efforts to

- produce intelligible speech,
- achieve normal pitch change and loudness,
- compensate for velopharyngeal incompetence by using the glottis to produce plosives and fricatives, and/or
- mask hypernasality and nasal emission. (Shipley & McAfee, 1998, p. 394)

Language

The co-occurrence of developmental disabilities in children with clefts is well-documented. In addition, children with clefts often have mild conductive hearing losses caused by the presence of fluid in the middle ear. Therefore, the child's receptive and expressive language should also be assessed. Research indicates that children with clefts have a lower mean length of utterance than do their peers. Also, the quality and quantity of their verbal language is lower than their peers' (Crowe, 1997). The reader is referred to the chapter on language disorders in preschool children for additional information on this topic.

Speech

Speech impairments related to cleft palate include resonance disorders, difficulty producing pressure consonants, and the use of compensatory articulation strategies (Moller & Starr, 1993). Articulation and phonology can be assessed using standard tests in these areas (see chapter on articulation and phonology). In addition to the articulation and phonology, the degree of velopharyngeal closure, airflow, and intraoral pressure must also be assessed (these are discussed elsewhere in this chapter). Thus, in addition to providing an inventory of sounds the client can and cannot produce, articulation testing may also indicate the adequacy of velopharyngeal closure (Haynes & Pindzola, 1998). Articulation tests that can be used to assess both include those listed in Table 12–3.

As in all instances of assessing articulation and phonology, the clinician should analyze the speech samples obtained, listening to speech in single-words, phrases, and connected speech. Overall intelligibility should be determined, along with an analysis of the articulatory and phonatory patterns the client uses. However, when assessing the speech of a child with craniofacial anomalies and/or velopharyngeal insufficiency, the clinician must also "distinguish speech errors that may be due to faulty velopharyngeal or other structural deviations from speech errors that are compensatory or developmental" (Haynes & Pindzola, 1998, p. 393).

Compensatory Articulation Strategies

"Compensatory articulation strategies are learned behaviors that clients with clefts sometimes use in an effort to compensate for velopharyngeal incompetence" (Shipley &

Table 12–3   Articulation tests useful in assessing velopharyngeal function

P-B Articulation Screening Test for Preschoolers

   (Van Demark and Swickard 1980)

   This is a 25-item single-word test of two phonemes, /p/ and /b/. The authors claim that velopharyngeal inadequacy is indicated when errors occur on at least 50 percent of the sounds tested.

Error Pattern Screening Articulation Test

   (Bzoch 1979; Bzoch, Kemker, and Wood 1984)

   The 31 words are purported to be useful in identifying gross substitution errors in children aged 3 and 4. Plosives, fricatives, affricates, glides, nasals, and blends are tested. Scoring involves assigning an error value to each sound. Sounds are scored as correct, indistinct from nasal emissions alone, distortion, simple substitution, gross substitution, or omission.

Bzoch Error Pattern Diagnostic Articulation Test

   (Bzoch 1979)

   The diagnostic test has four forms, each with a different set of 100 words. Tested are 67 consonants and 33 blends in the initial, medial, final positions of the words. This is the full-length version of the screening test previously listed and is constructed with the same properties.

Iowa Pressure Articulation Test (IPAT)

   (Templin and Darley 1969)

   This test consists of 43 words containing pressure consonants. The percentage of correct responses is said to reflect the severity of velopharyngeal incompetence.

The reading passage "The Picnic"

   (Wilson 1987)

   The 43 words from the IPAT are incorporated in the short paragraph called "The Picnic." Production of the test words therefore can be tested in reading, rather than the traditional single-word method.

Sentence articulation tests

   (Fletcher 1978; Van Demark 1964, 1966)

   These are two examples of informal tests at the sentence level, which may be more ecologically valid than single-word tests.

Articulation Protocol

   (McCabe and Bradley 1973)

   The protocol, with a 10–15 minute administration time, compares accuracy of articulated words in automatic speech, single words, sentences, reading, and conversation.

From *Diagnosis and Evaluation in Speech Pathology* (5th ed.) (p.384), by W. O. Haynes and R. H. Pindzola, 1998, Boston, MA: Allyn & Bacon. Copyright 1998 by Allyn & Bacon. Reprinted with permission.

McAfee, 1998, p. 395). Oftentimes, speech therapy is directed toward eliminating these compensatory patterns after surgical intervention has eliminated the physiological deficit. A list of these patterns is in Table 12–4.

Common articulatory substitutions are listed in Table 12–5.

Hypernasality and Nasal Emission

A variety of quality aberrations are possible in the speech of individuals with a cleft palate, but hypernasality and nasal emission caused by poor closure of the velopharyngeal port are the most frequently seen (Haynes & Pindzola, 1998). Frequently, this can be addressed surgically. If hypernasality persists as measured through subjective and objective assessments

TABLE 12–4 Compensatory articulation strategies	
Strategy	*Description*
Glottal stops	The vocal folds are used in an effort to produce plosive consonants.
Pharyngeal stops	Produced by lingual contact with the posterior pharyngeal wall
Mid-dorsum palatal stops	The mid-dorsum of the tongue makes contact with the mid-palate.
Pharyngeal fricatives	Produced by narrowing the pharyngeal airway through linguapharyngeal constriction. These are attempted substitutes for sibilant fricatives.
Velar fricatives	Fricatives are produced in the approximate place where /k/ and /g/ are normally produced.
Nasal fricatives	Excessive nasal emission is used as a substitute for consonants.
Posterior nasal fricatives	Produced when the velum or uvula approximates the posterior pharyngeal wall of the nasopharynx. The back of the tongue may elevate in an attempt to assist velopharyngeal closure.
Nasal grimaces	A narrowing of the nostrils produced in an attempt to control nasal emission and inefficient use of the air source.

Adapted from *Assessment in Speech-Language Pathology* (p. 395–396), by K. G. Shipley and J. G. McAfee, 1998, San Diego, CA: Singular Publishing Group. Copyright 1998 by Singular Publishing Group. Adapted with permission.

TABLE 12–5 Common articulatory substitutions in cleft palate speech
Substitution of /t/ for /k/, or vice versa
Substitution of /d/ for /g/, or vice versa
Substitution of /n/ for /t/ and /d/
Substitution of /n/ for /ŋ/, or vice versa
Phonemes /k/ and /g/ may be produced by contact of the back of the tongue and the posterior pharyngeal wall, or by substitution of /h/ for /k/ and /g/.
Labiodental and interdental phonemes may be produced bilabially.
Phonemes /t/ and /d/ may be produced interdentally.

Adapted from *Assessment in Speech-Language Pathology* (p. 396), by K. G. Shipley and J. G. McAfee, 1998, San Diego, CA: Singular Publishing Group. Copyright 1998 by Singular Publishing Group. Adapted with permission.

after the child has received primary surgery, it may be necessary to have a second surgical reconstruction of the velopharyngeal mechanism (Bzoch, 1997a).

Hypernasality may be noted during the production of glides, liquids, and vowels. If hypernasality is consistent, the client probably has velopharyngeal incompetence, with or without a cleft, and physiologic management is indicated. If it is inconsistent, or present only on the production of specific phonemes, the hypernasality is most likely a behavioral issue which will respond to speech therapy (see Treatment).

Nasal emission may be noted during the production of pressure consonants. The absence of velopharyngeal closure creates difficulty in developing sufficient intra-oral pressure to produce the pressure consonants (Shipley & McAfee, 1998). A list of words and phrases that can be used to assess velopharyngeal function is in Table 12–6.

TABLE 12-6 Pressure consonants

Have the patient repeat a series of words and short sentences containing the pressure consonants. Some examples are as follows:

/p/	paper Pass the pepper. Please put the supper up.	pepper papa's puppy	top up top
/b/	Bob baby's tub Baby's bib is by the tub.	baby baby's bib	bib the bear cub
/k/	cake Kathy's cake truck Katie's breakfast was cake.	hockey kid's breakfast	kick broke the
/g/	gave Give it here. Gary gave sugar to the dog.	forgot Go get the sugar.	hug big hog
/t/	two tabletop Terry took the top hat.	guitar top hotel	hat hit the light
/d/	day Dave did it. Dick was louder with David.	today Ted cried.	good good bread
/f/	fall feed father Fred carefully fed his calf.	laughter before relief	off half a loaf
/v/	view very evil Vicki loves to drive.	review every cover	five have to drive
/s/	sit Suzie said so. Sarah spilled the sausage by the box.	icy It's icy.	house It's rice.
/z/	zero Zack is lazy. Zack was too busy to choose.	busy Easy does it.	his those eyes
/ʃ/	ship ship-shape She washed a bushel of fish.	ashes wishy-washy	wish fresh radish
/ʒ/	visual beige corsage a casual corsage	usual visual pleasure	prestige usual prestige
/tʃ/	chalk child's chair Chip reached for the teacher's watch.	teacher richest butcher	batch each pitch
/θ/	thought thirsty father Thought I'd get a toothbrush for both.	birthday third birthday	bath through both
/ð/	they their father Their other brother likes to bathe.	father the leather	bathe They bathe.

From *Assessment in Speech-Language Pathology* (2nd ed.) (pp. 277–278), by K. G. Shipley and J. G. McAfee, 1998, San Diego, CA: Singular Publishing Group. Copyright 1998 by Singular Publishing Group. Reprinted with permission.

Bzoch (1997a) suggests testing for hypernasality by testing 10 vowels in a /b—t/context. Each word (beet, bit, bait, bet, bat, bought, boat, boot, but, Bert) is said with the nares occluded and with the nares unoccluded. If the individual has normal velopharyngeal closure, the clinician will not notice a shift in the productions in each of the two conditions. If the clinician does hear a shift, hypernasality is present.

Another simple test to administer is recommended by Mason and Grandstaff (1971) who assessed hypernasality by having their clients count from 60 to 100. According to Haynes and Pindzola (1998), the following observations with regard to resonance are noted in the counting procedure:

1. The 60 series of numbers may reveal velopharyngeal incompetence and nasal emission due to the frequent occurrence of the /s/ pressure phoneme.

2. The 70 series may reveal assimilative hypernasality owing to the embedded /n/ phoneme.

3. The 80 series should reveal normal or near-normal articulation and resonance.

4. The 90 series should sound normal when produced by a patient with hypernasality because of the frequent production of nasal consonants. The patient with hyponasality may display the articulatory substitution of d/n. (p. 383)

Velopharyngeal competence can also be assessed using a mirror placed below the nares. When the client speaks, the mirror will become cloudy if there is nasal emission. A nonglass mirror with a handle is available from the Floxite Company (Niagara Falls, NY 14303). Nasal emission can also be measured using the See-Scape, which is available from a variety of speech-language supply companies. A tube is placed in the tip of the client's nose, and the tube is attached to a cylinder with a light ball inside. If the client has nasal emission, the ball will rise in the tube when the client speaks.

If an articulation test is used to assess nasal emission, it is suggested that the clinician analyze the results using the following questions. These questions are suggested by Haynes and Pindzola (1998) based on the work of Morris and Smith (1962):

1. Does the speaker misarticulate fricatives, plosives, and affricates that have been demonstrated to require high intraoral breath pressure?

2. Do the misarticulations involve audible nasal emission?

3. Are there evidences of facial grimacing during the production of these consonants?

4. Does occluding the nostrils (preventing an air leakage) result in normal production of them? (p. 386)

Other videographic measures can also be used to assess velopharyngeal incompetence, particularly if the VPI is borderline and may not be picked up by the aforementioned measures. Videographic measures include cephalometry, cinefluorography, fiberoptic endoscopy, ultrasonography, tomography, CT scanning, and/or videofluoroscopy.

Modified Tongue Anchor Procedure

Developed by Fox and Johns (1970), the modified tongue anchor procedure is another method of assessing velopharyngeal function. The procedure as described by Shipley and McAfee (1992) is as follows:

1. Tell the client to "puff up your cheeks like this." Then puff up your cheeks and hold the air in the oral cavity to model the behavior.

2. Tell the client to stick out his or her tongue as you hold the anterior portion with a sterile gauze pad.

3. While you are holding the tongue, tell the client to puff up the cheeks again. Say "Puff up your cheeks again like you did the first time. I will help you by holding your nose so the air doesn't get out." Then gently pinch your client's nose closed.

4. Tell the client to continue holding the air in the cheeks as you release the nostrils.

5. As the nostrils are released, listen for nasal emission. Velopharyngeal seal is considered *adequate* if the air does not escape through the open nostrils. It is considered *inadequate* if air leaks out.

6. Complete a minimum of three trials to be sure the client understands the task and to verify your observations. (Shipley and McAfee, p. 279)

Cul-de-sac Resonance

Cul-de-sac resonance is a hollow vocal quality due to hyperfunction of the tongue. The clinician should have the client produce an open vowel such as /a/ so that the position of the tongue can be observed. In cul-de-sac resonance, the tongue will be retracted posteriorally in the oral cavity and oropharynx. Sometimes cul-de-sac resonance is exhibited by speakers who use a slow rate of speech, such as individuals with hearing impairment. The slower rate of speech may be caused by altered syllable durations, having a negative effect on voice quality and speech intelligibility. In these individuals, increasing the speaking rate may have a positive effect (Haynes & Pindzola, 1998).

In confirming the presence of cul-de-sac resonance, the clinician should have the client read word lists or sentences that are heavy with phonemes that encourage anterior placement of the tongue (and, thus, inhibit tongue retraction). Prather and Swift (1984) suggest the following phonemes: Tongue Tip Phonemes: /t/, /d/, /s/, /z/; Front Consonants: /w/, /hw/, /p/, /b/, /f/, /v/, /ɵ/, and /l/; Front Vowels: /i/, /I/, /e/.

Acoustic Measures

The presence of excessive nasality in speech is very difficult to establish perceptually. Therefore, one must rely on more objective measures to assess hypernasality. Measures of nasalance using a nasometer, and acoustic analysis of speech on a spectrogram can be used to get an objective measurement of velopharyngeal dysfunction in speech.

TREATMENT

In 1986, the American Cleft Palate Association (ACPA) reported that for patients with unilateral cleft lip and palate, lip repairs were performed between 4 and 10 weeks of age in 42% of the 186 teams that responded to their survey. After 10 weeks of age, 47% of the repairs were done, and the remaining 11% were done prior to 4 weeks of age. Repair of the soft and hard palates were done in synchrony between 6 and 18 months of age by 73% of the reporting teams (Bzoch, 1997b). These statistics reflect a trend toward earlier closure of cleft lips and cleft palates.

Bzoch (1997a) outlines the following treatment protocols for optimal standards of cleft palate care:

Shortly After Birth

Parents should be counseled by team members prior to hospital discharge regarding feeding, needed surgical correction of defects, and the importance of prelanguage stimulation.

First Year

Surgery to correct any clefts of the primary palate (cleft lip) should be performed, usually at 2 to 3 months of age.

Referral of complex cases to a complete craniofacial center for initial comprehensive evaluation and recommendations.

Early evaluation by a cleft palate team with recording of basic information, including details of the extent and classification of congenital abnormalities. Collection of pertinent baseline records.

Family genetic counseling.

Audiometric evaluations with referrals for otologic treatment and/or amplification and auditory training as indicated.

Counseling of parents on the basics of pragmatic language stimulation techniques and the norms of early speech and language development skills.

Pediatric dental evaluation with instruction in dental hygiene and treatment, including presurgical maxillary orthopedic appliances coordinated with initial lip cleft closure procedures in selected cases (usually combined clefts of both the primary and secondary palates).

Team re-evaluations followed by recommended treatment at or before 6 months and 12 months of age.

Second Year
12–18 Months

Complete closure of both the hard and soft palate structures by 12 months of age if possible. Recent extensive cephalometric research by Ross indicates that early complete palatal closures of unilateral complete clefts (repair prior to 12 months of age) result in better facial growth patterns than later complete closures.

Assessment of the adequacy of the velopharyngeal functions for speech from clinical behavioral observational tests and parental history and any possible instrumental tests by the speech and language pathologist over the first year following surgery.

Family counseling, as appropriate, relative to the patient's plan of treatment.

Audiological and otological monitoring of middle ear functioning and the presence of disease.

Development of a home-based speech and language stimulation program, if indicated during routine reevaluation team clinics.

Team re-evaluation at approximately 18 months of age.

Dental evaluation, with instruction and treatment as indicated.

18–24 Months

This is considered to be the most critical and rapid period of motor speech and expressive language skill development. Speech and language skill acquisition should be monitored as regularly as possible, but at a minimum of 6-month intervals; a direct speech and language therapy program is established as indicated.

Audiological monitoring with otologic treatment as needed.

Third Year

Usual respite from secondary surgical intervention.

Speech and language re-evaluations with recommendations for further diagnostic therapy to determine velopharyngeal adequacy to support further speech and language development or modify cleft palate speech gross substitution error patterns.

Audiological and otological examinations and treatment as needed.

Two complete team re-evaluations, including planning for implementation of possible dental, orthodontic, or secondary surgical palatal reconstruction.

Referral to an early educational setting outside the home (i.e., Head Start, pre-kindergarten, or day care centers) as deemed appropriate.

Fourth Year

Patients identified as having had complete primary reconstruction of palatal clefts with persistent clinical evidence of persistent velopharyngeal insufficiency for normal speech and language development from repeated clinical tests and developmental histories should usually be referred for secondary palatal reconstructive surgery or for a limited period of prosthetic speech appliance management. Cine- or videofluoroscopy and/or nasoendoscopy are advisable before proceeding with recommendations for secondary surgical or prosthetic correction of velopharyngeal insufficiency. Correction of velopharyngeal insufficiency for normal speech development should be identified and verified through objective instrumental means as early as possible.

Speech and language skill re-evaluations and implementation of speech and language therapy as needed.

Two team evaluations with implementation of the surgical, dental, hearing, and psychosocial and economic needs of the family and child should be provided.

Fifth Year

Team visit and re-evaluation at 6-month intervals.

Pediatric health care review with dental evaluation and treatment, possible first-phase orthodontic treatment or planning, speech and language evaluation and treatment as indicated, and correction of velopharyngeal insufficiency as needed.

Sixth Year

Speech and language therapy as required for each patient.

Pediatric dental evaluation and treatment.

Orthodontic casts, photographs, or cephalometric X-rays deemed necessary for evaluation and treatment planning or the efficacy of new surgical intervention procedures for complex or congenital craniofacial disorders.

Audiological and otological monitoring and treatment as needed.

Complete team re-evaluations at 6-month intervals for unresolved, more complex case studies.

Early School Age

Initial treatment should be completed (i.e., basic surgical, dental, pediatric medical care, and developmental speech and language and hearing problems should be eliminated or modified as possible).

Orthodontic and surgical treatment procedures are required, most often bone graft reconstructions of alveolar area clefts through bone grafts after two-third eruption of the permanent cuspids.

Early Adolescence

Treatment services may include lip revisions, rhinoplasties, alveoloplasties with bone grafts, routine speech and language re-evaluations with therapy as indicated, routine dental care, and mixed dentition orthodontic treatment as indicated by team evaluations.

Psychosocial counseling of each child born with cleft palate should be provided, as indicated by team clinic evaluations (pp. 36–37).

Feeding

A booklet entitled "Feeding an Infant with a Cleft" (1992) is available from the American Cleft Palate-Craniofacial Association (see Resources). Many children with cleft lip and/or palate feed normally and do not require supplemental nutrition. Some infants, particularly those with cleft lip will have trouble efficiently latching on to the nipple because of a poor lip seal. Children with cleft palate may also have feeding difficulties due to the inability to create a good suction to draw liquid from the nipple. Furthermore, liquid can be lost through the nose. Frequently, babies with cleft palate chew on the nipple instead of sucking on the nipple. Regardless of the type of trouble the infant is having, it is critical to provide feeding intervention to assist the parents. "Successful feeding removes one important source of parental anxiety and makes mothers and fathers more confident of their parenting skills, freeing them to relate to the child in a more relaxed way" (Crowe, 1997, p. 268).

Baby bottles should be made of soft plastic so that the feeder can squeeze the bottle slightly to assist in controlling the flow of the fluid. Mead Johnson has developed a Cleft Palate Nurser bottle and nipple set that is quite effective. Several nipples are also available for babies with cleft palate. To be effective, the nipple should be soft with either a cross cut or several extra holes to lessen the amount of suction needed to obtain the fluid. The Mead Johnson nipple has a cross cut and is longer than regular nipples, placing the fluid farther back on the tongue to facilitate swallowing. Also, the softness of the nipple combined with the cross cut facilitates the release of liquids when the baby uses a chewing motion instead of a sucking motion.

The Haberman Feeder is another feeding unit designed especially for babies who have cleft palate. The nipple on the Haberman Feeder retains the liquid once it has been sucked into the nipple; with normal nipples, the liquid flows back into the bottle. There is a slice-cut hole in the nipple which responds to the chewing motion of the infant. Also, depending on the infant's needs, the flow can be adjusted to come out in a slow, medium, or fast mode. The Haberman Feeder is available as follows:

Medela, Inc.
4610 Prime Parkway
P.O. Box 660
McHenry, IL 60051-0660
1-800-435-8316

The Mead Johnson Cleft Palate Nurser set is available from:

Mead Johnson Company
Nutritional Division
Evansville, IN 47721

The baby should be fed as upright as possible. The more upright the infant is, the more gravity can assist in pulling the liquid into the throat instead of the nose or ear canals. Children with cleft palate are at increased risk of ear infections. Therefore, avoiding the accumulation of fluid in the Eustachian tubes is critical in reducing the risk of ear infections. A slight chin tuck is also helpful in coordinating the suck and swallow motion.

When presenting the bottle to the infant with a cleft lip, it is helpful to hold the upper lip together to help create suction needed to guide fluid out of the nipple. For babies with cleft palate, gently holding the baby's cheeks forward helps to create a smaller space in the mouth and increases the oral contact with the nipple.

Pharyngeal Flap

Disadvantages of a pharyngeal flap include contracture (caused by a relatively poor blood supply), decreased palatal movement, obstruction, and pain. A pharyngeal flap should be made after previous tonsillectomy, following failure of primary palatal repair (15–20% will have VPI), velo-cardio-facial syndrome (if anatomy dictates), and failure of pharyngoplasty

(Burstein, F. D., 1999). Other problems associated with pharyngeal flaps include improper vertical positioning on the posterior pharyngeal wall, difficulty in revision and postoperative sleep apnea (Skolnick & McGall, 1972).

Velopharyngeal dysfunction (VPD) is a common sequela following cleft palate repair. VPD may also occur congenitally in children with intact palates, but with a large or hypotonic nasopharynx (Morris, 1973; Calnan, 1971). "VPD may cause defective velopharyngeal valving with incomplete separation of the oral and nasal cavities during speech, blowing, sucking, and swallowing" (Kasten et al, 1999, p. 3). The incomplete separation is known as velopharyngeal insufficiency (VPI). VPI results "in nasal air emission, and varying degrees of hypernasal resonance during speech" (Kasten et al., 1999, p. 3). There is a 20–30% incidence rate of VPI in patients with cleft palate, even with a palatal closure using any one of several viable techniques (Morris, 1973).

VPI has traditionally been corrected through pharyngeal flaps. However, recently, dynamic sphincter pharyngoplasty has become widely accepted as a means of surgical management of VPI. It has several advantages over pharyngeal flaps "including a dynamic port closure mechanism, freedom from the problem of flap contracture and ease of revision" (Kasten et al., 1999, p. 10).

Nonsurgical Treatment of Hypernasality

The use of speech appliances in the correction of hypernasality, though not as usual today as it was several years ago because of the improvement of complete early surgical reconstruction techniques, speech appliances, including palatal lift appliances and hard-palate obturators, still merit consideration in some cases. "Prosthetic speech appliances or the temporary use of hard-palate obturators to cover palatal fistulae offer an important alternative to surgical physical management for correcting velopharyngeal insufficiency in cases where surgery is not advisable" (Bzoch, 1997b, p. 93).

As stated previously, if the hypernasality is inconsistent and/or phoneme specific, speech therapy may be warranted. Phoneme-specific insufficiency is the type of velopharyngeal insufficiency most responsive to speech therapy. Phoneme-specific insufficiency actually can be regarded as an articulation disorder. Treatment could include acoustic feedback and feedback with pressure and/or airflow devices. Some clients with phoneme-specific insufficiency may have a tight velopharyngeal seal for all speech tasks except for those associated with /s/, /z/, /f/, and /v/. Sometimes affricates are also symptomatic. One intervention technique is described as follows:

> By using the /t/ phoneme in therapy to have the patient achieve velopharyngeal closure with the same tongue placement in a voiceless production, the therapist can use a slender applicator stick to groove the center of the tongue during the production of /t/. This will cause air to escape through the center of the tongue resulting in /s/ with the same velopharyngeal closure as achieved on /t/. (Shprintzen, 1989, p. 226)

Another method of intervention for phoneme-specific insufficiency is the use of nasopharyngoscopic biofeedback therapy. This type of therapy utilizes videoendoscopy whereby the client "can see his own velopharyngeal valving mechanism and alter the valving pattern during a 20–30-minute session" (Shprintzen, 1989, p. 226).

Social-Emotional Development

Concerns During the Prenatal and Infancy Stages

Social-emotional counseling depends on the age of the child. In fact, since some craniofacial anomalies can be detected before birth using sonography and amniocentesis, prenatal counseling may be indicated. According to Crowe (1997), the "basic stability of the mother and father plays a major role in their ability to seek the support they need and to plan ahead for the birth and care of their baby" (p. 265). Once the parents resolve their initial grief and shock, they should be helped in asking substantive questions, beginning to plan for treatment of their child, meeting the craniofacial team and understanding their roles, and acquiring knowledge and skills they will need after the birth of their baby. Parent-to-parent support groups can be of tremendous assistance during this time period.

During the early days of infancy, most parents want and need assistance from the professionals, including the speech-language pathologist. It is important to see the parents several times in the first few days after their baby's birth, and to set up parent-to-parent contact if that was not done prenatally. The earlier the parents have an opportunity to discuss their child's anomaly, the more quickly they will be able to accept the situation and begin to bond with their infant (Crowe, 1997). To facilitate the bonding, the speech-language pathologist (and other health-care professionals) should cuddle the baby, remarking on the other features of the baby (eyes, hair, hands, etc.), and let the parents see you enjoying their baby. The parents may need to be helped in responding to their baby rather than to the birth defect. Parents should be encouraged to smile at and vocalize to their babies, particularly since research shows that mothers of children with craniofacial disorders tend to smile and vocalize to their babies with less frequency than the mothers of babies born without impairments (Field & Vega-Lahr, 1984).

It is also important during the stage of infancy to deal with the here-and-now. Counseling should be "directed toward helping the parents cope with the situation as it exists rather than toward theoretical issues that may not apply to a specific case" (Crowe, 1997, p. 268). In other words, at this stage the parents should not be told more information than they need, or everything that could conceivably happen. They need to deal with the issues at hand, such as fear that may exist in relation to surgical management of the clefts. Probably the best approach is to deal with issues as they are brought up by the parents. For example, during the early infancy stage, some speech-language pathologists may want to discuss speech development. However, the parents' more immediate concerns are probably related to accepting the child, feeding the child, and dealing with medical and surgical intervention. Thus, it is probably better to wait until the parents bring up the issue of speech to discuss that topic.

Later in infancy, the focus in counseling may shift.

> After the acute anxieties associated with the birth, feeding, and provision of care have been alleviated and the baby is making progress, the task becomes one of following the infant's development, seeing that the parents are involved in the treatment program so that they are rigorous about keeping appointments, alerting the mother and father and other team members to new clinical needs should they arise, and providing additional clinical services as they are indicated. (Crowe, 1997 p. 271)

Since clinical visits may not be as frequent during late infancy, telephone counseling to maintain contact between clinical visits is strongly advised.

Concerns During Early Childhood

Concerns during early childhood include many that are shared with parents of children who do not have craniofacial anomalies: management and child rearing, developmental issues, expanding the child's world from a restricted to a broader environment. Two major concerns of parents of children with craniofacial anomalies that should be added to this list include monitoring and assisting in speech and language development, and preparing the child for hospitalizations and surgery.

In early childhood, the child is old enough to realize when a threatening situation has arisen. He may be frightened by the hospital environment, but he is probably too young to remember parental explanations and understand what will be happening. Waking up in a strange place with strangers in attendance can be traumatizing for the child. One thing that will help the child is to have the parents relaxed and as confident as possible, as these feelings can be transmitted to the child. The parents should have a clear understanding of the procedures that will take place before, during, and after the surgery. They should be informed in advance about the child's appearance following the surgery, and possible signs of discomfort and distress that their child may exhibit. The parents should be encouraged to bring a favorite stuffed animal (stuffed bears with "repaired" lips are available from the American Cleft Palate-Craniofacial Association) and books to the hospital. It is also helpful to have a surprise gift that the child can look forward to receiving after the surgery. They should plan to sit with their child, hold his hand, and talk quietly about going home soon.

As mentioned previously, another concern in early childhood is the speech and language development of the child. The speech-language pathologist should carefully monitor the child's cognitive, social, and communication development during this period. One-on-one counseling and group sessions for the parents may be helpful at this stage. The clinician should model effective techniques for facilitating speech and language. Also, it is important that the speech-language pathologist not assume that all speech delays are cleft-related delays. As already mentioned, developmental disabilities may accompany cleft lip and/or palate. Therefore, the possibility of an isolated expressive language problem needs to be considered. Also, receptive abilities and all other aspects of development should be carefully monitored. Parents should be helped to understand the nature of developmental delay and its relationship to chronologic and mental ages. It may be helpful to create a toy and book lending library, making suggestions to parents about items that are appropriate for their child's developmental age (Crowe, 1997).

The quantity and quality of verbal output by children with craniofacial anomalies is often reduced, as is the mean length of utterance. These children are frequently shy, withdrawn, inhibited, and delayed in verbal expression. Therefore, counseling related to psychosocial development is critical. It may be helpful for the parents to have contact with parents of older children with craniofacial anomalies so they can learn from their experiences. Also, parent groups reduce parental stress, which, according to some researchers, may be related to the child's development of social skills. The parents should also be encouraged to enroll their child in a regular preschool setting to facilitate social development.

Irwin and McWilliams (1974) developed a Creative Dramatics program to assist children with craniofacial anomalies to express their feelings and thoughts. The program consisted of 32 sessions. The first ten sessions included dramatic play, rhythmic activities, and pantomime. The next 14 sessions, the children acted out a structured story. Irwin and McWilliams found that, for the next eight sessions, the children spontaneously began to act out original stories, express their fears, and verbalize fantasies.

The School-Aged Child

Issues in dealing with school-aged children with craniofacial anomalies include independence, school progress, teacher evaluations, relationships with a larger group of peers, and adequacy of communication skills.

With regard to independence, children with craniofacial deficits often see themselves as less acceptable than their peers. Therefore, they may see themselves as needing more assistance from others, and as being sad and angry more frequently than their peers. Children with craniofacial anomalies frequently identify with passive and isolated children due to their own social inhibitions (Kapp-Simon, 1986). They may also have reduced personal and social self-concepts (Broder & Strauss, 1989). It is critical that the parents, teachers, and others look for special talents (drawing, acting, motor skills . . .) and reinforce the child for those abilities. Group counseling with role play, including non-impaired children, may also be of benefit. The child could be encouraged to join smaller groups of children such as Scouts and church youth groups, where adjustment may be easier than in a large classroom.

To assist in school adjustment, the speech-language pathologist should act as a liaison between the teacher and the parents if necessary. It has been found that there are fewer teacher-initiated conferences with parents of children with craniofacial anomalies. Therefore, the speech-language pathologist should definitely stay in regular contact with the teacher to maintain attention on the child's adjustment to school. The speech-language pathologist provides continuing education to the teacher(s) to educate them about the nature of the child's craniofacial disorders, and to update them on the cognitive, social, and communication status of the child. Also, it may be helpful to provide programming for the child's classmates to help them understand the nature of the child's anomalies and/or speech problems, and help them develop ways to relate to the child and include him in classroom and playground activities. Creative Dramatics as described under the Early Childhood section can also be helpful with the school-aged population.

It is also critical that the team that has been managing the child prior to and throughout school stay in contact with the school speech-language pathologist. This is necessary in order to insure that the school-based SLP understands the nature and extent of the child's anomalies, and the diagnostic and management history. This also helps to minimize the possibility of conflicting recommendations that could confuse the parents and child.

The Teenage Years

Concerns expressed by teenagers with craniofacial anomalies include the following: appearance; acceptance by peers; adapting to the physical changes of adolescence, in addition to further surgical and dental procedures related to the anomalies; increased interest in the nature and causes of their birth defects, and awakening concerns about their offspring; and plans beyond high school, including career counseling.

Teenagers may express the desire for additional surgical and orthodontic procedures to improve various aspects of their appearance, such as their profile, or their nose. They can also be taught the skillful use of make-up to minimize the overt appearance of scar tissue. They should be encouraged to join support groups, with the teens choosing the topics and directing the discussion. Frequent topics are genetic counseling, career and educational planning, and desires to be treated "just like everyone else." It may be helpful to have successful adults with clefts to address the group. Opportunities for social learning (social initiation, conversational skills, assertion, direct communication, active listening, problem solving, and conflict resolution) should also be addressed in group and one-on-one counseling. The use of Creative Dramatics is also helpful in this age group.

APPENDIX 12-A: CHECKLIST FOR THE ASSESSMENT OF CLIENTS WITH CLEFTS

Name: _____ Age: _____ Date: _____

Primary care physician: _____

Type of cleft: _____

Date of surgery: _____

Other conditions and medical history: _____

_____

_____

Examiner: _____

Oral-Facial Examination

Instructions: Administer a standard oral-facial examination. Additionally, make observations about the following oral-facial features. Check and circle each item noted. Include descriptive comments in the right-hand margin.

Comments

_____ Type of cleft: lip/palate/lip and palate (describe) _____

_____ Adequacy of cleft repair: good/fair/poor _____

_____ Other facial abnormalities: absent/present (describe) _____

_____ Submucosal cleft: absent/present _____

_____ Labial pits in lower lip: absent/present _____

_____ Labiodental fistulas: absent/present _____

_____ Alveolar fistulas: absent/present _____

_____ Palatal fistulas: absent/present _____

Comments

_____ Velar fistulas: absent/present _____

_____ Perceived length of velum: normal/short/long _____

_____ Perceived depth of nasopharynx: normal/shallow/deep _____

_____ Shape of the alveolar ridge: notched/cleft/wide/collapsed _____

_____ Notes from standard oral-facial examination _____

_____

_____

Assessment of Voice

Instructions: Evaluate the client's voice, paying particular attention to possible cleft-related problems. Check deficits that are present and indicate severity. Record additional notes in the right-hand margin.

 1 = mild
 2 = moderate
 3 = severe

Comments

_____ Pitch variation is reduced _____

_____ Vocal intensity is reduced _____

_____ Vocal quality is hoarse/harsh/breathy (circle) _____

_____ Vocal quality is strangled _____

_____ Client produces glottal stops in place of plosives and fricatives _____

_____ Client attempts to mask hypernasality and nasal emission _____

_____ Client strains voice to achieve adequate pitch change and loudness _____

_____ Client strains voice in attempt to increase speech intelligibility _____

Assessment of Resonance and Velopharyngeal Integrity

Instructions: Evaluate the client's voice, listening for the following qualities of resonance. Check each characteristic the client exhibits and indicate severity. Record additional notes in the right-hand margin.

     1 = mild

     2 = moderate

     3 = severe

                                                      Comments

_____ Hypernasality _____

_____ Nasal emission _____

_____ Cul-de-sac resonance _____

_____ Hyponasality _____

Instructions: Use the administration guidelines for the modified tongue anchor procedure described in this chapter. Check your observation below:

_____ Velopharyngeal function is adequate (no nasal emission)

_____ Velopharyngeal function is inadequate (nasal emission present)

_____ Further testing using objective instrumentation is necessary

Instructions: Ask the client to produce the pressure consonants /p/, /b/, /k/, /t/, /d/, /f/, /v/, /s/, /z/, /ʃ/, /ʒ/, /tʃ/, /ɵ/, and /ɚ/ (see Table 6 of this chapter for stimulus words and phrases), and listen for hypernasality and nasal emissions. Check the appropriate observations below:

_____ Velopharyngeal function is adequate (no nasal emission or hypernasality)

_____ Velopharyngeal function is inadequate (nasal emissions or hypernasality present)

_____ Further testing using objective instrumentation is necessary

_____ Nasal emissions and hypernasality are consistent

_____ Nasal emissions and hypernasality are inconsistent

Assessment of Articulation and Phonology

Instructions: Listen to the client's articulatory accuracy. Pay particular attention to the client's production of stop-plosives, fricatives, and affricates, which are most likely to be negatively affected by a cleft. Indicate severity and make additional comments in the right-hand margin.

> 1 = mild
> 2 = moderate
> 3 = severe

Comments

_____ Stop-plosive errors _____

_____ Fricative errors _____

_____ Affricate errors _____

_____ Glide errors _____

_____ Liquid errors _____

_____ Nasal errors _____

_____ Vowel errors _____

_____ Error patterns are consistent _____

_____ Error patterns are inconsistent _____

_____ Further assessment is recommended _____

Instructions: Check the following compensatory strategies the client uses during speech production and indicate severity. Make additional comments in the right-hand column.

> 1 = mild
> 2 = moderate
> 3 = severe

_____ Glottal stops _____

_____ Pharyngeal stops _____

_____ Mid-dorsum palatal stops _____

_____ Pharyngeal fricatives _____

Comments

_____ Velar fricatives _____

_____ Nasal fricatives _____

_____ Posterior nasal fricatives _____

_____ Nasal grimaces _____

Summary

Instructions: Check areas that require further assessment. Make additional comments in the right-hand margin.

Comments

_____ Articulation—Cleft-related _____

_____ Articulation—Non-cleft-related _____

_____ Cognition _____

_____ Hearing _____

_____ Language _____

_____ Velopharyngeal integrity _____

_____ Voice _____

CHAPTER THIRTEEN
Dementias

DEFINITION/DESCRIPTION

"Dementia is a debilitating condition that causes chronic and progressive deterioration in intellect, personality, and communicative functioning" (Payne, 1997, p. 101).

According to the American Psychiatric Association (1987), dementia is characterized by "impairment of short- and long-term memory, abstract thinking judgment, disturbances of higher cortical function, or personality changes that disturb normal functions, activities, or relationships" (Payne, 1997, p. 103).

Causes of Dementia

Degenerative changes caused by aging or a disease process can result in dementia. Multi-infarct disease (MID) is the second most common cause of vascular dementia. Trauma to the head can also produce dementia, as can infections and metabolic problems. Other etiologies include toxic factors, autoimmune disorders (i.e., rheumatoid arthritis, lupus, scleroderma, myositis), and poor nutrition. Psychiatric etiologies are also possible (ASHA, Dementia Grand Rounds, 1996).

Medications, depression, alcohol, benign tumors, and subdural hematomas can also cause memory loss. Therefore, it is critical that these factors be ruled out before using memory loss as a sign of possible dementia. Genetic factors involving chromosomes 21, 14, 19, and 1 have also been implicated as causative factors in dementia (ASHA, Dementia Grand Rounds, 1996).

Reversible And Irreversible Dementias

Dementias may be reversible or irreversible. Reversible dementias include those that arise in any of the following: depression, infection, drug interactions or toxicity, hearing and speech disorders, metabolic and endocrine disorders, intracranial masses, nutritional deficiencies, normal-pressure hydrocephalus, cardiopulmonary disorders, alcohol abuse, vitamin deficiencies, neurosyphilis, arteriosclerotic complications, and epilepsy (Payne, 1997; Golper, 1998).

Etiological factors in irreversible dementias include dementia of the Alzheimer's type, AIDS-related dementia, alcoholic dementia syndromes, Pick's disease, Parkinson's disease, multi-infarction diseases, cerebrocerebellar degenerations, supranuclear palsy, Binswanger's disease, Creutzfeldt-Jakob disease, Huntington's chorea, and Korsakoff's disease (Payne, 1997; Golper, 1998).

Cortical, Subcortical, and Mixed Dementias

"Cortical dementias occur in diseases with predominant degeneration in neocortical association areas with a relative sparing of subcortical structures" (Payne, pp. 102–103). In cortical dementias, motor speech is typically spared. The primary cortical dementias are Alzheimer's disease and Pick's disease.

"Subcortical dementias have pathologic alterations that affect the deep structures such as the basal ganglia, thalamus, and brain stem, with relative sparing of the cerebral cortex" (Payne, 1997, pp. 102–103). In the subcortical dementias, language comprehension and use are less impaired than they are in cortical and mixed dementias. According to Cummings and Bensen (1984) in Payne (1997):

> Subcortical dementia, unlike cortical dementia, has a clinical presentation of forgetfulness, slowing of mental processes, impaired ability to manipulate acquired knowledge, and personality and affective changes, including apathy and depression. Cortical dementia, in contrast, presents with deterioration of both verbal expression and auditory comprehension, indifference and disinhibition, and severe memory disorders. (p. 103)

Examples of subcortical dementias include AIDS dementia syndrome, Parkinson's disease, Huntington's disease, and progressive supranuclear palsy (Payne, 1997).

In subcortical dementias, there is typically a motor disturbance accompanying the dementia, with the motor disturbances preceding the associated dementia. Patients with subcortical dementia typically will demonstrate dysarthria, gait disturbances, weak vocal intensity, and difficulties with the rate of speech. They may also have difficulties with articulation and pitch (Davis, 1993). Finally, depression is more common in patients with subcortical dementias. Typically, the mood remains relatively normal in cortical dementias (Lass, McReynolds, Northern, & Yoder, 1988).

Mixed dementias include multi-infarct disease (vascular dementia), Binswanter's disease, Creutzfeldt-Jakob disease, and Korsakoff's disease (Payne, 1997). Table 13–1 offers a comparison of cognitive functions in cortical and subcortical dementias.

Dementias Other Than Alzheimer's Disease

Dementias other than Alzheimer's disease include those associated with Pick's disease, progressive supranuclear palsy, and Parkinson's disease. Pick's disease is a frontal lobe

TABLE 13-1 Comparison of impaired cognitive functions in cortical and subcortical dementias	
Cortical Dementia	*Subcortical Dementia*
Aphasia	Psychomotor retardation
Poor abstraction abilities	Forgetfulness
Agnosia	Cognitive dilapidation
Amnesia	Impaired insight
Acalculia	Poor strategy formulation
Visuospatial disturbances	

disease with an early onset of dementia. Progressive supranuclear palsy is also a frontal lobe dementia.

Parkinson's Disease

Dementia associated with Parkinson's disease is irreversible, and it is a subcortical dementia. Approximately 30% of patients with Parkinson's disease develop dementia similar to Alzheimer's. Up to 40 to 50% of patients with Parkinson's disease suffer from problems with word-finding, cognition, and memory. If the dementia occurs early in the disease process, involvement of the brain may be more extensive with degenerating neurons, creating an "extended" form of Parkinson's disease (Duvoisin, Golbe, Mark, Sage, & Walters, 1996). These problems typically occur later in the disease process and in older patients with Parkinson's disease. Nonetheless, the symptoms are still milder than those associated with Alzheimer's disease.

Similarly, confusion may be a problem, although it is sometimes difficult to determine whether the confusion is related to the disease process or is a side effect of the anti-parkinsonian medications that are taken by many of the patients (Duvoisin et al., 1996).

Huntington's Disease

Huntington's disease, or Huntington's chorea, is another neurological disease that is frequently associated with subcortical dementia. Chorea, a dominant sign of Huntington's disease, is defined by Hegde as "irregular, spasmodic, jerky, complex, rapid, and involuntary movements of the limb and facial muscles" (Hegde, 1996, p. 242). Genetic in origin, Huntington's disease affects men and women equally and has been identified in children as young as 4 years of age.

In the early stages, the patient undergoes gradual changes in behavior and personality. The changes can include depression, anxiety, and irritability. Emotional outbursts are common. The patient may have a false sense of superiority, be suspicious, and show complaining behaviors and nagging. The patient may have problems with abnormal motor movements that resemble fidgeting. Speech becomes disorganized, and problems with memory, executive functions, and judgment may be seen (Hegde, 1996).

Advanced symptoms include a worsening of the deficits that appeared early in the disease process. Chorea becomes generalized, and intellect deteriorates. The patient will have attention deficits, confusion, and disorientation. Language impairments frequently associated with dementia also appear and progress to the profoundly impaired level. Hyperkinetic dysarthria, which is characterized by involuntary movements, disorders of loudness and rate, interruptions in phonation, and abnormal muscle tone, is also found. Death typically occurs within 10 to 20 years after onset (Vinson, 1999).

Pick's Disease

Pick's disease resembles Alzheimer's disease in its symptoms, but not in its etiology. Pick's disease is a "progressive neurologic disease associated with a gradual decrease in brain mass, especially in the temporal and frontal lobes" (Hegde, 1996, p. 333). Early symptoms include changes and deterioration in social behaviors. Patients may display uninhibited mannerisms, such as making offensive comments and telling inappropriate jokes. They often repeatedly engage in meaningless and ritualistic behaviors. Patients with Pick's disease also display intellectual disturbances similar to those seen in patients with Alzheimer's disease. They, too, develop impaired judgment. Another common symptom in the early stages is the development of excessive eating and an accompanying weight gain (Hegde, 1996).

In the later stages of Pick's disease, the patient continues to demonstrate a progressive deterioration of intellectual functioning. Echolalia and meaningless repetition of phrases is common. Naming problems accompanied by circumlocution also are common (Hegde, 1996). In contrast to the person with Alzheimer's disease, the patient with Pick's disease is more likely to show a deterioration in the form of language (morphology, syntax, and phonology) than in the content of language. Auditory agnosia is common.

As the disease progresses, anomia and impaired speech fluency become evident, and the patient demonstrates symptoms consistent with a primary progressive aphasia. However, language comprehension and nonverbal cognition frequently are preserved (Payne, 1997). Typically, the patient's condition progresses to a point of mutism, total disorientation, and confusion (Hegde, 1996).

Multi-Infarction Diseases

Approximately 20% of patients diagnosed as having some form of senile dementia will have multi-infarction disease. This disorder typically is the result of several small strokes involving areas that extend throughout the cortex, resulting in the loss of blood flow to the damaged areas (Boone & Plante, 1993). Based on this disease process, multi-infarction diseases (MIDs) often are referred to as vascular dementia. MIDs are characterized by the "loss of intellectual functioning due to significant cerebrovascular disease and repeated infarctions" (Payne, 1997, p. 128). The etiology is frequently hypertension with arteriosclerosis. The patient may have a history of stroke with a sudden onset of mental decline and an uneven decline of other functions (Payne, 1997). Impulse control and personality also are affected in most cases (Tonkovich, 1988). Payne (1997) notes that "neurological characteristics are multiple areas of softening of brain tissue and may involve possible pathological alterations in cerebral blood vessels" (p. 128). The presence of multiple infarcts resulting in damaged subcortical structures is sometimes referred to as Binswanger's disease (Hegde, 1996).

Cognition in MID is characterized by inconsistent memory lapses and gradual intellectual loss (Payne, 1997). Memory, abstract thinking, and judgment frequently are affected (Tonkovich, 1988).

Language disorders in MID are dependent on the site of the lesion or lesions. For example, if the lesion is in the left middle cerebral artery, the clinician can expect to see aphasia, apraxia, and dementia. If the lesion is in the right middle cerebral artery, visuospatial disorders are common. When the lesion occurs in the posterior middle artery, the patient typically displays fluent aphasia, and alexia with agraphia (Payne, 1997).

Alzheimer's Disease

The term "Alzheimer's disease" is used synonymously with the terms Alzheimer's Dementia, Senile Dementia of the Alzheimer's type, and Dementia of the Alzheimer's type. Alzheimer's disease accounts for 50% of all dementias. According to Guilmette, Alzheimer's disease is "a progressive disease process that results in a gradual but insidious decline in a person's cognitive, behavioral, and adaptive functioning" (Guilmette, 1997, pp. 26–27). "The underlying neuropathology is the development of high numbers of neurofibrillary tangles (tangles of fine fibers in cell bodies) and senile plaques (extracellular byproducts of neuronal degeneration)" (Guilmette, 1997, p. 27). In Alzheimer's disease, there is parietal loss of metabolic activity (ASHA, 1996). Granulovacuolar degeneration and amyloid plaques have also been noted, and it is suspected that a loss of neurotransmitters may also play a causal role (Payne, 1997).

There are several risk factors associated with dementia of the Alzheimer's Type. These are delineated in Table 13–2.

Early warning signs of any dementia are listed in Table 13–3.

Stage-Associated Changes in Alzheimer's Disease

Alzheimer's disease typically consists of three overlapping stages: early or mild, middle or moderate, and late or severe (Payne, 1997). Early stage symptoms are usually limited to

TABLE 13–2 Risk factors associated with Alzheimer's disease
Family history of dementia
Family history of Down syndrome
Family history of Parkinson's disease
Late onset of depression
Head injury
Hypothyroidism
Maternal age greater than 40 years when patient was born

Adapted from "Mental Status and Aging: Cognition and Effect," by D. J. Johnson, 1997, in *Aging and Communication* (p. 80), by B. B. Shadden and M. A. Toner (Eds.), Austin, TX: Pro-Ed. Copyright 1997 by Pro-Ed.

TABLE 13–3 Early warning signs of any dementias
Recent memory loss that affects job skills
Difficulty performing familiar tasks
Problems with language (word-finding difficulties)
Disorientation of time and space
Poor or decreased judgment
Problems with abstract thinking
Misplacing things
Changes in mood or behavior
Changes in personality or depression
Loss of initiative

From "Dementia" Grand Rounds, by ASHA, 1996 (videotape), Rockville, MD. Copyright 1996 by American Speech-Language-Hearing Association.

TABLE 13-4	**Effects of dementing illnesses on communication**

EARLY STAGES

Sounds:	Used correctly.
Words:	May omit a meaningful word, usually a noun, when talking in sentences. May report trouble thinking of the right word. Vocabulary is shrinking.
Grammar:	Generally correct.
Content:	May drift from the topic. Reduced ability to generate series of meaningful sentences. Difficulty comprehending new information. Vague.
Use:	Knows when to talk, although may talk too long on a subject. May be apathetic, failing to initiate a conversation when it would be appropriate to do so. May have difficulty understanding humor, verbal analogies, sarcasm, and indirect and nonliteral statements.

MIDDLE STAGES

Sounds:	Used correctly.
Words:	Difficulty thinking of words in a category. Anomia in conversation. Difficulty naming objects. Reliance on automatisms. Vocabulary noticeably diminished.
Grammar:	Sentence fragments and deviations common. May have difficulty understanding grammatically complex sentences.
Content:	Frequently repeats ideas. Forgets topic. Talk is about events of past or trivia. Fewer ideas.
Use:	Knows when to talk. Recognizes questions. May fail to greet. Loss of sensitivity to conversational partners. Rarely corrects mistakes.

LATE STAGES

Sounds:	Generally used correctly, but errors are not uncommon.
Words:	Marked anomia. Poor vocabulary. Lack of word comprehension. May make up words and produce jargon.
Grammar:	Some grammar is preserved, but sentence fragments and deviations are common. Lack of comprehension of many grammatical forms.
Content:	Generally unable to produce a sequence of related ideas. Content may be meaningless and bizarre. Subject of most meaningful utterances is the retelling of a past event. Marked repetition of words and phrases.
Use:	Generally unaware of surroundings and context; insensitive to others. Little meaningful use of language. Some patients are mute. Some are echolalic.

From "Management of Neurogenic Communication Disorders Associated with Dementia," by K. A. Bayles, 1986, in *Language Intervention Strategies in Adult Aphasia* (3rd ed.) (p. 542), by R. Chapey (Ed.), Baltimore: Williams & Wilkins. Copyright 1986 by Williams & Wilkins. Reprinted with permission.

short-term memory loss. Middle stage symptoms may include "a deterioration in speech and communication, particularly naming, verbal fluency, spelling, comprehension, and the meaningfulness of speech" (Guilmette, 1997, p. 27). Later symptoms include "deficits with perceptual functioning, reasoning, problem solving, abstract thinking, and apraxia" (Guilmette, 1997, p. 27). A more comprehensive list of the effects of dementia on communication at each stage appears in Table 13–4.

Individuals with Alzheimer's disease also undergo behavioral and emotional changes, including depression, agitation, apathy, restlessness, and irritability (Guilmette, 1997). Behavioral characteristics are listed by stage in Table 13–5.

TABLE 13-5 **Behavioral characteristics of the three primary stages in progression of Alzheimer's disease**

FIRST STAGE: 2 to 4 years leading up to, and including, diagnosis

Dominant Symptom(s)—recent memory loss

Behavioral Indicators:

- progressive forgetfulness and difficulty with routine chores
- confusion related to directions, decisions, and memory management; may arrive at wrong time or place; constantly checks calendar
- loss of initiative and spontaneity
- disorientation with respect to time and place
- loses objects often, or forgets they are lost
- changes in mood, personality, and judgment
- repetitive actions and statements common

SECOND STAGE: 2 to 10 years following diagnosis (longest stage)

Dominant Symptom(s)—increasing memory loss, confusion, and shorter attention span

Behavioral Indicators:

- wandering and restlessness, particularly in late afternoon and evening
- problems recognizing close friends and/or family
- difficulty with thought organization and logical thinking
- increased irritability, fidgeting, and/or teariness
- occasional muscle twitching or jerking
- becoming sloppy, for example, in dressing behaviors and eating skills
- sleeps often but also awakens frequently at night and wanders ("sundowners")
- perceptual-motor problems noted for basic ADLs* and IADLs* (sitting, setting table)
- increase in paranoia and suspicion
- inability to read signs, write name, perform basic mathematical operations
- impulse control impaired with associated inappropriate behaviors
- changes in appetite
- needs full-time supervision

THIRD STAGE: 1 to 3 years

Dominant Symptom(s)—unable to recognize family members or self in mirror

Behavioral Indicators:

- capacity for self-care diminished severely, with total assistance required for bathing, dressing, eating, and toileting
- oral communication disappears, leading to mutism, although groans, screams, and grunts may persist in some patients
- swallowing problems, loss of weight (even with proper diet) (may lead to emaciation)
- bowel and bladder incontinence
- attempts to put everything in mouth; compulsion for touching
- other medical problems may emerge, such as skin infections or seizures
- sleeps more, becomes comatose; eventually dies

*ADL, Activities of Daily Living; IADL, Instrumental Activities of Daily Living

DSM CRITERIA FOR DEMENTIA OF THE ALZHEIMER'S TYPE

A. The development of multiple cognitive deficits manifested by both

   (1) memory impairment (impaired ability to learn new information or to recall previously learned information)

   (2) one (or more) of the following cognitive disturbances:

   (a) aphasia (language disturbance)

   (b) apraxia (impaired ability to carry out motor activities despite intact motor function)

   (c) agnosia (failure to recognize or identify objects despite intact sensory function)

   (d) disturbance in executive functioning (i.e., planning, organizing, sequencing, abstracting)

B. The cognitive deficits in Criteria A1 and A2 each cause significant impairment in social or occupational functioning and represent a significant decline from a previous level of functioning.

C. The course is characterized by gradual onset and continuing cognitive decline.

D. The cognitive deficits in Criteria A1 and A2 are not due to any of the following:

   (1) other central nervous system conditions that cause progressive deficits in memory and cognition (e.g., cerebrovascular disease, Parkinson's disease, Huntington's disease, subdural hematoma, normal-pressure hydrocephalus, brain tumor)

   (2) systemic conditions that are known to cause dementia (e.g., hypothyroidism, vitamin B_{12} or folic acid deficiency, niacin deficiency, hypercalcemia, neurosyphilis, HIV infection)

   (3) substance-induced conditions

E. The defiicts do not occur exclusively during the course of a delirium.

F. The disturbance is not better accounted for by another Axis I disorder (e.g., Major Depressive Disorder, Schizophrenia)

Code based on type of onset and predominant features:

With Early Onset: if onset is at age 65 years or below

   290.11 With Delirium: if delirium is superimposed on the dementia

   290.12 With Delusions: if delusions are the predominant feature

   290.13 With Depressed Mood: if depressed mood (including presentations that meet full symptom criteria for a Major Depressive Episode) is the predominant feature. A separate diagnosis of Mood Disorder Due to a General Medical Condition is not given.

   290.10 Uncomplicated: if none of the above predominates in the current clinical presentation

With Late Onset: if onset is after age 65 years

  290.3 With Delirium: if delirium is superimposed on the dementia

  290.20 With Delusions: if delusions are the predominant feature

  290.21 With Depressed Mood: if depressed mood (including presentations that meet full symptom criteria for a Major Depressive Episode) is the predominant feature. A separate diagnosis of Mood Disorder Due to a General Medical Condition is not given.

  290.0 Uncomplicated: if none of the above predominates in the current clinical presentation (DSM, p. 142)

DSM-IV DIAGNOSTIC CRITERIA FOR DEMENTIA DUE TO OTHER GENERAL MEDICAL CONDITIONS

A. The development of multiple cognitive deficits manifested by both

  (1) memory impairment (impaired ability to learn new information or to recall previously learned information)

  (2) one (or more) of the following cognitive disturbances:

    (a) aphasia (language disturbance)

    (b) apraxia (impaired ability to carry out motor activities despite intact motor function)

    (c) agnosia (failure to recognize or identify objects despite intact sensory function)

    (d) disturbance in executive functioning (i.e., planning, organizing, sequencing, abstracting)

B. The cognitive deficits in Criteria A1 and A2 each cause significant impairment in social or occupational functioning and represent a significant decline from a previous level of functioning.

C. There is evidence from the history, physical examination, or laboratory findings that the disturbance is the direct physiological consequence of one of the general medical conditions listed below.

D. The deficits do not occur exclusively during the course of a delirium.

DSM-IV Coding for Dementias

- 294.1   Dementia Due to HIV disease
  Coding note: Also code 042 HIV infection affecting central nervous system on Axis III.

- 294.1   Dementia due to Head Trauma
  Coding note: Also code 854.00 head injury on Axis III

- 291.1   Dementia due to Parkinson's Disease
  Coding note: Also code 332.0 Parkinson's disease on Axis III

- 294.1   Dementia due to Huntington's Disease
  Coding note: Also code 333.40 Huntington's disease on Axis III

- 291.1   Dementia due to Pick's Disease
  Coding note: Also code 331.1 Pick's disease on Axis III

- 291.1   Dementia due to Creutzfeldt-Jakob Disease
  Coding note: Also code 046.1 Creutzfeldt-Jakob disease on Axis III

- 294.1   Dementia due to . . . [Indicate the General Medical Condition not listed above]
  For example, normal-pressure hydrocephalus, hypothyroidism, brain tumor, vitamin B_{12} deficiency, intracranial radiation
  Coding note: Also code the general medical condition on Axis III (DSM, pp. 151–152)

ASSESSMENT

As with other disorders, the first step in assessment is to get a good case history. A suggested format for a case history for elderly persons with cognitive-language deficits is found in Table 13–6.

Initially, blood tests and a CT scan should be done to exclude other problems such as tumor, blood clots, or stroke. Findings related to dementia of various neuroimaging techniques are delineated in Table 13–7.

SPEECH-LANGUAGE PATHOLOGY ASSESSMENT

When assessing an individual who is suspected of having declining cognition and/or language, the clinician should examine the relationship between the patient's pre-morbid and post-morbid status to determine how much the patient's cognition and/or language have changed. According to Carramazza and Hillis (1991), one of the purposes of assessment is to determine how the aforementioned factors will be involved in setting treatment outcomes and goals. Payne lists the following objectives of the speech-language assessment for a patient diagnosed with dementia:

1. Obtain the most reliable historic information from medical records and from persons in the patient's support network about the patient and all cultural dynamics in the patient's life;

2. Differentiate the language and cognitive deficits associated with dementia from the other types of language diosrders associated with aging neuropathologies;

3. Differentiate the language and cognitive deficits associated with dementia from other types of behavioral changes from depression or confusion, and other forms of treatable dementia;

4. Determine if dementia is primarily cortical, subcortical, or mixed and how the dementia has affected language;

TABLE 13-6 Case history format for elderly persons with cognitive-language deficits

Name:

Dementia Diagnosis:

Primary Disease Entity:

Secondary Disease Entity:

Onset of Problem:

Date of Case History:

Primary Informant and Relationship to Patient:

Additional Informants and Relationships:

Interviewer:

SECTION I: MEDICAL HISTORY

1. History of stroke or significant cardiovascular or cerebrovascular disease; current status.
2. History of dementia of the Alzheimer's type: current status.
3. Types of medications and side-effects; current status.
4. History of alcohol use; current status.
5. History of progressive or chronic motor disorders; current status (Parkinson's disease, Huntington's disease, supranuclear palsy; or other motor disorder).
6. History of seizures; current status.
7. Ambulation and gait.
8. Hearing or visual disturbances.
9. Head trauma.
10. Activities of daily living; instrumental activities of daily living.

SECTION II: CURRENT COGNITIVE AND COMMUNICATION STATUS

1. Functional and pragmatic skills in verbal expression, understanding spoken language, reading, and writing.
2. Memory loss.
3. Behavioral changes and characteristics.
4. Depression.
5. Disorientation.

SECTION III: PSYCHOSOCIAL PARAMETERS

Ethnicity	Family arrangements	Education
National origin	Exercise patterns	Communication needs
Living arrangements	Degree and source of emotional stress	Communication style
Native language	Past patterns of illness	Leisure activities
Occupation	Preferred approaches to treatment	Special interests
Socioeconomic status	Perceptions of cause of illness	Perception of health status
Significant family and friends		

SECTION IV: SUMMARY OF NEUROIMAGING AND NEUROPSYCHOLOGICAL TEST DATA

From *Adult Neurogenic Language Disorders: Assessment and Treatment* (pp. 144–145), by J. C. Payne, 1997, San Diego, CA: Singular Publishing Group. Copyright 1997 by Singular Publishing Group. Reprinted with permission.

TABLE 13–7 Brain imaging: morphological and functional findings	
Test	*Findings*
CT scan	Atrophy
	Ventricular enlargement
	Focal lesions
MRI	Atrophy
	Ventricular enlargement
	Focal lesions
	Better at finding small lesions in white matter
	Cerebral blood flow
SPECT	Cerebral blood flow
	Receptor density (neurochemical measurements)
PET*	Cerebral blood flow
	Energy metabolism
	Transmitter activity

Note: PET scans are still used only in research; they are not used clinically at this time.

ASHA, Dementia Grand Rounds (1996)

5. Ascertain where the patient's language deterioration is in relation to the progression of the dementia;

6. Diagnose the patient's residual abilities as a starting point for therapy;

7. Evaluate the patient's communicative needs in the daily living environment;

8. Determine the level of support and reinforcement that can be expected from family members and others in the support network;

9. Synthesize the patient's age, gender, disease onset, severity, and deficits in order to arrive at a tentative statement of prognosis;

10. Ascertain whether there are any barriers to the patient's compliance with recommended treatment approaches;

11. Target appropriate and reasonable goals for therapy. (Payne, 1997, p. 140)

Neuropsychological Assessment

Assessment of dementia should last 90–120 minutes. Areas of neuropsychological assessment include cognition, behavior, function (how patient puts together cognition and activities of daily living), and quality of life. Efforts should be made to differentiate dementia from aphasia, confusion, depression, and right hemisphere syndrome (Hegde, 1996). All these conditions can mimic dementia and must be ruled out before a diagnosis of dementia can be made. (See Tables 13–8, 13–9, 13–10, and 13–11.)

A multimodality approach is recommended, including the auditory modality, the visual modality, and the tactile and verbal modalities as well. A motor speech evaluation addressing the following areas should also be done: respiration, phonation, articulation, oral musculature, resonance, and prosody.

TABLE 13-8 Dementia or aphasia?

Dementia	Aphasia
Onset mostly is slow	Onset mostly is sudden
Bilateral brain damage	Damage in the left hemisphere
Diffuse brain damage in most cases	Focal brain lesions in most cases
May be moody, withdrawn, and agitated	Mood usually is appropriate, though depressed or frustrated at times
Cognition is mildly or severely impaired, but better language skills until later stages	Impaired language, but generally intact cognition
Memory is impaired to various degrees, often severely	Memory typically is intact
Behavior often is irrelevant, socially inappropriate, and disorganized	Behavior generally is relevant, socially appropriate, and organized
Mentally confused and disoriented to time and space	Mentally alert and oriented to time and space
Disorientation to self in later stages	No disorientation to self
Progression of deterioration from semantic to syntactic to phonologic performance	Semantic, syntactic, and phonologic performance simultaneously impaired
Fluent until dementia becomes worse	Fluent or nonfluent
Relatively poor performance on spatial and verbal recognition tasks	Relatively better performance on spatial and verbal recognition tasks
Relatively poor story retelling skills	Relatively better story retelling skills
Relatively poor description of common objects	Relatively better description of common objects
Relatively poor silent reading comprehension	Relatively better silent reading comprehension
Relatively poor pantomimic expression	Relatively better pantomimic expression
Relatively poor drawing skills	Relatively better drawing skills

From *Pocketguide to Assessment in Speech-Language Pathology* (pp. 158–159), by M. N. Hegde, 1996, San Diego, CA: Singular Publishing Group. Copyright 1996 by Singular Publishing Group. Reprinted with permission.

TABLE 13-9 Dementia or the language of confusion?

Dementia	Confusion
Degenerative diseases more common causes	Traumatic brain injury and toxic and metabolic disturbances are the most common causes
Reduced range and variety of word usage	No significant problems in word usage
Slow onset	Generally more abrupt onset
Disorientation to time, place, and person only in more advanced stages	Disoriented to time, place, and persons
Progressive worsening of symptoms	More rapid, positive changes in symptoms

From *Pocketguide to Assessment in Speech-Language Pathology* (pp. 159–160), by M. N. Hegde, 1996, San Diego, CA: Singular Publishing Group. Copyright 1996 by Singular Publishing Group. Reprinted with permission.

TABLE 13-10 Dementia or depression (pseudodementia)?

Dementia	Pseudodementia
Imprecise onset date	More precise onset date
Family members often do not know about the symptoms	Family members know about the symptoms
Slow progression of symptoms	Rapid progression of symptoms
No or rare history of psychiatric problems	History of psychiatric problems
Patients do not complain of cognitive problems in detail	Patients complain of cognitive problems
Patients try to conceal their problems	Patients highlight their disability, failure, sense of distress
Patients struggle to perform	Patients make no or little effort to perform even simple tasks
Social skills often preserved until the later stages	Loss of social skills
Attentional deficits and poor concentration	No attentional deficits, good concentration
Patient's response to orientation tests is confusion	Patient's response to orientation tests is "don't know"
More severe loss for recent events more severe than that for remote events	The same degree of memory loss for both recent and remote events
Generalized memory problems	Selective memory problems
Consistent difficulty in performing the same task	Variability in performing the same task

Note: Pseudomentia is dementia-like symptoms associated with depression; the differentiating characteristics summarized here are based on Wells (1980).

From *Pocketguide to Assessment in Speech-Language Pathology* (pp. 160–161), by M. N. Hegde, 1996, San Diego, CA: Singular Publishing Group. Copyright 1996 by Singular Publishing Group. Reprinted with permission.

TABLE 13-11 Dementia or right hemisphere problems?

Dementia	Right Hemisphere Problems
Significant problems in naming, especially generative naming	Only mild problems in naming, reading, and writing
Significant problems in auditory comprehension	Mild problems in auditory comprehension
Left-sided neglect not a diagnostic feature	Left-sided neglect a diagnostic feature
Prosodic defects less severe	Significant prosodic defect
	Inappropriate humor
May retell stories without context or location	May retell only nonessential, isolated details of stories (no integration)
Pragmatic impairments less striking until the later stages	Pragmatic impairments more striking (eye contact, topic maintenance, etc.)
Significant linguistic deficits except for syntactic and phonological skills, which also decline in later stages	Pure linguistic deficits are not dominant

From *Pocketguide to Assessment in Speech-Language Pathology* (pp. 161–162), by M. N. Hegde, 1996, San Diego, CA: Singular Publishing Group. Copyright 1996 by Singular Publishing Group. Reprinted with permission.

Cognitive factors that should be assessed in patients suspected of having Alzheimer's or any other type of dementia should focus on the following:

1. Arousal (Is the patient awake?)

2. Attention arousal (Is the patient lethargic?)

3. Selective attention (Can the patient shift from one task to another?)

4. Cognitive effort

5. Perception

6. Memory time span: How long does memory last?
   Iconic: memory that lasts longer than one second
   Immediate
   Recent
   Long-term

7. Language

8. Praxis

9. Visuospatial

10. Executive functions

Standardized Assessment Tools

A standard aphasia battery, including such tests as the Western Aphasia Battery or the Boston Diagnosis of Aphasia Exam, should be completed. It should be noted that the Western Aphasia Battery has been standardized for dementia.

Assessment Battery for Comprehension in Dementia Cognitive Capacity Screening Examination (Jacobs, Bernard, & Delgado, 1977)

This test takes approximately 10–20 minutes to administer. The test uses 30 items to test "orientation, concentration, attention, mental control, language (including concept formation), and short term memory" (Golper, p. 139).

Galveston Orientation and Amnesia Test (Levin, O'Donnell, & Grossman, 1979)

The Galveston test is used primarily with patients with traumatic brain injury to evaluate "the major spheres of orientation (time, place, and person) and memory functions" (Golper, p. 139).

Mini-Mental State Examination (MMSE) (Folstein, Folstein, & McHugh, 1975)

The MMSE takes approximately 15–20 minutes to administer. The test is a "brief questionnaire with items related to orientation, registration (short-term memory), attention, calculation, language (naming, repeating, reading, writing), and drawing" (Golper, p. 137). The test is used for screening and to probe decline in progressive dementing illnesses.

Arizona Battery for Communication Disorders of Dementia
(Bayles & Tomoeda, 1993)

The Arizona Battery for Communication Disorders of Dementia can be used to assess mild to moderate dementia. It can also be used to document the progression of dementia over time. The Arizona Battery assesses episodic memory (words and stories), word learning lists, linguistic expression, linguistic comprehension, and visuospatial construction (Haynes & Pindzola, 1998). It consists of 14 subtests, and four of the subtests can be used as a screening tool (Hegde, 1996).

The Communication Profile: A Functional Survey (Payne, 1994)

The Communication Profile is based on the patient's self-report, or the report of his caregiver(s). The test measures "26 items for everyday understanding, reading, speaking, and writing skills on a 5-point scale of importance to daily living" (Payne, 1997, p. 148).

The Middlesex Elderly Assessment of Mental State (MEAMS)

The Middlesex Elderly Assessment of Mental State test is easy to administer and score, and is not dependent on intelligence. The MEAMS can be used to differentiate between functional and organic illness. Subtests include orientation, naming, remembering pictures, spatial construction, unusual views, and verbal fluency.

Functional Assessment of Communication Skills for Adults (ASHA FACS)
(Payne, 1994)

The ASHA FACS can be used as a self-reporting, or caregiver-reporting tool. It "measures four assessment domains: social communication, communication needs, reading, writing, and number concepts, and daily planning on a 7-point scale of communication independence" (Payne, 1997, p. 148).

The F-A-S Word Fluency Test (Borkowski, Benton, & Spreen, 1967)

The F-A-S Word Fluency Test assesses phonemic associations, requiring the patient to generate words that start with a specific phoneme. Word generation tasks typically show degeneration in the early stages. Categorization is most predictive of Alzheimer's.

Functional Communication Profile (FCP) (Sarno, 1969)

The FCP rates communicative behavior in daily situations based on 45 examples. It includes rating of movement, speaking, and understanding on a 3-point scale (Payne, 1997).

The Discourse Abilities Profile (Terrel & Ripich, 1989)

The Discourse Abilities Profile is also standardized for use with patients with Alzheimer's disease. On this test, the patients typically do best on the conversation subtest, perhaps because it is the most structured. The next best performance is on procedural discourse. They do the worst on the narrative subtest, which is most discriminative between Alzheimer's and normal aging changes.

Global Deterioration Scale (Reisbert, Ferris, DeLeon & Crook, 1982)

The Global Deterioration Scale rates dementia on a 7-point rating scale (Hegde, 1996).

Short Portable Mental Status Questionnaire (SPMSQ) (Pfeiffer, 1975)

The SPMSQ involves asking a patient a series of nine questions, such as the following: (Golper, 1998, pp. 137–139)

What is the date today?

What day of the week is it?

What is the name of this place?

Who is president of the United States?

The patient is also asked to subtract 3 from 20 and to keep subtracting 3 from each new number. The degree of cognitive impairment is based on the number of errors on the test.

Communication Abilities in Daily Living (CADL) (Holland, 1989)

The CADL consists of 68 items divided into 10 categories to measure functional daily activities. The 10 categories are role-playing, social convention, speech acts, divergences, context use, deixis, sequential relationships, nonverbal relationships, nonverbal symbolism, reading/writing/calculation, and humor/metaphor/absurdity. The CADL scoring is based on a 3-point scale.

Revised Edinburgh Functional Communication Profile (EFCP) (Wirz, Skinner, & Dean, 1990)

The EFCP is based on a 5-point scale to determine how effectively a patient uses communication functions for greeting, acknowledging, responding, requesting, and initiating.

In summary, there are a wide variety of assessment devices that can be used to determine the cognitive and language status of elderly patients. They can also be used to differentially diagnose between dementia and other disorders commonly associated with the elderly population. In addition, Bayles et al. (1989) suggest that the patient be given a test of reading comprehension. The results of this type of testing can be used to differentially diagnose dementia from aphasia. The information gained from a carefully taken history, rating scales completed by the patient and/or caregiver(s), and assessment tools can be used to plan what type of intervention will take place, and what functional outcomes will be targeted.

TREATMENT

Intervention with patients with dementia will involve, as in many disorders, an interdisciplinary team. This team will be composed of specialists in medicine, dentistry, nutrition, nursing, psychiatry, neuropsychology, speech-language pathology, and other rehabilitation specialists. Involvement of the speech-language pathologist in treatment typically revolves around developing strategies to maximize communication given the client's existing skills, and teaching the family and significant others to use these strategies. The speech-language pathologist also "monitors changes in communicative status as the disease progresses, provides cognitive-language stimulation therapy to enable the patient to maintain skills for as long as possible, and gives information and counseling to the patient and the patient's caregiving network" (Payne, 1997, p. 153).

General management strategies include helping the patient and his family to establish a simple and consistent routine. This will help the patient remember things that must be done on a daily basis, such as taking prescribed medications. Also, the patient should be taught to use simple reminders to manage the memory problems. These reminders can include notes, alarms, and reminders from family and/or caretakers. Patients can also be taught to make lists of daily tasks. Personal belongings should be kept in specific, invariable spots to assist in locating them (keys, glasses, remote controls, pens, etc.). It is also important, particularly in the middle and late stages, that the patient wear an ID bracelet or carry a card that contains personal identification information, the phone number of a family member, and the name of a health care professional (Hegde, 1996).

Behaviorally, the FOCUSED program as described in an ASHA videotape titled *Dementia Grand Rounds* (1996) is one approach to therapy for patients with dementia. The FOCUSED program is based on six modules, which are described as follows:

Module 1: Characteristics and pathology of AD
             Making the diagnosis of AD
             Language comprehension and processes
             Differentiate between Alzheimer's and aphasia

Module 2: Description of memory and memory processes
             Memory and depression in normal aging vs. AD

Module 3: Importance of communication in AD

Module 4: Seven FOCUSED strategies (see Table 13–12)

Module 5: Language stages of AD (review Module 2)
             Communication goals and approaches at each stage (role-play)
             Give laminated FOCUSED card

Module 6: Optional
             Cultural considerations in the workplace (people of one culture taking care of people from another culture).

There are also some medications available for use with patients with dementia. Cognex (tacrine), which is taken four times a day, was the first drug approved for use with patients with Alzheimer's. Generally, drugs offer symptomatic treatment, with cognitive and behavioral improvement being the primary goals. Aracept can be taken once a day and has fewer side effects than Cognex, which can cause liver damage. Cognex and Aracept both improve symptoms of memory and attention.

To summarize, the speech-language pathologist will be involved in the treatment of patients with dementia, particularly during the early stages when it is important to develop and teach strategies that can facilitate memory in activities of daily living. The speech-language pathologist will be involved in counseling the patient and/or his caregivers, and in monitoring the patient's status as the dementia progresses.

TABLE 13-12 The strategies associated with the FOCUSED acronym

F = Face

Face the person with AD directly

Call his or her name

Touch the person

Gain and maintain eye contact

O = Orient

Orient the person with AD to the topic by repeating key words several times

Repeat and rephrase sentences

Use nouns and specific names

C = Continue

Continue the same topic of conversation for as long as possible

Restate the topic throughout the conversation

Indicate to the person with AD that you are introducing a new topic

U = Unstick

Help the person with AD become "unstuck" when he or she uses a word incorrectly by suggesting the intended word

Repeat the sentence the person said using the correct word

Ask, "Do you mean . . . ?"

S = Structured

Structure your question so that the person with AD will be able to recognize and repeat a response

Provide two simple choices at a time

Use yes/no questions

E = Exchange

Keep up the normal exchange of ideas we use in everyday conversation

Keep conversations going with comments such as, "Oh, how nice," or "That's great!"

Do *not* ask "test" questions

Give the person with AD clues as to how to answer your questions

D = Direct

Keep sentences short, simple, and direct

Put the subject of the sentences first

Use and repeat nouns (names of persons or things) rather than pronouns (he, she, it, their, etc.)

Use hand signals, pictures, and facial expressions

From American Speech-Language-Hearing Association (1996). *Dementia Grand Rounds* (videotape). Rockville, MD: American Speech-Language-Hearing Association.

CHAPTER FOURTEEN
Dysarthria

DEFINITION/DESCRIPTION

Caruso and Strand (1999b) cite Darley, Aronson, and Brown in defining dysarthria as "a group of motor speech disorders that result from deficits in muscular control of the speech mechanism due to central or peripheral nervous system damage. The speech problem, then, is due to an abnormal neuromuscular state of the muscles (e.g., paralysis, atrophy, spasticity) or the resulting disruption of movement of those muscles (e.g., weakness or incoordination)" (Caruso & Strand, 1999b, p. 13). There are five types of dysarthria: flaccid, spastic, ataxic, hyperkinetic, and hypokinetic (in Parkinson's disease). Ataxic dysarthria is characterized by a drawing out and blurring of speech, much as one sounds when using "drunken speech." In ataxic dysarthria, the lesion is in the cerebellum or in the input and output pathways (Cannito & Marquardt, 1997).

The speech of a person with hyperkinetic dysarthria (too much movement) is typically characterized by vocal harshness, articulatory imprecision, and prosodic abnormalities. It is caused by a lesion in the extrapyramidal system. Hyperkinetic dysarthria can be categorized as a quick form or a slow form. The most common types of the quick form are chorea (articulatory incompetence, resonatory incompetence, prosodic insufficiency and excess), myoclonus (sudden, jerking, unsustained muscle contractions), and tic disorders (rapid, stereotyped, brief, nonpurposeful movements). The most common types of the slow form are athetosis (writhing movements), dystonias (neurogenic disorders of muscle tone affecting posture and movement), and dyskinesia (movement characterized by slowness) (Zraick & La Pointe, 1997).

Movements of the muscles involved in articulation, resonance, phonation, and respiration are problematic for individuals with dysarthria. This results in reduced speed and strength, decreased range of motion, and, periodically, uncoordinated movement. These deficits create speech characterized by problems with rate control, use of imprecise consonants and vowel distortions, and hypernasality. They may also cause respiratory and phonatory deficiencies (Caruso & Strand, 1999b).

Hypokinetic dysarthria is typically associated with Parkinson's disease as well as Wilson's disease and progressive supranuclear palsy. The speech is characterized by a reduction in the mobility of the oral musculature and structures used for speech. It, too, is caused by a lesion in the extrapyramidal tract. A system for classifying dysarthria based on the neurophysiologic system is in Table 14–1.

The term "developmental dysarthria" may be used to describe children who have normal neuroradiologic examinations, yet exhibit soft signs for which no specific diagnosis can be

Table 14–1   Dysarthria classifications

Type	Site of Lesion	Possible Causes	Primary Speech Characteristics
Flaccid	Lower motor neuron	Viral infection Tumor CVA Congenital conditions Disease Palsies Trauma	Hypernasality Imprecise consonants Breathiness Monopitch Nasal emission
Spastic	Upper motor neuron	CVA Tumor Infection Trauma Congenital condition	Imprecise consonants Monopitch Reduced stress Harsh voice quality Monoloudness Low pitch Slow rate Hypernasality Strained-strangled voice Short phrases
Mixed (flaccid and spastic)	Upper and lower motor neuron	Amyotrophic lateral sclerosis Trauma CVA	Imprecise consonants Hypernasality Harsh voice quality Slow rate Monopitch Short phrases Distorted vowels Low pitch Monoloudness Excess and equal stress Prolonged intervals
Ataxic	Cerebellar system	CVA Tumor Trauma Congenital condition Infection Toxic effects	Imprecise consonants Excess and equal stress Irregular articulatory breakdowns Distorted vowels Harsh voice Loudness control problems Variable nasality
Hypokinetic	Extrapyramidal system	Parkinsonism Drug-induced	Monopitch Reduced stress Monoloudness Imprecise consonants Inappropriate silences Short rushes of speech Harsh voice Breathy voice
Hyperkinetic	Extrapyramidal system	Chorea Infection Gilles de la Tourette syndrome Ballism Athetosis CVA Tumor Dystonia Drug-induced Dyskinesia	Imprecise consonants Distorted vowels Harsh voice quality Irregular articulatory breakdowns Strained-strangled voice Monopitch Monoloudness

From *Assessment in Speech-Language Pathology: A Resource Manual* (pp. 287–288), by K. G. Shipley and J. G. McAfee, 1992, San Diego, CA: Singular Publishing Group. Copyright 1992 by Singular Publishing Group. Reprinted with permission.

made. These soft signs include hyponasality, or delayed gross or fine motor control. These children are not specifically impaired in the area of execution, programming, or sensori-motor planning, but they exhibit speech characteristics similar to dysarthria. Other children have dysarthria caused by congenital neurophysiological problems, such as cerebral palsy, or neurological diseases or trauma (Caruso & Strand, 1999b).

ASSESSMENT

Based on the work of McNeil and Kennedy (1984), Strand and McCauley (1999) outlined several purposes for assessment of motor speech disorders in children. These purposes are delineated in Table 14–2.

As in all assessments, the initial component should be a complete history. The history should help the clinician in deciding which tasks in the actual evaluation to have the client complete. Also, while gathering the case history, the clinician should be an astute observer and note the following: presence of tremors, fasciculations, or other involuntary move-ments; general muscle tone; postural control; quality of voice; general appearance; and asymmetries of the orofacial area (Kent, 1997). This should be followed by a complete oral-facial assessment, including observing the structures at rest and during sustained phonation (see chapter on articulation and phonology). Kent (1997) then recommends an orosensory evaluation, particularly in clients who have Parkinson's disease, trigeminal nerve damage, oral apraxia, localized cerebral lesions, head injury, or any severe motor involvement of the orofacial system. Orosensory examination should consist of light static touch, kinetic touch, temperature, and double-simultaneous touch. In light static touch, the patient identifies the presence or absence of tactile stimulation, and in kinetic touch the patient describes (or gestures) the direction of the moving stimulus. Testing of temperature sensitivity consists of touching the patient with test tubes filled with warm or cold water and having the patient identify which is which. Finally, in double-simultaneous touch, the client identifies whether he is being touched in one or two places (Kent, 1997).

TABLE 14–2 Purposes for assessment

Detect or confirm a problem

Differential diagnosis

Classify

Determine neuropathology

Specify severity, prognosis

Determine treatment focus

Make decisions regarding number and length of sessions, stimuli, tasks, etc.

Establish if criteria for treatment termination or change has occurred

Measure change that occurs as a result of treatment

From "Assessment Procedures for Treatment Planning in Children with Phonologic and Motor Speech Disorders," by E. A. Strand and R. J. McCauley, 1999, in *Clinical Management of Motor Speech Disorders in Children* (p. 74), by A. J. Caruso and E. A. Strand (Eds.), New York: Thieme Medical Publishers. Copyright 1999 by Thieme Medical Publishers. Reprinted with permission.

A variety of non-speech tasks should be performed, including the following: tongue protrusion, baring teeth, smile, pucker lips, cough, puff cheeks, touch nose with tongue tip, touch chin with tongue tip, touch corner of mouth with tongue tip, blow, suck, bite lip, bite tongue, lick lips, move tongue from corner to corner of mouth, mastication, swallow (Kent, 1997).

The client should be asked to perform these tasks as isolated movements and repetitive movements. For more information and elaboration, the reader is referred to Kent (1997).

The client should then participate in a series of speech tasks, including the following:

- phonation duration (sustained vowel after maximal inspiration)
- friction duration (sustained production of /s/ and /z/
- assessment of the fundamental frequency
- sound pressure range (sustained /a/ from soft to loud)
- sustained /a/ from high pitch to low pitch (or vice versa)
- diadochokinetic rate
- routine automatic speech (counting, simple greetings)
- repetition of words and phrases
- tasks requiring language formulation (naming, describing a picture, retelling a story, etc.) (Kent, 1997)

While the client is participating in the above tasks, his intelligibility should be evaluated, as well as vocal quality, fluency, and prosody.

In assessment of an individual to determine the presence of dysarthria, a complete examination of the oral-facial mechanism is mandatory. In addition, a speech sample should be collected that features both spontaneous speech and the reading of a passage such as the Grandfather Passage or the Rainbow Passage (see Appendix A). Published tests that can be used in the diagnosis of dysarthria include the following:

- *Assessment of Intelligibility of Dysarthric Speakers* (Yorkston, Beukelman, & Traynor, 1984)
- *Frenchay Dysarthria Assessment* (Enderby, 1983)
- *Ling's Phonetic Level Speech Evaluation* (Ling, 1976)
- *Assessment of Phonological Processes—Revised* (Hodson & Paden, 1983)

The evaluation of neurogenic speech disorders may involve the use of specialized instrumentation to test the physiologic and acoustic parameters of the patient's speech. These tests are described in the chapter on voice and resonance disorders. It also may be necessary to complete an evaluation of the patient's ability to use an augmentative/alternative communication device (Golper, 1998, p. 3).

When evaluating a child for the presence of a motor speech disorder, some of the following questions and observations may be helpful:

Is the child able to achieve adequate volume for speech?

Is vocal quality breathy, harsh, or strained-strangled?

Is there instability in the phonation (i.e., fluctuation in intensity or frequency)?

TABLE 14-3 Questions to address when observing the child at rest, during eating, and during play
Can the child maintain lip seal when drinking liquids?
Does the child have full jaw opening during crying or laughter?
Is there full lateral tongue movement during chewing?
Does the child increase muscle tension for plosing during vocal play?
Is there any asymmetry of the lips or facial muscles at rest?
Can the child achieve good volume for laughter or crying (indicating good respiratory support)?

From "Assessment Procedures for Treatment Planning in Children with Phonologic and Motor Speech Disorders," by E. A. Strand and R. J. McCauley, 1999, in *Clinical Management of Motor Speech Disorders in Children* (p. 89), by A. J. Caruso and E. A. Strand (Eds.), New York: Thieme Medical Publishers. Copyright 1999 by Thieme Medical Publishers. Reprinted with permission.

Are there voice breaks?

Does the child exhibit stridor when taking air in or blowing air out?

Can the child achieve good laryngeal adduction during a cough? (Caruso & Strand, 1999b, pp. 92–93)

Other questions to address are indicated in Table 14–3.

TREATMENT

In dysarthria, the primary problem is the weakness of the muscle. Therefore, therapy should address improving the strength of the muscles. However, Liss et al. (1994) stress the need to increase strength through neural adaptation as opposed to muscle fiber change. Specifically, Liss et al. believed that the greatest strength changes would occur "when the training occurs in the position(s) that the movement operates through" (Hageman, 1997). For example, "if the target was tight lip closure to prevent leakage during eating, then push against resistance in the closed position while allowing the jaw to move" (Hageman, 1997, p. 199).

Dworkin proposed that respiration and resonation should be addressed first, followed by phonation, then articulation and prosody. Others (Rosenbek, LaPointe, Netsell) respect the components, but say the hierarchy should be individualized to the patient. Zraick and LaPointe (1997) suggest the following hierarchy of respiration subsystem treatment exercises:

1. Muscle relaxation and postural adjustment
2. Air pressure generation
3. Prolonged inhalations/exhalations
4. Quick breathing
5. Inhalatory/exhalatory synchronization
6. Isolated sound productions
7. Connected speech breathing

Yoss and Darley suggest the following treatment hierarchy:

- If there is a coexisting oral apraxia, begin with mirror work and imitation of various tongue and lip movements.

- Have the child imitate sustained vowels, with exaggerated lip movement and range of movement of the mandible.

- Have the child imitate visible consonants, then pair them with all vowels in either CV or VC combinations.

- Make use of diphthongs paired with consonants to introduce stress and intonational patterns, accompanied by visible movements of some kind to accentuate the changes in placement of the articulators.

- Move on to imitation of CVC shapes. Use rhyming words (real and nonsense) in minimal pairs, again with some type of body movement to accent stress patterns.

- Extend sequencing efforts by using carrier phrases. Incorporate consonant cluster words and continue using stress patterns.

- Introduce awareness of self-monitoring of spontaneous speech as early as possible in therapy, often necessitating slowing of rate. (Caruso & Strand, 1999, p. 116)

Some functional outcome statements for pediatric therapy are listed in Table 14–4.

Finally, Guilmette (1997) proposes the following therapy suggestions: large muscle group training prior to fine movements; provide compensations; "emphasize functional and overlearned tasks"; monitor frustration, depression, motivation levels (Guilmette, 1997, p. 46).

TABLE 14–4 Functional outcome statements

1. Your child attempts to say words.
2. Your child understands what you say to him or her.
3. Your child is successful at communicating his or her needs to others by speaking.
4. Your child is successful at communicating his or her needs to others without speaking (by using nonverbal means such as sign language, gestures, facial expressions, communication devices, etc.).
5. Your child is successful at communicating with other children of a similar age.
6. Your child is able to talk without stuttering (at home, school, or in new situations).
7. How much of your child's speech can an unfamiliar listener understand?

From "Motor Speech Disorders in Children: Definitions, Background, and a Theoretical Framework," 1999, in *Clinical Management of Motor Speech Disorders in Children* (p. 389), by A. J. Caruso and E. A. Strand (Eds.), New York: Thieme Medical Publishers. Copyright 1999 by Thieme Medical Publishers. Reprinted with permission.

CHAPTER FIFTEEN
Dysphagia in Adults

DEFINITION/DESCRIPTION

Sometimes dysphagia occurs concomitantly with a communication disorder, and sometimes it does not. Regardless, the assessment and treatment falls within the scope of practice of speech-language pathologists (ASHA, 1987). In the "Ad Hoc Committee on Dysphagia" report, ASHA (1987) defined dysphagia as follows:

> Dysphagia is a swallowing disorder characterized by difficulty in oral preparation for the swallow or in moving material from the mouth to the stomach. Subsumed in this definition are problems in positioning food in the mouth and in the oral manipulation preceding the swallow including suckling, sucking and mastication.

The speech-language pathologist functions as part of a team, which typically includes a radiologist, a pulmonary physician, a gastroenterologist, a nutritionist, an otolaryngologist, and a nurse.

According to Logemann (1998a), the acute care population of adult patients with dysphagia represents a comprehensive list of etiological factors, including the following: stroke; head injury; spinal cord injury; progressive neurological diseases (e.g., Parkinson's disease); motor neuron disease; multiple sclerosis; Alzheimer's disease; head and neck cancer; and systemic diseases (e.g., rheumatoid arthritis, scleroderma, dermatomyositis) (Logemann, 1998a).

It is also important to differentiate between symptoms and dysfunction. "The anatomic and/or neuromuscular dysfunctions are the actual disorders leading to the symptom for which treatment is designed" (Logemann, 1998b, p. 71). Swallowing disorders can be caused by a mechanical problem or a neurological problem. In mechanical disorders, the innervation (central and most peripheral) is intact, but the structures needed to accomplish swallowing are not. Mechanical disorders may be secondary "to combinations of deglutitory muscle loss and loss of the motor and sensory innervations to those muscles" (Groher, 1997, p. 73). Most patients with mechanical swallowing problems have had removal or reconstruction of oral, pharyngeal, laryngeal, or esophageal structures because of cancer. Other causes of mechanical dysphagia include acute inflammations, trauma, macroglossia, pharyngoesophageal diverticulum, cervical spine disease, nasoenteric tubes, and tracheostoma tubes. There are numerous causes of neurogenic dysphagia. These are outlined in Table 15–1.

Dysphagia can occur in the oral, pharyngeal, laryngeal, and/or esophageal stages of the swallow. Oral dysphagia relates to disorders in the mastication of the food, the formation of a bolus by mixing the food with saliva, and the anterior to posterior transit of the bolus as it is positioned for the swallow. This positioning for the oral phase of the swallow triggers

TABLE 15-1 Causes of neurogenic dysphagia	
Stroke	Multiple sclerosis
Traumatic brain injury	Neoplasms and other structural disorders
Cerebral palsy	Poliomyelitis and postpolio syndrome
Dementia, including Alzheimer's disease	Infectious disorders
Parkinson's disease	Guillain Barré syndrome and other polyneuropathies
Progressive supranuclear palsy	Myasthenia gravis
Huntington's disease	Myopathy
Wilson's disease	Iatrogenic oral/pharyngeal dysphagia
Torticollis	Age-related changes
Motor neuron disease	Psychogenic dysphagia

From "Neurologic Disorders of Swallowing" by D. W. Buchholz, 1997, in *Dysphagia: Diagnosis and Management* (p. 44), by M. E. Groher (Ed.), Boston: Butterworth-Heinemann Publishers. Copyright 1997 by Butterworth-Heinemann Publishers. Reprinted with permission.

the pharyngeal swallow. During the pharyngeal swallow, "the anterior portion of the tongue is retracted and depressed, mastication then ceases, and respiration is inhibited. Retraction of the tongue and its elevation against the hard palate force the bolus into the upper part of the pharynx" (Groher, 1997, p. 17). The posterior movement of the tongue drives the bolus into the pharynx and elevates the entire larynx, pulling it upward and forward. The elevation of the larynx depresses the epiglottis to protect the airway. The airway is also protected by the cessation of respiration, which allows the vocal cords to close off the trachea. When the cricopharyngeus muscle relaxes, the bolus is propelled into the esophagus. Peristaltic actions of the esophagus direct the bolus into the stomach (Groher, 1997).

ASSESSMENT

Many patients who have dysphagia do not seek help because of specific complaints related to swallowing. Rather, a related problem that is a subjective complaint may be their first reason for consulting a physician or a speech-language pathologist. These are summarized by Miller (1997) as follows:

1. *Complaints about food sticking in the throat:* Patients who complain about food sticking in the throat oftentimes have some obstructive condition such as a tumor, a web, or a stricture that interferes with the passage of solid food through the esophagus or throat.

2. *Obstruction:* While this could be related to the strictures described above, it is also possible that the patient has a neurological condition resulting in muscle incoordination and/or weakness. In these cases, the obstruction is often at the site of the cricopharyngeus or the pharyngoesophageal area.

3. *Nasal regurgitation:* Patients should be asked whether they have episodes of fluid or food moving into the nasal cavity (instead of into the throat), and, if so, how frequently. Occasional episodes are usually of no concern. However, frequent episodes could be indicative of "some malfunction of the palatal and upper pharyngeal mechanism" (Groher, 1984, p. 88).

4. *Mouth odor:* Mouth odor can be caused by gastric reflux, poor hygiene, dental disease, periodontal disease, oral retention of food (incomplete oral phase of the swallow), or oral-mucosal lesions. Another cause is Zenker's pharyngoesophageal diverticulum, or the formation of small sacs in which food can become trapped and create a foul odor.

5. *Aspiration:* Aspiration can occur in a variety of disorders but is most frequently associated with neuromuscular swallowing disorders. The patient will typically complain of frequent coughing and/or choking while eating. The patient should also be questioned with regard to the entry of food and/or liquids into the windpipe.

6. *Gastroesophageal reflux:* Typically, patients will report gastroesophageal reflux as episodes of heartburn. Reflux is a common occurrence, but frequent episodes should be explored, possibly by a gastroenterologist. Reflux can be symptomatic of a hiatal hernia. Reflux has the potential to be quite problematic because it can lead to aspiration of stomach contents, irritation of the esophageal mucosa, dysfunction of esophageal muscles and sphincter actions, and ulceration of the laryngeal mucosa.

7. *Speech and voice:* Speech and swallowing share many of the same neurological, muscular, and anatomic bases, so swallowing disorders may be accompanied by changes in the voice. Frequent complaints are hoarseness (which may be associated with reflux), and loss of voice (temporary). If the patient complains of weakness, or slurring of his speech, the etiology could be neurological. Inflammatory and neoplastic disorders are also commonly shared in people who have speech and/or voice disorders associated with dysphagia.

8. *Pain:* Pain accompanying swallowing (odynophagia) is usually related to neoplasms, mechanical obstructions in the pharynx, or infection. It may also be associated with an esophageal motor disorder.

9. *Weight loss:* Weight loss may be caused by impaired nutrition associated with dysphagia. If the patient is having difficulty swallowing, he may reduce his nutritional intake, resulting in weight loss.

10. *Pneumonia:* A patient who has recurrent pneumonia should be assessed for aspiration. Typically, this is associated with weakness of the swallowing mechanism, or with neuromuscular incoordination. Other etiological factors associated with deficits in swallowing include an inability to protect the airway, vocal cord paralysis, mechanical obstruction of the deglutitory tract, and reflux.

In patients who present with any of the above complaints, dysphagia assessment will, for most patients, consist of a screening followed by a complete assessment of the patient's oral motor functions and swallowing abilities. A sample of a checklist of items for a dysphagia screening is in Table 15–2. The assessment should include a review of the patient's nutritional and hydration status.

Prior to seeing a patient who has been referred for dysphagia assessment, the speech-language pathologist should carefully review the patient's medical records, focusing on the medical diagnosis, current medications, surgical history (recent and remote), trauma, or neurological damage. The clinician should also review any notes from an otolaryngologist or a neurologist. Special note should be made as to whether or not the patient has a history of tracheostomy or mechanical ventilation, and the conditions and length of that support. History of gastrointestinal problems should be documented, as well as that of any stroke or

TABLE 15–2 Checklist of items for dysphagia screening

Screening should be quick (less than 15 minutes), easy, and inexpensive

Check appropriate box for each item

Yes	No	
☐	☐	1. History of recurrent pneumonia
		2. Diagnosis of
☐	☐	• partial laryngectomy
☐	☐	• oral resection
☐	☐	• full course of radiation to head or neck
☐	☐	• anoxia
☐	☐	• Parkinson's disease
☐	☐	• motor neuron disease (e.g., Werdnig-Hoffman disease)
☐	☐	• myasthenia gravis
☐	☐	• bulbar polio
☐	☐	• anterior cervical spinal fusion
☐	☐	• brainstem stroke
☐	☐	• Guillain-Barré
☐	☐	• laryngeal trauma
☐	☐	3. History of prolonged or traumatic intubation or emergency tracheostomy
☐	☐	4. Severe respiratory problems
☐	☐	5. Gurgly voice, cry
☐	☐	6. Coughing before, during, and/or after swallowing
☐	☐	7. Poor awareness and poor control of secretions
☐	☐	8. Infrequent swallowing (less than one saliva swallow in 5 minutes)
☐	☐	9. Constant copious chest secretions
		10. If patient is eating, observe eating. If patient is not eating, observe saliva swallowing. Identify any of these, particularly if they change during or immediately after a meal:
☐	☐	• breathing difficulty
☐	☐	• increased secretions
☐	☐	• voice changes (gurgly sound)
☐	☐	• multiple swallowing per bolus
☐	☐	• reduced laryngeal lifting on swallow
☐	☐	• throat clearing
☐	☐	• coughing
☐	☐	• significant fatigue

Note: Items 1 through 4 should be obtained from brief chart review. Items 5 through 10 require brief patient observation.

From *Evaluation and Treatment of Swallowing Disorders* (2nd ed.) (p. 103), by J. A. Logemann, 1998, Austin, TX: Pro-Ed. Copyright 1998 by Pro-Ed. Reprinted with permission.

head injury. Finally, any incidence of prior dysphagia, including the surrounding circumstances (non-oral nutritional support and nutritional status) and the resolution, should be noted. In addition, the clinician should check for the presence of any advance directives related to the administration of nutrition and hydration in the event the patient is incompetent to make those decisions.

Initially, patients may be seen for a brief bedside screening in which the oral and pharyngeal stages of the swallow are evaluated. This screening should consist of the following determinations: "(1) general level of alertness; (2) general secretion levels in the mouth, throat, and chest; (3) awareness of secretions, as exhibited by attempts to wipe away drooling, throat clearing, or coughing and attempts to clear chest secretions; (4) vocal quality (i.e., hoarse or gurgly); (5) history of any pneumonia; (6) obvious reduction in oromotor control; (7) history of neurologic insult or other neurologic or structural damage; and (8) medical diagnosis" (Logemann, 1998a, p. 19). Miller summarizes the components of a comprehensive evaluation for dysphagia as outlined in Table 15–3.

Patients who exhibit difficulty initiating the pharyngeal swallow or who have problems with any of the other neuromotor aspects of swallowing should receive an in-depth evaluation, including a modified barium swallow. If the problem is in the oral cavity, a complete bedside assessment should be performed to identify the precise problem and to initiate therapy (which may include a modified diet) (Logemann, 1998a).

TABLE 15–3   Comprehensive evaluation for dysphagia

Factors Influencing Swallowing	*Methods of Assessment*
Oral Phase	
Mental status, judgment	Screen orientation, language, visual-motor perception, and memory
Muscles of facial expression	Examine for symmetry at rest and during movement
Muscles of mastication	Palpate and gently resist movement
Mucous membranes	Inspect
Dentition	Inspect
Lingual muscles	Inspect at rest and on protrusion; resist movement
Orofacial sensation	Subjective; identify stimulus qualities
Pharyngeal Phase	
Palatopharyngeal closure	Observe at rest and during phonation; stimulate gag reflex
Pharyngeal constriction	Stimulate gag; motion radiography, electromyography
Extrinsic laryngeal muscles	Palpate larynx during swallow, auscultation
Intrinsic laryngeal muscles	Indirect laryngeal inspection or fiberoptic examination
Cricopharyngeus muscle	Motion radiography
Esophageal Phase	
Morphology of the esophagus	Motion radiography and endoscopy
Esophageal motility	Manometry and motion radiography
Gastroesophageal sphincter function, hiatal hernia, and reflux	Manometry, motion radiography, gastroesophageal scintiscanning, acid perfusion, pH monitoring, endoscopy, and biopsy

From "Evaluation of Swallowing Disorders," by R. Miller, 1984, in *Dysphagia: Diagnosis and Management* (p. 170), by M. E. Groher (Ed.), Boston: Butterworth-Heinemann Publishers. Copyright 1997 by Butterworth-Heinemann Publishers. Reprinted with permission.

A complete bedside clinical assessment should follow the initial screening when so indicated. Logemann lists competencies that are needed by the speech-language pathologists prior to initiating a bedside screening and/or assessment for dysphagia:

> (1) knowledge of the range of normal oral anatomy and range, pattern, and coordination of lips, tongue, jaw, and palate, and (2) the various screening procedures and their appropriateness for various patients, and skills in: (a) eliciting and evaluating oromotor actions for speech and non-speech tasks in various types of patients, and (b) auditory recognition of normal and abnormal articulation and voice. (Logemann, 1998a, p. 25)

A description of the oral cavity assessment for dysphagia is in Table 15–4.

In addition to inpatients, outpatients with idiopathic dysphagia comprise a portion of the caseload for speech-language pathologists. In these cases, the speech-language pathologist should assess the patient's voice, speech, and respiratory functions, and evaluate the oral and pharyngeal stages of the swallow. Referrals should then be made to a physician to determine the underlying cause of the patient's dysphagia (Logemann, 1998a). In many cases, these patients have had "neurologic damage or undiagnosed neurologic disease including brainstem stroke, motor neuron disease, Parkinson's disease, Guillain-Barré, multiple sclerosis, or brainstem tumor" (Logemann, 1998a, p. 18).

TABLE 15–4 Oral cavity assessment for dysphagia
Symmetry at rest
Presence of scar tissue
Dentition
Presence and status of oral secretions
Strength, coordination, and range of motion of lips
Strength, coordination, and range of motion of tongue
Strength, coordination, and range of motion of palate
Function of tongue and lips during spontaneous swallows
Frequency of spontaneous swallows (count swallows in a 5-minute period)
Patient's ability to hold breath for 1, 3, 5, and 10 seconds (to determine patient's ability to tolerate swallowing interventions during treatment; note any stress or difficulty)
Vocal quality and respiratory control during sustained production of /o/
Symmetry of pharyngeal wall motion (elicit gag to observe)
Laryngeal function
Posturing while eating a meal (unless NPO)
Placement of food in the mouth when eating
Signs of aspiration while eating

Neurogenic Dysphagia

The first step in evaluation of neurogenic dysphagia includes taking a thorough history of the patient. When obtaining the history, the clinician should pay particular attention to the temporal pattern of the symptoms. If the symptoms had a sudden onset, the etiology is likely to be a stroke. In contrast, dysphagia associated with myopathy and motor neuron disease typically is gradually progressive (Buchholz, 1997).

Another important step in the diagnosis of neurogenic dysphagia is the distinguishing between pseudobulbar and bulbar palsy. Each of these syndromes is associated with specific diseases. Both bulbar and pseudobulbar palsy result in dysphagia and dysarthria. However, bulbar palsy is a lower motor neuron disorder characterized by weakness in the muscles supplied by the medulla, fasciculations, muscle atrophy, and decreased reflexes. Disorders associated with bulbar palsy include motor neuron disease (amyotrophic lateral sclerosis), myasthenia gravis, Guillain-Barré syndrome, polio, and polymyositis. A comparison of paralytic dysphagia and pseudobulbar dysphagia is in Table 15–5.

Pseudobulbar palsy is a disorder of the upper motor neurons. It is characterized by weakness of the tongue, the pharynx, the larynx, and the face. Patients also exhibit impairment of voluntary functions, with incoordination being out of proportion to the muscle weakness. They also have spasticity and hyperactive gag and jaw jerk reflexes. The speech of these individuals is slow and effortful, with a strained vocal quality. They may also exhibit signs of upper motor neuron problems in their limbs, with signs of hyperreflexia and spasticity. Etiologies of upper motor neuron disorders include motor neuron disease, multiple sclerosis, traumatic brain injury, and bilateral hemispheral strokes (Buchholz, 1997).

Guillain-Barré Syndrome

Guillain-Barré syndrome is a polyneuropathy characterized by "immune-mediated demyelination of peripheral and cranial nerves" (Buchholz, 1997, p. 53). The demyelination may result in subacute weakness and sensory loss affecting the oral cavity, the pharynx, and the larynx. Frequently, the swallowing problems are the first symptoms, with generalized weakness and paralysis following 24–48 hours later (Logemann, 1998). Typically, patients spontaneously recover, although mechanical ventilation and tube feeding may be part of

TABLE 15–5 Differences between pseudobulbar dysphagia and paralytic dysphagia

Factor	Paralytic Dysphagia	Pseudobulbar Dysphagia
Pathology	Lower motoneuron	Upper motoneuron
Swallow reflex	Absent or very weak	Present, slow, or uncoordinated
Intellect	Intact	May be impaired
Oral strength	Poor	May be normal or uncoordinated
Affect	May be labile	Lability is common
Speech	Flaccid dysarthria	Spastic, hypokinetic, or hyperkinetic dysarthria

From "General Treatment of Neurologic Swallowing Disorders" (Chapter 9), by R. M. Miller and M. E. Groher, 1997, in *Dysphagia: Diagnosis and Management* (p. 229), by M. E. Groher (Ed.), Boston: Butterworth-Heinemann Publishers. Copyright 1997 by Butterworth-Heinemann Publishers. Reprinted with permission.

the treatment process. Because these patients are often compromised with regard to their respiratory system, swallowing maneuvers that affect the duration of airway closure should not be implemented until the respiratory system has improved. These patients benefit from gentle range of motion and resistance exercises, use of the supraglottic swallow, and the Mendelsohn maneuver (again, once the respiratory control is improved and stabilized) (Logemann, 1998).

Other Polyneuropathies

Unlike Guillain-Barré syndrome, most polyneuropathies do not involve the cranial nerves. They typically "affect axons in a length-dependent fashion, such that any resulting weakness is predominantly in the distal limbs" (Buchholz, 1997, p. 53). Polyneuropathies are often associated with alcohol abuse or diabetes, and rarely do they result in oral/pharyngeal dysphagia. However, they can affect esophageal functioning if there is involvement of the small unmyelinated nerve fibers that typically mediate autonomic functions. This would include the "vagal branches that innervate the myenteric plexus and regulate distal esophageal motility" (Buchholz, 1997, p. 53), resulting in esophageal dysphagia.

Multiple Sclerosis

Multiple sclerosis (MS) is characterized by "immune-mediated demyelination of nerve fibers in the brain and spinal cord that can result in dysphagia" (Buchholz, 1997, p. 50). Typically, dysphagia occurs when the demyelination affects the corticobulbar tracts or the brain stem pathways involved in regulating swallowing. Individuals with multiple sclerosis often report disturbances in taste sensation in addition to the motor dysfunction of the pharynx and the oral cavity (Buchholz, 1997).

MS patients exhibit assorted swallowing disorders depending on whether the lesions affect single or multiple cranial nerves. The most common findings, based on a study at Northwestern University Medical School, are "delayed pharyngeal swallow and reduction in pharyngeal wall contraction" (Logemann, 1998, p. 337). Treatment is often centered around thermal-tactile stimulation, which heightens sensory input. The improved sensation leads to improvement in triggering the pharyngeal stage of the swallow. Patients with MS who develop dementia and/or cognitive impairments benefit from the implementation of compensatory strategies (Logemann, 1998).

Poliomyelitis and Postpolio Syndrome

"Acute paralytic poliomyelitis is a viral infection that predominantly affects lower motor neurons" (Buchholz, 1997, p. 51). It usually involves the brainstem, resulting in dysphagia. Although poliomyelitis is rare today, there are approximately 250,000 survivors of polio in the United States, with 20% of the survivors complaining of residual dysphagia (Buchholz, 1997). Oral stage dysphagia is characterized by "reduced lingual control of the bolus in chewing and a disturbed pattern of lingual bolus propulsion" (Logemann, 1998, p. 323). Pharyngeal problems include nasal regurgitation caused by reduced velopharyngeal closure, reduced pharyngeal contraction, and unilateral pharyngeal paralysis (Logemann, 1998).

Postpolio syndrome (PPS) is characterized by progressive fatigue, muscle wasting, weakness, and pain. These symptoms typically appear decades after the original infection. Most patients with PPS exhibit "unilateral and bilateral pharyngeal wall weakness, reduced tongue base retraction, and reduced laryngeal elevation resulting in reduced closure of the laryngeal vestibule" (Logemann, 1998, p. 336). As a result of these problems, the patient may have pharyngeal residue following the swallow, putting him or her at risk for aspiration. Since aggressive exercises to treat the swallowing problems will frequently result in muscular fatigue, the teaching of compensatory strategies is the best approach to therapy (Logemann, 1998).

Amyotrophic Lateral Sclerosis (ALS)

ALS results in degeneration of the motor neurons in the spinal cord, the brainstem, and the brain. A progressive disease, ALS typically results in death within 5 years of onset. The disease may involve upper motor neurons or lower motor neurons, or both upper and lower motor neurons. "Upper motor neuron features include spasticity, incoordination, and increased reflexes, whereas lower motor neuron features include muscle wasting, fasciculations, and decreased reflexes" (Buchholz, 1997, p. 50).

Dysphagia complications are prevalent, and may be among the first symptoms, with the patient being diagnosed after seeking medical help for the dysphagia. This is particularly true in patients with corticobulbar involvement. Patients with corticospinal involvement may not show signs of dysphagia until several years following their diagnosis. In fact, in these individuals, weight loss may be the earliest sign of the presence of dysphagia.

Early signs in those patients with corticobulbar involvement typically center on the oral stage of the swallow, with the patient having difficulty lateralizing with the tongue to facilitate chewing and difficulty maintaining a controlled bolus. Initially, the patient may have more difficulty with thick foods, and gradually start to avoid them. Lip closure may also be affected, with the patient exhibiting drooling and spillage of food and liquids from the mouth.

As the disease progresses, the patient may have difficulty triggering the pharyngeal phase of the swallow, with resultant aspiration of food and liquid into the airway on subsequent inhalations. Aspiration from pharyngeal and oral residue is also problematic, even in the early stages of ALS (Logemann, 1998).

Treatment in the early stages can include thermal-tactile stimulation to enhance oral sensation. However, in the later stages, this is ineffective. Typically, the patient shifts to thinner consistencies and liquids. This is acceptable as long as there is airway protection. However, tube feeding may be necessary when the patient can no longer protect the airway (Logemann, 1998).

Parkinson's Disease

Parkinson's disease "involves progressive degeneration of neurons in a number of subcortical and brain stem regions, especially the dopamine-producing neurons of the substantia nigra in the midbrain" (Buchholz, 1997, p. 48). Initial symptoms of Parkinson's disease include tremor at rest, impairment of gait (unstable, shuffling gait), reduced limb movements, and monotone speech. Dysphagia is associated with all three phases of the swallowing process. In fact, aspiration pneumonia is a leading cause of death in patients with Parkinson's disease (Buchholz, 1997; Logemann, 1998).

Based on her own experiences with patients with Parkinson's disease, Logemann (1998, p. 335) describes the sequence of problems in swallowing as follows:

> The progression of swallowing dysfunction in the patient with Parkinson's disease begins with reduction in tongue base retraction and the repetitive rocking-rolling motion of the tongue. Triggering of the pharyngeal swallow may then become delayed. As the disease progresses, the reduction in tongue base movement and pharyngeal contraction may worsen, and laryngeal elevation and closure during swallowing may also become inadequate. A cricopharyngeal dysfunction may also occur.

She also points out that there is tremendous variability in the presence of dysphagia symptoms in patients with Parkinson's disease. Some patients, even in the advanced stages, do not exhibit severe swallowing problems.

Stroke

According to Buchholz (1997), stroke is probably the most common cause of neurogenic dysphagia. Twenty-five percent to 50% result in temporary dysphagia, while in other patients it is a major factor in post-stroke morbidity. This post-morbidity is usually associated with malnutrition and respiratory complications.

Both unilateral and bilateral strokes can result in dysphagia, but there are large differences in the oral and pharyngeal stages of the swallow when the two types of strokes are compared. "It has been reported that left-sided lesions tend to predominantly impair the oral phase and that right-sided strokes are more likely to compromise pharyngeal function and result in aspiration" (Buchholz, 1997, pp. 44–45). A summary of swallowing disorders based on site of lesion is delineated in Table 15–6.

TABLE 15–6 Swallowing disorders by site of lesion

Site	Swallowing Patterns
Unilateral medulla stroke (lower brainstem)	Functional oral control; significant impairment of triggering pharyngeal swallow; poor neuromotor control of pharyngeal swallow; residue in valleculae and pyriform sinuses
Pontine stroke (high brainstem)	Severe hypertonicity; delay in triggering of pharyngeal swallow, or absent pharyngeal swallow; unilateral spastic pharyngeal wall paralysis or paresis; reduced laryngeal elevation; severe cricopharyngeal dysfunction
Subcortical stroke	Mild delays in oral transit time; mild delays in triggering pharyngeal swallow; mild to moderate impairment in timing of neuromuscular components of the pharyngeal swallow; possible aspiration
Cerebral cortex stroke; anterior left hemisphere	Apraxia of swallow ranging from mild to severe; possible oral apraxia; delay in initiating oral swallow; no tongue motion in response to bolus; mild oral transit delays; mild delays triggering pharyngeal swallow
Cerebral cortex stroke; right hemisphere	Mild oral transit delays; pharyngeal swallow delays; delayed laryngeal elevation; aspiration

Based on information in "Neurologic Disorders of Swallowing," by D. W. Buchholz, 1997, in *Dysphagia: Diagnosis and Management* (pp. 37–72), by M. E. Groher (Ed.), Boston: Butterworth-Heinemann Publishers. Copyright 1997 by Butterworth-Heinemann Publishers; and *Evaluation and Treatment of Swallowing Disorders,* by J. A. Logemann, 1998, Austin, TX: Pro-Ed. Copyright 1998 by Pro-Ed.

Brainstem strokes result in dysphagia when any of the following are involved: medullary swallowing centers, trigeminal nuclear complexes, nuclei ambigui, corticobulbar tracts, hypoglossal nuclei, or nuclei tracti solitarii. Small brainstem strokes are difficult to document, even with MRI; therefore, many cases of undiagnosed dysphagia may be related to brainstem strokes. Because of the proximity of the brainstem tracts and nuclei, however, it is not unusual to find disturbances in voice, balance, eye movements, and limb movements.

Stroke-related dysphagia may be missed on an initial examination. However, if a patient demonstrates any of the following, a videofluorographic swallowing study should be done prior to having the patient eat: dysphonia, reduced level of consciousness, abnormal gag reflex; and difficulty managing secretions or food.

The swallowing study can help with decision making related to treatment and management of dysphagia in the post-stroke patient. Frequently, patients with post-stroke dysphagia will experience some spontaneous recovery within days to months, minimizing the need for intervention (Buchholz, 1997).

Mechanical Dysphagia

Acute Inflammations

Acute inflammations that contribute to dysphagia are nonspecific reactions secondary to traumatic insults, chemical irritants, fungi, bacterial agents, or viral agents. In and of themselves, acute inflammations rarely cause significant dysphagia, or dysphagia that lasts over a long period of time. However, they may complicate dysphagia caused by other disorders. Early identification is important because, typically, acute inflammations can be medically treated before they interfere significantly with the oral intake of food. Examples of inflammation include herpes simplex (viral), abscesses, cavities, infection following the extraction of a tooth, lingual tonsillitis, epiglottitis, and acute pharyngitis. Inflammations can also occur in reaction to prolonged and/or excessive use of phenol, some mouthwashes, anesthetic throat lozenges, and aspirin (Groher, 1997).

Macroglossia

An enlarged tongue can negatively affect the propulsion of the bolus in the oral stage of the swallow. Macroglossia may occur "secondary to lymphatic obstruction, secondary to surgery or irradiation, hypothyroidism, mongolism, amyloid deposits, and lymphangiomatous or hemangiomatous processes" (Groher, 1997, p. 78).

Pharyngoesophageal Diverticulum

Also referred to as Zenker's diverticulum, this is an "abnormal muscular outpouching that forms from either above the cricopharyngeal muscle through Killian's dehiscence or below through Laimer's triangle" (Groher, 1997, p. 78). In some patients, this outpouching is associated with esophageal disease. Small diverticuli are usually of no consequence. However, when enlarged, the diverticuli can result in regurgitation of undigested food, feelings of fullness in the neck, bad breath, weight loss, and nocturnal coughing resulting in aspiration (Groher, 1997).

Cancer

Problems secondary to cancer are the leading causes of mechanical dysphagia. They can affect the oral, pharyngeal, laryngeal, and esophageal stages of the swallowing process. Generally speaking, if less than 50% of a structure is excised, it should not significantly interfere with deglutition. However, Groher (1997) warns that this is only a guideline; there is extreme variability among patients due to "preoperative and postoperative health, psychological reaction to the disability, and ability to learn adaptive swallowing techniques" (p. 79).

In addition to the loss of structural function, the clinician needs to be concerned about the loss of sensation in the oral, pharyngeal, and laryngeal structures secondary to surgery, chemotherapy, and irradiation. The effects of sensation deficits can be seen in the patient's efforts to form and control a bolus during the oral stage of the swallow.

Oral lesions may involve the mandible, the maxilla, the floor of the mouth, the anterior tongue, and submental structures (Groher, 1997; Logemann, 1998). Disorders of these structures can affect both the oral and pharyngeal stages of the swallow because of "difficulty with mastication, formation and retention of a bolus, and anteroposterior transport" (Groher, 1997, p. 81). These patients will also be at risk for aspiration. Generally speaking, patients with resections of the tongue often respond fairly well to the development of compensatory movements. However, when there is resection of other structures in conjunction with resection of the tongue, the prognosis is not as promising.

Fleming (1978) defined a hemilaryngectomy as including "unilateral resection of the vocal fold, vestibular fold, ventricle, and superior laryngeal nerve with preservation of the epiglottis" (Groher, 1997, p. 86). Patients who have a hemilaryngectomy may experience some initial dysphagia. Generally speaking, these patients regain their ability to eat orally (Leonard et al., 1972; Weaver and Fleming, 1978). However, Schoenrock and his associates (1972) found that the larynx did not elevate evenly on the excised side, resulting in persistent aspiration in several of their patients. Also, irradiation, chemotherapy, or other complications may negatively affect the recovery of oral feeding.

Weaver and Fleming (1978) describe a supraglottic laryngectomy as typically including resection of "both vestibular and aryepiglottic folds and one or both superior laryngeal nerves" (Groher, 1997, p. 88). Dysphagic complications are common, especially in the first 2–4 weeks following the supraglottic laryngectomy. Aspiration occurs in some patients.

> The eventual severity and duration of dysphagia beyond this period appears to be highly variable, however, partly because not all supraglottic resections remove identical structures, some patients develop postsurgical complications, and some receive either preoperative or postoperative irradiation. While a small majority eventually do swallow with minimal aspiration, resections that compromise the arytenoid cartilages and extend into the piriform sinus and tongue base create significant and sometimes persisting dysphagia. (Groher, 1997, p. 88)

Total laryngectomy can also result in dysphagia. In many of these cases, the cricopharyngeal muscle does not perform as it did preoperatively. Many patients who undergo laryngectomy can tolerate a soft diet after approximately two weeks postoperatively. However, the use of irradiation appears to slow down the recovery process. Irradiation can contribute to a drying of the secretions of the mouth, leading to reduced flow of saliva, and may also result in areas of inflammation that may interfere with swallowing. Many of the patients complain of having difficulty with meats and larger-sized boli. Persistent complaints of dysphagia should be monitored carefully, because they could be the initial signs of a recurrence of the cancer (Groher, 1997).

Tracheostoma Tubes

According to Arms, Dines, and Tinstman (1974), when a tracheostoma tube is in place, the patient is at greater risk for aspiration. Tracheostoma tubes restrict normal elevation of the larynx during the swallowing process. Thus, the glottal protection created by the elevation is lost. In Groher's experience (1997), when a tracheostomy is paired with surgical resection of the head and neck, there is compromised deglutition in addition to the added risk of aspiration. Overinflated cuffed tracheostoma tubes create the risk of an obstructed esophagus caused by pressure placed on the tracheoesophageal wall. These patients are also at risk for aspiration due to spillover of the food that cannot enter the esophagus (Groher, 1997; Logemann, 1998).

Assessment Tools

Ultrasound

The use of ultrasound is limited to visualization of the oral cavity. It cannot be used to examine the pharyngeal stage of the swallow caused by the mix of muscle, bone, and cartilage in the pharynx. With regard to the oral cavity, ultrasound can be used to visualize functioning of the tongue in the oral cavity during swallowing. It can also be used as a biofeedback technique during therapy for oral tongue functioning (Logemann, 1998b).

Blue Dye Test

In the Blue Dye Test, the clinician gives the patient thin liquids, thick liquids, and pureed and mechanical soft foods. However, all the foods and liquids have been dyed blue to enable the clinician to distinguish between the ingested materials and body secretions. The Blue Dye Test is particularly useful in patients who have a tracheostomy. "If the patient loses food out of the tracheostomy during or after a swallow or for a period of time after eating, aspiration is indicated and the need for videofluorographic or definitive diagnostic study identified" (Logemann, 1998, p. 25).

Fiberoptic Endoscopic Examination of Swallowing (FEES)

The purpose of FEES is to observe the condition of the oral cavity and pharynx before and immediately following a swallow with no X-ray exposure. It cannot be used to visualize the oral stage of the swallow, but it does provide assessment of the pharyngeal stage of swallowing. A fiberoptic laryngoscope is placed through the nasal cavity with the tip of the laryngoscope being positioned posterior to the uvula. In this position, the pharynx can be viewed "before the pharyngeal swallow triggers and again when the pharynx relaxes after the swallow" (Logemann, 1998b, p. 54). A rigid scope can also be used, but the patient cannot swallow when the rigid scope is in the mouth.

A disadvantage to videoendoscopy is that the actual swallow cannot be viewed because the pharyngeal structures close around the scope during the swallow. However, the structures prior to and immediately following the swallow can be compared, and inferences about the swallow mechanism can be made. An advantage is that videoendoscopic or FEES evaluations can be recorded on videotape for further evaluation and review. It provides "an excellent superior view of the pharyngeal anatomy, including the relationship between the epiglottis, airway entrance, valleculae, aryepiglottic folds, and pyriform sinuses" (Logemann, 1998b, p. 58). In addition, the patient's ability to do a supraglottic and super-supraglottic swallow can be visualized (prior to the actual swallow) (Logemann, 1998a).

Videofluoroscopy

Videofluoroscopy is an extremely effective tool in the evaluation of the oral and pharyngeal stages of swallowing in the patient who is exhibiting symptoms of dysphagia. Using a standard videotape recorder attached to the fluoroscopic equipment, the image can easily be recorded. Therefore, since videofluoroscopic images can be stored on videotape, it also can be used to evaluate the effectiveness of treatment by comparing studies done pre- and postintervention. Videofluoroscopy can be used to image "(1) oral activity during chewing and the oral stage of swallowing, (2) the triggering of the pharyngeal swallow in relation to position of the bolus, and (3) the motor aspects of the pharyngeal swallow" (Logemann, 1998b, pp. 60–61).

According to Logemann,

> The types of swallows introduced during the videofluorographic study should be selected based on two characteristics: (1) the bolus characteristics that create systematic changes in normal swallowing, including increases in volume and viscosity, as well as (2) the types of stimuli the clinician believes may improve the patient's swallow physiology and thereby eliminate aspiration or significant residue. Since we know that bolus volume and viscosity can cause significant changes in normal swallow physiology, the typical modified barium swallow includes presentation of two to three swallows of 1 ml, 3 ml, 5ml, 10 ml, and cup drinking of thin liquids, as tolerated. Similarly, because bolus viscosity creates significant changes in normal swallow physiology, the patient is typically given thin liquids, pudding-type material, and something requiring mastication such as a Lorna Doone cookie. (Logemann, 1998a, pp. 25–26)

Also, the clinician can use a modified barium swallow to assess the effects of therapeutic changes such as variations in thickness and viscosity, postural changes, and amount changes to see whether there is any change in the swallow function.

Logemann (1998a) also describes the expected outcomes of a modified barium swallow. Specifically, the clinician should be able to identify the anatomic and/or physiologic dysfunctions during the oral and pharyngeal stages of the swallow, and delineate the cause-and-effect relationships of the physiology to the patient's symptoms. The clinician can also test treatment strategies during the study that will allow the identification of procedures to improve the pharyngeal swallow and identify the conditions under which the patient can eat safely. As part of delineating these procedures, the speech-language pathologist can identify the need for non-oral nutrition or supplements due to possible aspiration. Finally, the procedure can be used to determine the need for reassessing the patient (Logemann, 1998a).

Cervical Auscultation

Cervical auscultation can be used to determine the status of a patient's pharyngeal stage of swallowing, as well as its most common dysfunction symptom, aspiration. The clinician places a stethoscope, a small microphone, or an accelerometer against the patient's neck and listens for the sounds of swallowing and respiration. It is possible for the clinician to determine the phase of respiration during which the patient swallows. Actually, there are very few sounds associated with swallowing. However, there is a distinct "click" when the eustachian tube opens up and a "clunk" when the upper esophageal sphincter opens (Logemann, 1998a; Logemann, 1998b).

The advantages of cervical auscultation include the fact that it is noninvasive, equipment is easily available, prolonged sampling periods can be obtained, and there is no need for radiation or contrast studies. The problem with cervical auscultation is that findings have not yet been standardized. Different stethoscopes have different acoustic characteristics. There is no direct visualization of the swallowing mechanism, and there is somewhat limited ability to detect aspiration (Arvedson & Rogers, 1998).

Electromyography (EMG)

Electromyography is a study of the muscles of swallowing through the placement of suction cup, hooked-wire, or surface electrodes. The most frequently used electrodes in swallowing studies are the surface electrodes. EMG can be used to study the muscles of the mouth and of the laryngeal mechanism. It has been shown that electrical activity of the swallowing muscles begins early in the swallow. Therefore, "surface EMG of these muscles has been used as a marker of the onset of swallow" (Logemann, 1998b, p. 63).

In addition to being used as a diagnostic tool, EMG can be used as a biofeedback technique for patients involved in swallowing therapy.

Electroglottography (EGG)

Electroglottography is typically used to track the movement of the vocal folds. It can also be used to track laryngeal elevation, which provides information about the "onset and termination of a pharyngeal swallow" (Logemann, 1998b, p. 64). In addition, like EMG, EGG can be used as a biofeedback system, providing information on the extent and duration of laryngeal elevation during a swallow.

Pharyngeal Manometry

A bolus passes through the pharyngeal stage of the swallow in 0.5–1 second. Therefore, any measurement of the pharyngeal stage must be sensitive to the rapid changes of the pharyngeal mechanism during the swallowing process. Pharyngeal manometry uses solid-state pressure sensors to measure the pressure changes during the pharyngeal swallow.

Pharyngeal manometry allows measurement of intrabolus pressures and the timing of the pharyngeal contractile wave. Pharyngeal manometry also enables indirect examination of the relaxation of the cricopharyngeal muscle by identification of the drop in pressure at the upper sphincter (as measured by a sensor in the sphincter) in relation to the opening of the upper sphincter as seen on videofluorography. (Logemann, 1998b, p. 65)

At this time, pharyngeal manometry is not used as a standard procedure in the diagnosis of swallowing disorders. It is an invasive procedure, and the need to combine it with video-fluoroscopy requires equipment coordination and personnel that exceed that available in most clinics (Logemann, 1998b).

Esophageal Stage Studies

Normally, food progresses through the esophagus in 8–20 seconds via peristaltic action that pushes the bolus through the esophagus until it enters the stomach via the lower esophageal sphincter (Logemann, 1998b).

Esophageal motility studies include scintigraphy, 24-hour pH probes, esophageal manometry, and upper GI radiological series. Scintigraphy involves having the patient eat an egg and toast (or similar food) laced with radioisotopes. The progress of the isotopes through the digestive system is monitored by a gamma camera, confirming or denying the presence of motility and reflux problems in the gastrointestinal tract. The scans can be repeated up to several hours, so delayed emptying of the GI tract and delayed reflux (and subsequent aspiration if present) can be visualized.

Scintigraphy can also be used to measure the amount of aspiration and residue, "but the physiology of the mouth and pharynx is not visualized so that the dysfunctions causing the residue and aspiration are not identified" (Logemann, 1998b, p. 61). While a routine procedure for measuring esophageal and gastrointestinal motility, scintigraphy for studying the oropharynx is not a standard clinical tool (Logemann, 1998b).

A common problem associated with esophageal motility deficits is gastroesophageal reflux disease (GERD). Gastroesophageal reflux is the returning of stomach contents into the esophagus. Modified barium studies are not very effective at showing gastroesophageal reflux. Therefore, a patient with GERD and/or suspected esophageal motility disorders should be referred to a gastroenterologist for further evaluation and treatment (Logemann, 1998b).

Protocols for Dysphagia Assessment

The Clinical Evaluation of Dysphagia (CED)

The CED was developed at the Rehabilitation Institute of Chicago by Cherney, Pannell, and Cantiere in 1994. When a patient is at high risk for aspiration, a prefeeding assessment is done. The prefeeding assessment includes taking a complete history and observing the oral, pharyngeal, and laryngeal functions and structures. The specific areas of assessment are outlined in Table 15–7.

Once the preassessment is complete, the clinician can decide whether to proceed with oral feedings. If the patient can tolerate at least one food consistency, evaluation of the status of the patient's dysphagia can be done.

TABLE 15-7 Prefeeding assessment areas of focus on the Clinical Evaluation of Dysphagia (CED)

1. Medical and nutritional status
2. Respiratory status
3. History of aspiration
4. Type and size of tracheostomy (if present)
5. Level of responsiveness
6. Behavioral characteristics
7. Current feeding methods
8. Positioning
9. Observations of oral motor, pharyngeal, and laryngeal functioning
10. Presence or absence of involuntary and elicited cough
11. Gag reflex
12. Voluntary swallow
13. Other observations
14. Response to stimulation
15. Recommendations and goals

Adapted from *Diagnosis and Evaluation in Speech Pathology* (5th ed.) (pp. 309–310), by W. O Haynes and R. H. Pindzola, 1998, Boston: Allyn and Bacon. Copyright 1998 by Allyn and Bacon. Adapted with permission.

The Fleming Index of Dysphagia

The Fleming Index of Dysphagia was developed by Fleming and Weaver in 1987. It is a computerized index. The patient is asked a series of questions and prompts, and the answers are put into the computer. Each answer is given an impact score, which is combined with program codes and severity ratings to "determine the severity of the dysphagia, the urgency for treatment, and suggestions for patient management" (Haynes & Pindzola, 1998, p. 309).

The BELZ Dysphagia Scale

The BELZ Dysphagia Scale was developed by Longstreth in 1986. The BELZ uses a 0–3 scale and rates 12 different categories. These are outlined in Table 15–8.

TABLE 15-8 Twelve categories rated on the BELZ Dysphagia Scale

1. Clinical swallowing evaluation
2. Otolaryngology examination
3. Cognition/communication status
4. Physical status
5. Pulmonary function
6. Chest X-ray
7. Videofluoroscopic evaluation of swallowing physiology
8. Tracheostomy tube status
9. Diet consistency
10. Tube feeding
11. Respiratory tract treatments
12. Gastrointestinal function

Adapted from *Diagnosis and Evaluation in Speech Pathology* (5th ed.) (p. 309), by W. O Haynes and R. H. Pindzola, 1998, Boston: Allyn and Bacon. Copyright 1998 by Allyn and Bacon. Adapted with permission.

THERAPY FOR SWALLOWING DISORDERS IN ADULTS

Miller and Groher (1997) write that "it is important that the dysphagia specialist become familiar with the clinical pathologic mechanisms of certain disease processes. This should include a thorough understanding of effects on the neuromuscular system, clinical course and expected prognosis, changes that medical or surgical intervention can bring, and potential effects on the patient's learning skills. The interaction of these factors should determine the proper approach to management" (p. 223). Because most patients with dysphagia follow an individual sequence and time table with regard to symptomology, any discussion of treatment should be used only as a guideline and should not be generalized.

One of the first steps in therapy is to establish a viable communication system. Many patients with symptoms of dysphagia may have difficulty producing intelligible speech, or speech may be very tiring. Therefore, an alternative means of communication may need to be implemented. The patient needs to be able to express his needs and wishes with regard to eating in order for a dysphagia treatment program to be successful.

Therapy for swallowing disorders can be direct and indirect. Direct therapy measures should not be used with patients who cannot comprehend and follow directions, or with fatigued patients. In direct therapy, food and/or liquids are used to change the swallow physiology.

> Direct therapy procedures include swallowing maneuvers that are voluntary neuromuscular controls applied to selected aspects of the oropharyngeal swallow. There are four swallow maneuvers: (1) the supraglottic swallow, (2) the super-supraglottic swallow, (3) the effortful swallow, and (4) the Mendelsohn maneuver. (Logemann, 1998a, p. 32)

Indirect therapy is done without food or liquid to minimize the risk of aspiration and its associated sequelae. In indirect therapy, the clinician introduces exercises for the muscle groups used in swallowing and practices specific neuromuscular elements of the swallow (Logemann, 1998a).

Logemann (1998b) states that a number of factors need to be taken into consideration when determining whether to start a dysphagia treatment program:

1. Diagnosis: Some patients (e.g., stroke victims) may regain their swallowing ability with only a few compensation methods being suggested. Others (e.g., motoneuron disease patients) may not be able to tolerate strengthening exercises due to muscle fatigue. Patients with dementia may not be able to follow instructions. Thus, one must know the diagnosis of the patient to determine whether therapy is appropriate, and, if so, what type of therapy will be provided.

2. Prognosis: Patients with sudden-onset damage (e.g., stroke, head trauma, spinal cord injury) or structural damage (e.g., from surgery, irradiation, gunshot wounds, trauma) may benefit from a regimen of therapy. Patients with progressive neuromuscular diseases or other degenerative processes such as dementia may be appropriate patients in the early stages of their disorders, but cease to benefit from treatment in the later stages.

3. Reaction to compensatory strategies: If a patient responds to the use of compensatory strategies, and spontaneous recovery is probable, it may be best to re-evaluate the patient after 3–4 weeks of using compensatory methods than to start an active treatment program.

4. Severity of the patient's dysphagia: Some patients cannot take any food or liquid (other than their own saliva) by mouth. If these patients do not respond to compensatory measures, indirect therapy may be warranted.

5. Ability to follow directions: Some swallowing maneuvers taught in therapy require complex directions that the patient must be able to comprehend. Compensatory measures are often controlled by the caregiver, so it may be possible to implement them even if the patient is unable to follow directions.

6. Respiratory function: The airway closes briefly during a normal swallow. However, patients who have compromised respiratory systems may not be able to tolerate even that brief closure. Thus, if the respiratory function of the patient has been affected, it may be necessary to postpone some procedures until the respiratory status of the patient has improved.

7. Availability of caregiver support: Some patients may need reminders to practice their swallowing maneuvers, and others may need assistance from a caregiver. As with all therapies, the clinician should spend time with the caregiver to determine the extent of support he or she is able to offer.

8. Patient motivation and interest: To succeed in resuming oral feedings, the patient must be motivated enough to participate in the therapy procedures on a regular basis.

Diet

Diet can consist of solids, semisolids, pureed foods, and liquids. Depending on the type of lesion the patient has, the nutritionist and speech-language pathologist can make a dietary plan for each individual patient.

Patients with lower motoneuron disease may have difficulty controlling pureed foods and liquids. Because of weakness of the oral musculature, they may find it difficult to form a bolus and trigger the swallow reflex. They tend to do best with a semisolid diet that has enhanced flavoring, temperature, and texture that can serve as cues to stimulate chewing and swallowing. Solids may become obstructed because of malfunctioning of the cricopharyngeus muscle, so softer foods and liquids will pass into the esophagus more easily than the solids (Miller & Groher, 1997).

A chart delineating food consistencies that are appropriate and inappropriate based on the type of swallowing disorder is found in Table 15–9.

Oral and Non-Oral Feedings

Logemann (1998b) points out two major parameters that affect the decision as to whether a patient can tolerate oral feedings: time needed to swallow a bolus, and the risk of aspiration.

> If the radiographic study indicates that it takes the patient more than 10 seconds for oral and pharyngeal transit time combined to swallow every

TABLE 15–9 Easiest food consistencies and foods to be avoided by patients with each swallowing disorder[a]

Swallowing Disorder	Easiest Food Consistencies	Food Consistencies to Avoid
Reduced range of tongue motion	Thick liquid	Thick foods
Reduced tongue coordination	Thick liquid	Thick foods
Reduced tongue strength	Liquid	Thick, heavy foods
Delayed pharyngeal swallow	Thick liquids and thicker foods	Thin liquids
Reduced airway closure	Pudding and thick foods	Thin liquids
Reduced laryngeal movement contributing to cricopharyngeal dysfunction	Liquid	Thicker, higher viscosity foods
Reduced pharyngeal wall contraction	Liquid	Thicker, higher viscosity foods
Reduced tongue base posterior movement	Liquid	Higher viscosity foods

[a]These consistency categories are necessarily rather gross as we still do not have any definitions of the viscosity ranges that delineate the various food consistencies.

From *Evaluation and Treatment of Swallowing Disorders* (p. 184), by J. A. Logemann, 1998, Austin, TX: Pro-Ed. Copyright 1998 by Pro-Ed. Reprinted with permission.

> consistency of food attempted, but there is no aspiration, the patient may feed by mouth but will need a nonoral feeding to supplement oral feedings and to provide adequate nutrition and hydration. (Logemann, 1998b, p. 195)

Initially, the non-oral feeding may be through a nasogastric tube. However, if the treatment is expected to last longer than 3–4 weeks, the physician may want to do a gastrostomy or jejunostomy tube for the supplemental feedings. Factors to consider in deciding what type of non-oral feeding to use include "(1) the patient's gastrointestinal history, (2) the cost of feedings and insurance coverage, (3) the patient's behavior, (4) the patient's preference, and (5) the patient's medical diagnosis" (Logemann, 1998b, p. 195).

As mentioned previously, the presence of aspiration may also be an indicator that the patient needs a non-oral feeding method. In 1980, Logemann and her colleagues found that patients who were aware that they were unable to swallow any consistency of food with less than 10% aspiration would stop oral feedings voluntarily because of the discomfort of the frequent coughing. On the other hand, patients who were unaware of their aspiration would continue to attempt oral feedings (Logemann, 1998b).

Specific Treatment Procedures

Postural Techniques

Before implementing postural changes, the clinician must first be aware of the patient's physiologic and/or anatomic disorders related to swallowing. Only then can the proper postural compensations be offered. In Table 15–10, postural adaptations to facilitate swallowing are delineated.

Disorder Observed on Fluoroscopy	Posture Applied	Rationale
Table 15-10 Postural techniques successful in eliminating aspiration or residue resulting from various swallowing disorders and the rationale for their effectiveness		
Inefficient oral transit (Reduced posterior propulsion of bolus by tongue)	Head back	Utilizes gravity to clear oral cavity
Delay in triggering the pharyngeal swallow (Bolus past ramus of mandible, but pharyngeal swallow not triggered)	Chin down	Widens valleculae to prevent bolus entering airway; narrows airway entrance; pushes epiglottis posteriorly
Reduced posterior motion of tongue base (Residue in valleculae)	Chin down	Pushes tongue base backward toward pharyngeal wall
Unilateral laryngeal dysfunction (Aspiration during swallow)	Head rotated to damaged side; chin down	Places extrinsic pressure on thyroid cartilage, increasing adduction
Reduced laryngeal closure (Aspiration during swallow)	Chin down; head rotated to damaged side	Puts epiglottis in more protective position; narrows laryngeal entrance; increases vocal fold closure by applying extrinsic pressure
Reduced pharyngeal contraction (Residue spread throughout pharynx)	Lying down on one side	Eliminates gravitational effect on pharyngeal residue
Unilateral pharyngeal paresis (Residue on one side of pharynx)	Head rotated to damaged side	Eliminates damaged side from bolus path
Unilateral oral and pharyngeal weakness on the same side (Residue in mouth and pharynx on same side)	Head tilt to stronger side	Directs bolus down stronger side
Cricopharyngeal dysfunction (Residue in pyriform sinuses)	Head rotated	Pulls cricoid cartilage away from posterior pharyngeal wall, reducing resting pressure in cricopharyngeal sphincter

From *Evaluation and Treatment of Swallowing Disorders* (p. 199), by J. A. Logemann, 1998, Austin, TX: Pro-Ed. Copyright 1998 by Pro-Ed. Reprinted with permission.

Typically, postural modifications are temporary compensations until the patient's swallow improves. However, some patients with structural changes or severe neurological conditions may need to use the postural changes permanently.

Sensory Awareness

"Techniques to improve oral sensory awareness prior to a swallow are generally utilized in patients with swallow apraxia, tactile agnosia for food, delayed onset of the oral swallow, reduced oral sensation, or delayed triggering of the pharyngeal swallow" (Logemann, 1998b, p. 201). The sensory sensation is offered before the patient initiates a swallow in order to alert the central nervous system that a swallow is impending. Logemann (1998b, p. 201) lists six different sensation awareness techniques:

1. Increasing downward pressure of the spoon against the tongue when presenting food in the mouth

2. Presenting a sour bolus

3. Presenting a cold bolus

4. Presenting a larger volume bolus (3 ml or more)

5. Presenting a bolus requiring chewing

6. Thermal-tactile stimulation

The two most commonly used sensory stimulation techniques to trigger the pharyngeal swallow are thermal-tactile stimulation and the suck-swallow procedure. Thermal-tactile stimulation is accomplished by "vertically rubbing the anterior faucial arch firmly, four or five times, with a size 00 laryngeal mirror (which has been held in crushed ice for several seconds) in advance of the presentation of a bolus and the patient's attempt to swallow" (Logemann, 1998b, p. 201). The sensory stimulation increases oral awareness and alerts the cortex and brainstem to expect a quicker triggering of the pharyngeal swallow once the oral stage of the swallow has been initiated.

The suck-swallow is a reflex that normalizes around 6 months of age. However, an exaggerated suck-swallow movement (increased vertical tongue-jaw sucking movements with the lips closed) may trigger a pharyngeal swallow (Logemann, 1998b).

Effortful Swallow

The effortful swallow is used when there is reduced posterior movement of the base of the tongue, with the belief being that the effortful swallow will increase movement of the posterior base of the tongue during the pharyngeal stage of the swallow (Logemann, 1998b). Effortful swallows can be monitored using EMG as a biofeedback device so the patient can visualize the differences in muscle action when using a normal swallow and an effortful swallow (Groher, 1997). During the effortful swallow and during the Mendelsohn maneuver (described below), the duration of the closure of the airway is affected as a side effect of the procedure.

The Mendelsohn Maneuver

The Mendelsohn maneuver is "designed to improve the extent and duration of laryngeal elevation during the swallow and thus to improve the duration and width of cricopharyngeal opening during deglutition" (Logemann, 1998b, p. 63). It can easily be measured using EMG as a biofeedback procedure. The recordings from surface electrodes can be viewed on an oscilloscope screen to reflect the onset and duration of laryngeal elevation (Logemann, 1998b).

The Supraglottic Swallow

The supraglottic swallow voluntarily modifies the airway closure duration by closing the vocal folds before the swallow and during the swallow. This action protects the airway and prevents aspiration.

The procedure requires that the patient be relatively relaxed, alert, and able to follow instructions. The procedure should be practiced while swallowing saliva before the patient is given food to swallow. The procedure can be practiced at bedside prior to giving the patient food and performing the procedure using videofluoroscopy.

The patient is given something to swallow but told to hold it in his mouth while the following directions are being given:

1. Take a deep breath and hold your breath.

2. Keep holding your breath and lightly cover your tracheostomy tube (if a tracheostomy is present).

3. Keep holding your breath while you swallow.

4. Immediately after your swallow, cough. (Logemann, 1998, p. 217)

Patients who have an extended partial laryngectomy or who have bilateral adductor paralysis may have a gap in the glottic closure. Therefore, they may not be able to achieve complete airway protection using the supraglottic swallow. In these cases, it may be necessary to give adduction exercises prior to practicing the supraglottic swallow.

Also, some patients may hold their breath by stopping chest wall movement, and not achieve airway closure. For these patients, Logemann suggests modifying the instructions by telling the patient to "Inhale and then exhale slightly; hold the breath and swallow while holding the breath" (1998, p. 217). An alternative instruction is to have the patient inhale, then say "ah." The patient should then be instructed to stop voicing but to continue holding his breath. This, too, should result in glottal closure (Logemann, 1998).

It is critical to note that the sequence of events follows that of a normal swallow with two major exceptions. The first is that the patient exhales following the swallow instead of inhaling. If the patient were to inhale, he would aspirate. The second difference is that the swallow occurs at the beginning of the exhalation phase of respiration, not at the end. This timing permits an "adequate amount of pulmonary air to help clear the laryngeal aditus. Another swallow must follow to clear any materials pooled in the pharyngeal recesses" (Groher, 1997, p. 276).

The supraglottic swallow can also be used with patients who have reduced tongue mobility or reduced tongue bulk. These patients frequently use chin elevation (head extension) to move the bolus into the pharynx. When assessing these patients, the clinician should give the patient a small amount (1–3 ml) of liquid on a spoon. As the patient moves the liquid into the pharynx, he should be observed "to determine whether (1) the pharyngeal swallow triggers on time and (2) airway closure is sufficient to protect the airway" (Logemann, 1998, p. 218). If the pharyngeal swallow triggers normally, and there is sufficient airway closure, the patient can be given 5 to 10 ml of liquid in a cup and taught the following sequence:

1. Hold the breath tightly.

2. Put the entire 5 to 10 ml of liquid in the mouth.

3. Continue to hold the breath and toss the head back, thus dumping the liquid into the pharynx as a whole.

4. Swallow two to three times or as many times as needed to clear the majority of the liquid *while continuing to hold the breath.*

5. Cough to clear any residue from the pharynx. (Logemann, 1998, p. 218)

The Super-Supraglottic Swallow

Like the supraglottic swallow, the super-supraglottic swallow also modifies the airway closure duration during the swallow. This swallow procedure closes "the entrance to the airway voluntarily by tilting the arytenoid cartilage anteriorly to the base of the epiglottis before and during the swallow and closing the false cords tightly" (Logemann, 1998, p. 219). The patient is instructed to inhale and hold his breath very tightly and to bear down. He is then told to keep holding his breath and bearing down as he swallows. When the swallow is finished, the patient is to cough (Logemann, 1998). Patients who have undergone a supra-glottic laryngectomy and others who have reduced closure of the entrance to the airway may find this procedure useful. The super-supraglottic swallow facilitates swallowing in three ways:

1. It tilts the arytenoid cartilage forward to make contact with the base of the tongue in place of the missing epiglottis.

2. It improves the retraction of the tongue base, the anterior tilt of the arytenoid cartilage, and the adduction of the false vocal folds.

3. It facilitates the rate of laryngeal elevation at the initiation of the swallow.

In conclusion, a variety of diagnostic and therapeutic procedures are available to assess and treat dysphagia in the adult population. To explore each of these procedures is beyond the scope of this book. The reader is referred to the writings of Groher and Logemann (see References) for more complete descriptions of these procedures.

CHAPTER SIXTEEN
Fluency Disorders

DEFINITION/DESCRIPTION

A dysfluency is anything that disrupts the smooth flow of speech. This would include word-finding problems found in aphasia and groping behaviors characteristic of apraxia (Shipley & McAfee, 1992). Every speaker has, at one time or another, experienced some dysfluencies, and this is normal. In Table 16–1 Haynes and Pindzola (1998) summarize the work of Adams in differentiating between normal dysfluency and stuttering.

However, the major focus of this chapter is on stuttering. The major types of stuttering are listed in Table 16–2.

Typically, stuttering has an onset prior to 6 years of age. There have been many theories as to the cause of stuttering, but no one theory has predominated over the years. Stuttering basically consists of brief part-word repetitions and prolongations. The problems may be more pronounced at the beginning of words and in more complex and less frequently used words and phrases. It can be "eliminated or remarkably reduced in a variety of conditions: speaking while alone, choral speaking, singing, prolonged or slow speaking, talking in time to rhythm, or under masking conditions" (Haynes & Pindzola, 1998, p. 221).

Table 16–1	Adams' guidelines for distinguishing between the normally disfluent child and the incipient stutterer	
Criterion	**Normally Disfluent**	**Incipient Stutterer**
Total frequency (all types)	9 or fewer disfluencies per 100 words	10 or more disfluencies per 100 words
Predominate type	Whole-word and phrase repetitions, interjections, and revisions	Part-word repetitions, audible and silent prolongations, and broken words
Unit repetitions	No more than 2 unit repetitions ("b-b-ball")	At least 3 repetitions ("b-b-b-ball")
Voicing and air flow	Little or no difficulty starting or sustaining voicing or air flow; continuous phonation during part-word repetitions	Frequent difficulty in starting or sustaining voicing or air flow; heard in association with part-word repetitions, prolongations, and broken words; more-effortful disfluencies
Intrusion of the schwa	Schwa not perceived ("ba-ba-baby")	Schwa often perceived ("buh-buh-buh-baby")

From *Diagnosis and Evaluation in Speech Pathology* (5th ed) (p. 228), by W. O Haynes and R. H. Pindzola, 1998, Boston: Allyn and Bacon. Copyright 1998 by Allyn and Bacon. Reprinted with permission.

TABLE 16-2 Major types of stuttering	
Repetitions:	part-word, whole-word, phrases
Prolongations:	sound/syllable prolongations, silent prolongations
Interjections:	sound/syllable interjections, whole word interjections, phrase interjections
Silent Pauses:	a silent duration within speech considered abnormal
Broken Words:	a silent pause within words
Incomplete Phrases:	grammatically incomplete utterances
Revisions:	Changed words, ideas

From *Clinical Methods and Practicum in Speech-Langauge Pathology* (2nd ed.) (p. 324), by M. N. Hegde and D. Davis, 1995, San Diego, CA: Singular Publishing Group. Copyright 1995 by Singluar Publishing Group. Reprinted with permission.

DSM-IV DIAGNOSTIC CRITERIA FOR 307.0 STUTTERING

A. Disturbance in the normal fluency and time patterning of speech (inappropriate for the individual's age), characterized by frequent occurrences of one or more of the following:

(1) sound or syllable repetitions

(2) sound prolongations

(3) interjections

(4) broken words (e.g., pauses within a word)

(5) audible or silent blocking (filled or unfilled pauses in speech)

(6) circumlocutions (word substitutions to avoid problematic words)

(7) words produced with an excess of physical tension

(8) monosyllabic whole-word repetitions (e.g., "I-I-I-I see him")

B. The disturbance in fluency interferes wtih academic or occupational achievement or with social communication.

C. If a speech-motor or sensory deficit is present, the speech difficulties are in excess of those usually assoicated with these problems.

Coding note: If a speech-motor or sensory deficit or a neurological condition is present, code the condition on Axis III.

ASSESSMENT

The first step in stuttering assessment is to take a complete history. The history should include a written history by the client (or his parents if a minor), an interview with the client, and information from other professionals if available. Contributing factors should be addressed. This would include any medical or neurological problems the client may have, and noting the family history since there appears to be a familial component to stuttering. Background about the development of the disorder should also be noted.

The assessment process should then move to an oral-facial examination to rule out any neurological disorders such as apraxia and dysarthria. The next steps include a hearing screening, a speech sample, and tests for stimulability.

The speech sample can consist of spontaneous conversation, or asking a client to describe pictures or tell a brief story for 2–3 minutes. Since some individuals are dysfluent in some situations and not others, it may be worthwhile to collect a speech sample in several different situations and/or sites. The sample(s) should then be analyzed for the frequency of different types of stuttering, the total number of dysfluencies, the duration of the specific instances of stuttering, associated motor behaviors (secondary behaviors), and rate of speech (Shipley & McAfee, 1992).

A form for recording the frequency count for dysfluencies is in Appendix 16–A. The frequency count should then be used to determine the dysfluency indexes. There are three types of indexes: Total Dysfluency Index, Individual Types of Dysfluencies Index, and percentage of each type on the Total Dysfluency Index. To calculate the Total Dysfluency Index, follow these procedures:

1. Count the total number of words in the speech sample.

2. Count the total number of dysfluencies in the speech sample.

3. Divide the total number of dysfluencies by the total number of words.

To calculate the Individual Types of Dysfluencies Index, one would count the number of specific types of dysfluencies (for example, the number of prolongations) and divide that number by the total number of words in the speech sample (and convert the answer to a percentage). Finally, the Total Dysfluency Index is used to reflect the percentage of each dysfluency type in the speech sample. In this case, one divides the number of specified dysfluencies by the total number of dysfluencies in the speech sample, then changes the resultant number to a percentage. In addition, prolongations can be timed.

Finally, the client's feelings, attitudes, and reactions to his speech should be discussed with the client. If the client is a child, the parents' reactions, attitudes, and feelings should also be determined. The parent can complete the form in Appendix 16–B by changing "I" to "My child." The form in Appendix 16–C can help to decipher specific instances in which the stutterer has trouble.

All this information should be taken into consideration to determine whether therapy is to be undertaken.

TREATMENT

Haynes and Pindzola (1998) propose four different treatment options:

1. *Environmental treatment:* This treatment option consists of modification of the daily environment through the significant others. The clinician and significant others work to structure the environment to facilitate fluency. In this format, the significant others meet regularly with the clinician to discuss the modifications and their results and to plan new modifications if so warranted. Some of these modifications may include how the

significant others react to the stuttering instances. Clinicians can also give instructions in altering the pace and organization of the client's environment. The clinician does not work directly with the client. This approach is particularly applicable to young children who stutter.

2. *Combined environmental therapy with direct, modified therapy:* Also appropriate for use with children, this approach may use individual therapy, but in all likelihood will also include group therapy. In therapy, conditions known to typically reduce stuttering (e.g., choral speaking, singing, speaking to a rhythm) are implemented so that the client experiences easy, fluent speech. In addition, if the client is a child and has a language delay, this issue is also incorporated into therapy. Sometimes, improving the child's linguistic abilities will result in improvement of the stuttering behaviors as well.

3. *Combined environmental therapy with direct therapy:* Depending on the extent of the stuttering and the age of the client, individual and/or group therapy may be used. In direct therapy, the clinician deals directly with the stuttering behaviors, targeting specific treatment techniques to improve the stuttering. These techniques include, among others, rate control, airflow management, easy onset, slow speech, breathy speech, and soft glottal attack. The environmental manipulations continue to be a part of this approach (Haynes & Pindzola, 1998).

4. *Direct therapy:* This is similar to combined environmental therapy with direct therapy, except that no environmental manipulations are done. The therapy focuses on mastering the strategies and techniques used to establish fluency. This technique is useful if the client's stuttering has progressed to a point that environmental manipulation is no longer therapeutic, or if there are no significant others who can actively participate in modifying the environment (Haynes & Pindzola, 1998).

Description of therapy techniques:

1. *Regulated breathing and continuous airflow:* The clinician should model the breathing style for the client. First, inhale through the nose, taking a slightly deeper breath than is typical for regulated breathing, and a deeper breath for continuous airflow. Exhale a small amount of air through the mouth prior to initiating phonation. Use a slow, gentle, soft initiation of phonation after the exhalation has started. Using the same approach, work through words, phrases, and sentences. Gradually withdraw the modeling (Hegde, 1996).

2. *Continuous phonation:* The purpose of this approach is to maintain phonation throughout the utterance. It may be combined with prolonged speech, airflow management, and gentle phonatory onset. The client is instructed to maintain phonation throughout the utterance, slightly blurring the word boundaries. The clinician should begin with short phrases and progress to longer sentences (Hegde, 1996).

3. *Gentle phonatory onset:* This involves the use of "soft, easy, slow, and relaxed initiation of sounds as against harsh, abrupt, and tensed initiation" (Hegde, 1996, p. 249). It may be combined with airflow management and/or rate reduction.

4. *Rate reduction:* The client is encouraged to use a speech rate that is slower than his baseline rate. First, establish the baseline rate in terms of the number of syllables or words per minute. Model the reduction of rate by prolonging vowels (as opposed to

increasing pause durations). Ask the client to imitate the prolonging of vowels to reduce his rate of speech. Gradually withdraw the modeling. If the client is not successful, combine the rate reduction with delayed auditory feedback.

5. *Delayed auditory feedback:* Delayed Auditory Feedback (DAF) is a widely used method of controlling stuttering, although it tends to produce unnatural-sounding speech. The client "hears his own speech after a delay introduced by a mechanical device" (Hegde, 1996, p. 241). The client typically wears the device (although desktop versions are available). The clinician and client should experiment with different delays to find one that produces stutter-free speech (usually around 250 milliseconds of delay). The client should begin with responding to questions from the clinician using 2–3 word phrases or short sentences. If the client still stutters, try using single words or oral reading until he gets used to the delayed feedback. The client should use slow, prolonged speech with the DAF. Gradually move up to sentences and conversational speech, then begin to reduce the amount of feedback in 50-millisecond intervals (or less if the client is unable to maintain stutter-free speech). When the client is no longer using the delay, work toward developing prosodic speech. Offer booster sessions when necessary (Hegde, 1998).

6. *Counseling:* Counseling is an indirect therapy procedure that can be combined with any other approaches to therapy. The clinician should be an empathetic, noncritical listener. The client should be allowed to explore and express his feelings about his stuttering and his expectations regarding therapy. There are numerous checklists (see Appendix 16–B) available in which a client can mark those situations that create the most problems and/or anxieties with regard to his speech. The items checked off can serve as a "jumping off" point at which to begin the discussion of his speech. Help the client to concentrate on his strengths and positive feelings. Together, the clinician and the client should explore actions that create and negate stuttering behaviors and discuss ways to eliminate or reduce those behaviors that contribute to the stuttering (Hegde, 1996).

APPENDIX 16–A: FREQUENCY COUNT FOR DYSFLUENCIES

Name: _____ Age: _____ Date: _____

Examiner: _____

Instructions:
Make a check (√) on the appropriate line each time the corresponding dysfluency is produced.

Repetitions   Totals

   Part-word _____

   Whole-word _____

   Phrase _____

Prolongations

   Sound _____

   Silent _____

Interjections

   Sound/syllable _____

   Whole-word _____

   Phrase _____

Silent Pauses _____

Broken Words _____

Incomplete Phrases _____

Revisions _____

From *Assessment in Speech-Language Pathology* (p. 231), by K. G. Shipley and J. G. McAfee, 1992, San Diego, CA: Singular Publishing Group. Copyright 1992 by Singular Publishing Group. Used with permission.

APPENDIX 16–B: THE MODIFED S-SCALE[1]

Instructions: Answer the following by circling "T" if the statement is generally true for you, or circle "F" if the statement is generally false for you. If the situation is unfamiliar or rare, judge it on an "If it was familiar . . . " basis.[2]

1. T F I usually feel that I am making a favorable impression when I talk.
2. T F I find it easy to talk with almost anyone.
3. T F I find it very easy to look at my audience while talking in a group.
4. T F A person who is my teacher or my boss is hard to talk to.
5. T F Even the idea of giving a talk in public makes me afraid.
6. T F Some words are harder than others for me to say.
7. T F I forget all about myself shortly after I begin to give a speech.
8. T F I am a good mixer.
9. T F People sometimes seem uncomfortable when I am talking to them.
10. T F I dislike introducing one person to another.
11. T F I often ask questions in group discussions.
12. T F I find it easy to keep control of my voice when speaking.
13. T F I do not mind speaking before a group.
14. T F I do not talk well enough to do the kind of work I'd really like to do.
15. T F My speaking voice is rather pleasant and easy to listen to.
16. T F I am sometimes embarassed by the way I talk.
17. T F I face most speaking situations with complete confidence.
18. T F There are few people I can talk with easily.
19. T F I talk better than I write.
20. T F I often feel nervous while talking.
21. T F I often find it hard to talk when I meet new people.
22. T F I feel pretty confident about my speaking abilities.
23. T F I wish I could say things as clearly as others do.
24. T F Even though I knew the right answer, I have often failed to give it because I was afraid to speak out.

---

[1]From "Stuttering therapy: The relation between changes in symptom level and attitudes," by G. Andrews and J. Cutler, 1974, *Journal of Speech and Hearing Disorders, 39*, pp. 312–319. Copyright 1974 by ASHA. Reprinted with permission.

[2]Note that items 4, 5, 6, 9, 10, 14, 16, 18, 20, 21, 23, and 24 are presumed to be true for people who stutter; the other items are presumed to be false.

APPENDIX 16–C: ASSESSMENT OF ASSOCIATED MOTOR BEHAVIORS

Name: _____ Age: _____ Date: _____

Examiner: _____

Instructions:

Check all associated motor behaviors the client exhibits. Use the right hand column to describe behaviors or record frequency counts.

Eyes

_____ blinking _____

_____ shutting _____

_____ upward movement _____

_____ downward movement _____

_____ vertical movement _____

_____ other (specify) _____

Nose

_____ flaring _____

_____ dilation _____

_____ wrinkling _____

_____ other (specify) _____

Forehead

_____ wrinkling/creasing _____

_____ other (specify) _____

Head

_____ shaking _____

_____ upward movement _____

_____ downward movement _____

_____ lateral movement to the right _____

_____ lateral movement to the left _____

_____ other (specify) _____

Lips

_____ quivering _____

_____ pursing _____

_____ invert lower lip _____

_____ other (specify) _____

Tongue

_____ clicking _____

_____ extraneous movement _____

_____ other (specify) _____

Teeth

_____ clenching _____

_____ grinding _____

_____ clicking _____

_____ other (specify) _____

Jaw

_____ clenching _____

_____ opening _____

_____ closing _____

_____ other (specify) _____

Neck

_____ tightening _____

_____ twitching _____

_____ upward movement _____

_____ downward movement _____

_____ lateral movement to right _____

_____ lateral movement to left _____

_____ other (specify) _____

Fingers

_____ tapping _____

_____ rubbing _____

_____ clenching _____

_____ excessive movement _____

_____ clicking _____

_____ other (specify) _____

Hands

_____ fist clenching _____

_____ wringing _____

_____ splaying _____

_____ other (specify) _____

Arms

_____ excessive movement _____

_____ banging against side _____

_____ banging against leg _____

_____ jerky movement _____

_____ tensing _____

_____ other (specify) _____

Leg

_____ tensing _____

_____ kicking _____

_____ rapid movement _____

_____ other (specify) _____

Breathing

_____ speaking on little air _____

_____ unnecessary inhalation _____

_____ jerky breathing _____

_____ audible inhalation _____

_____ audible exhalation _____

_____ dysrhythmic _____

_____ other (specify) _____

Others (describe) _____

_____

_____

_____

_____

From _Assessment in Speech-Language Pathology_ (pp. 234–237), by K. G. Shipley and J. G. McAfee, 1992, San Diego, CA: Singular Publishing Group. Copyright 1992 by Singular Publishing Group. Used with permission.

CHAPTER SEVENTEEN
Hearing Loss

DEFINITION/DESCRIPTION

Conductive Hearing Loss

The loss that occurs as the result of any interference with the transmission of sound from the external auditory meatus to the inner ear is called a conductive hearing loss. In a conductive hearing loss, there is no problem with the inner ear. Rather, the sound vibrations are not sent to the cochlea, and the cochlea is not stimulated (Northern & Downs, 1974). In conductive losses, sounds transmitted by bone conduction are within normal limits. Oftentimes, conductive hearing losses are associated with the presence of otitis media and otitis media with effusion. Thus, conductive hearing losses are frequently treated medically (antibiotics and decongestants) and surgically (the insertion of PE tubes). Some conductive losses resolve spontaneously, although "some residual of the pathologic condition may remain for long periods of time" (Northern & Downs, 1974, p. 31). In adults, otosclerosis and ear canal collapse are the most common etiological factors in conductive hearing losses. Other causes include external otitis (inflammation of the external auditory meatus), aural atresia (closing of the external auditory meatus), and stenosis of the external auditory canal (Shipley & McAfee, 1998).

Sensorineural Hearing Loss

Sensorineural hearing losses are caused by damage to the sensory end organ or the cochlear hair cells. They are also the result of damage to the acoustic (VIII) nerve. With the use of electrocochleography, differentiation between a sensory loss and a neural loss can be determined. Since the problem in a sensorineural loss is with the inner ear, sounds transmitted by air conduction and by bone conduction are almost the same (within 10 dB of each other). In other words, you do not see the air-bone gap that is apparent in conductive or mixed hearing losses. Unlike conductive hearing loss, sensorineural hearing losses are irreversible (Northern & Downs, 1974).

Causes of sensorineural hearing loss include ototoxicity caused by drugs (including certain antibiotics and drugs containing high levels of aspirin), infections (i.e., meningitis or maternal rubella), and genetic factors. When syphilis is contracted during birth, or if the baby is deprived of oxygen during the birth process, a sensorineural hearing loss may result. Age-related changes and presbycusis also can be etiological factors in sensorineural hearing loss. Individuals suffering from Ménière's disease may also exhibit a sensorineural loss. The loss from Ménière's disease is typically a unilateral hearing loss associated with tinnitus and vertigo (Shipley & McAfee, 1998).

There are three characteristics typically associated with sensorineural hearing loss. The first one is shouting or talking in a loud voice. Because the individual with a sensorineural hearing loss does not hear his own voice (or the voices of others) normally, he may speak with increased volume. Some people learn to regulate their speech volume.

A second characteristic is poor word discrimination ability. Because there is a loss of nerve fiber, speech is distorted, and the individual has difficulty with word discrimination tasks. Individuals with sensorineural hearing loss typically have better hearing in the lower frequencies. Because many consonants contain high-frequency information, the person with a sensorineural hearing loss may not be able to hear and discriminate between consonant sounds. Because vowels contain low-frequency information, they are not as problematic for the individual (Roeser & Downs, 1988).

Recruitment is the third characteristic of sensorineural hearing loss. Recruitment is "an abnormal, rapid growth in loudness once the threshold of hearing has been crossed. After the signal is intense enough to be perceived, any further increase in intensity may cause a disproportionate increase in the sensation of loudness" (Roesser & Downs, 1988, p. 15). This is why people with sensorineural hearing loss have more difficulty hearing in noisy surroundings than do people with conductive hearing loss or normal hearing.

Mixed Hearing Loss

A mixed hearing loss is a combination of a conductive loss and a sensorineural loss. In a mixed hearing loss, both bone and air conduction are affected, although typically the bone conduction is better than the air conduction. The sensorineural component of a mixed hearing loss results in the presence of speech distortion, even if the speech is amplified. The bone conduction audiogram is the best predictor of the amount of the speech distortion.

Central Auditory Processing Disorder

A central auditory processing disorder is the result of damage "somewhere along the auditory nerve or within the cochlear nuclei" (Shipley & McAfee, 1998). As a result, the client will have difficulty localizing sound and understanding speech. Many patients also complain of tinnitus. Typically, the hearing acuity is within normal limits.

Conservative estimates are that 3–5% of the school-age population have some degree of a central auditory processing disorder. Furthermore, Holston (1992) believes that a higher percentage of central auditory processing disorders occurs in children with learning disabilities than in the general population. The prevalence figures may be low because many children with learning disabilities are not referred for central auditory processing testing. Auditory processing refers to "auditory processing that begins at the level of the cochlear nuclei in the brain stem, ascending ultimately to the cortex" (Wallach & Butler, 1994, p. 383).

> Individuals with central auditory processing problems have normal hearing acuity and intelligence, but are unable to process auditory information effectively. Most authorities report that central auditory processing disorders

cause difficulties in detection, interpretation, and categorization of sounds and that these problems may be cue to some type of dysfunction in lower or higher level cortical processes. (Vinson, 1999, pp. 184–185)

Language-based learning disabilities, dyslexia, attention deficit disorder, attention deficit disorder with hyperactivity, and central auditory processing disorders often present with similar symptomatology. Thus, it is advisable to rule out central auditory processing deficits before proceeding with the diagnosis and treatment of these other disorders. It should be pointed out that any of these disorders may co-occur with central auditory processing disorders.

Retrocochlear Pathology

According to Bess and Humes (1995), retrocochlear pathology "involves damage to the nerve fibers along the ascending auditory pathways from the internal auditory meatus to the cortex. This damage is often, but not always, the result of a tumor" (Shipley & McAfee, 1998, p. 405). Tests of speech recognition, auditory brainstem response (ABR) tests, and other auditory evoked potentials can be used to identify retrocochlear pathology. Typically, these individuals "perform poorly on speech recognition tasks, particularly when the speech signal is altered by filtering, adding noise, and so forth" (Shipley & McAfee, 1998).

Prelingual and Postlingual Hearing Loss

Prelingual and postlingual refer to the timing of the hearing loss. Hearing loss that is sustained before the child develops language is known as prelingual hearing loss. Hearing loss that occurs after the child develops language is called a postlingual hearing loss. It is critical that a prelingual hearing loss be diagnosed as early as possible so that early intervention can begin and help the child take advantage of any residual hearing he may have. According to Crystal and Varley (1993), 95% of children born deaf have some residual hearing. Early intervention includes proper amplification, environmental stimulation, and training the child to use his residual hearing.

The effects of hearing loss are dependent on the following factors:

> the type of loss; the dB levels and frequencies affected; age of onset; the client's age when the loss was diagnosed; previous intervention (e.g., therapy or educational placement, type of intervention, communication mode); medical intervention (e.g., ongoing, sporadic, etc.); the client's intelligence; the client's motivation; the client's general health; care and stimulation provided by caregivers. (Shipley & McAfee, 1998, p. 406)

The severity of a hearing loss is based on the levels (in decibels) at which the client responds to a pure tone. These levels are depicted in Table 17–1.

In addition to testing hearing acuity, the audiologist and speech-language pathologist should both be involved in testing central auditory processing, which measures how well the client processes information received through the auditory modality.

TABLE 17-1 Hearing thresholds and severity of hearing loss	
Average Hearing Level (in dB)	*Severity of Hearing Loss*
–10 to 15	**Normal hearing**
16–25	**Slight hearing loss**
26–40	**Mild hearing loss**
41–55	**Moderate hearing loss**
56–70	**Moderately severe hearing loss**
71–90	**Severe hearing loss**
91+	**Profound hearing loss**

From "Uses and Abuses of Hearing Loss Classification," by J. G. Clark, 1981, *Asha, 23*, pp. 493–500. Copyright 1981 by the American Speech-Language-Hearing Association. Reprinted with permission.

ASSESSMENT

The Audiogram

On an audiogram, the most frequently used symbols when thresholds are established are:

X = left ear, unmasked, air conduction (earphones)

O = right ear, unmasked, air conduction (earphones)

☐ = left ear, masked, air conduction (earphones)

Δ = right ear, masked, air conduction (earphones)

> = left ear, unmasked, bone conduction (mastoid)

< = right ear, unmasked, bone conduction (mastoid)

] = left ear, masked, bone conduction (mastoid)

[= right ear, masked, bone conduction (mastoid)

A variety of other symbols are also used depending on whether or not the patient responds and the type of stimulus. These are depicted in Table 17–2.

Screening

Screening can be used to rule out possible hearing loss but not to reach a diagnosis of hearing loss. A typical screening is done at 20 dB or 25 dB at 1000 Hz, 2000 Hz, and 4000 Hz. It is recommended that children be screened at 15 dB at 500 Hz, 1000 Hz, 2000 Hz, 4000 Hz, and 8000 Hz so that the clinician does not miss a mild loss. ASHA regulations also require tympanometry as part of a hearing screening protocol.

Pure Tone Audiometry

Pure tone audiometry can be done by air conduction or by bone conduction. In air conduction testing, the tones are presented either by earphones or in a sound field setting. In both

TABLE 17-2 Symbols commonly found on audiograms

Recommended set of symbols for those cases when thresholds are measured.

Response

MODALITY	EAR		
	LEFT	UNSPECIFIED	RIGHT
AIR CONDUCTION—EARPHONES			
UNMASKED	X		O
MASKED	☐		△
BONE CONDUCTION—MASTOID			
UNMASKED	>	∧	<
MASKED	]		[
BONE CONDUCTION—FOREHEAD			
UNMASKED		∨	
MASKED	⌈		⌉
AIR CONDUCTION—SOUND FIELD	✳	$	∅
ACOUSTIC—REFLEX THRESHOLD			
CONTRALATERAL	⊃		⊂
IPSILATERAL	⊢		⊣

Recommended set of symbols for those cases when no responses are elicited.

No Response

MODALITY	EAR		
	LEFT	UNSPECIFIED	RIGHT
AIR CONDUCTION—EARPHONES			
UNMASKED	X↘		↙O
MASKED	☐↘		↙△
BONE CONDUCTION—MASTOID			
UNMASKED	⌇	⇡	⌇
MASKED	⌇↓		⌊
BONE CONDUCTION—FOREHEAD			
UNMASKED		∨	
MASKED	⌊		⌋
AIR CONDUCTION—SOUND FIELD	✳↘	$↓	∅
ACOUSTIC—REFLEX THRESHOLD			
CONTRALATERAL	⊃↓		↓⊂
IPSILATERAL	⊢↓		↓⊣

From "Guidelines for Audiometric Symbols," *Asha* (April, 1991, Supplement No. 2), *32*(4), pp. 25–30. Copyright 1991 by the American Speech-Language-Hearing Association. Reprinted with permission.

cases, the client sits in a soundproof audiometric booth and attends to the presentation of a tone that is either constant or pulsed. The audiologist typically starts presenting the tone around 30 dB and increases the decibels in 10 dB increments, or lessens the decibels in 5 dB increments until a threshold of responsiveness is established. The tones are presented at 125 Hz, 250 Hz, 500 Hz, 1000 Hz, 2000 Hz, 4000 Hz, and 8000 Hz. The results of the testing are recorded on an audiogram that reflects at which decibels the client responded to each tone.

In bone conduction testing, the signals are presented at the same frequencies at varying decibel levels until a bone conduction threshold is established. The difference is in the presentation of the tone. In bone conduction testing, a single bone conduction oscillator is placed behind the ear on the mastoid bone. In bone conduction testing, both inner ears (cochlea) are stimulated simultaneously. If a hearing loss is present, it may be necessary to mask the ear that is not being tested. The results of the bone conduction testing are scored on the audiogram with the air conduction testing.

Tympanometry

Tympanometry is used to test middle ear function. Specifically, the "purpose of tympanometry is to determine the point and magnitude of greatest compliance of (mobility) of the tympanic membrane" (Shipley & McAfee, 1998, p. 416). On a tympanogram, the Y axis (the vertical axis) is used to measure compliance, and the X axis (the horizontal axis) is used to measure pressure (in mm H_2O).

Tympanograms are classified on the basis of pressure, compliance, and shape.

Pressure is shown by the location of the peak. A normal peak can mean otosclerosis, ossicular chain discontinuity, tympanosclerosis, or a cholesteatoma in the attic space. No peak, or a flat line, indicates a perforated tympanic membrane.

Compliance is shown by the height of the peak. Increased amplitude reflects an eardrum abnormality or ossicular chain discontinuity. A reduced amplitude is indicative of otosclerosis, tympanosclerosis, tumors, or serous otitis media. A normal amplitude indicates eustachian tube blockage or early acute otitis media.

Shape is shown by the slope of the peak. Reduced slope is indicative of otosclerosis, ossicular chain fixation, otitis media with effusion, or a tumor. Increased slope is seen in cases of eardrum abnormality or ossicular chain discontinuity. If the shape is not smooth, this could indicate vascular tumors, patulous eustachian tube, ossicular chain discontinuity, or an eardrum abnormality.

Types of Tympanograms

Tympanograms are of one of the following types:

Type A = Normal pressure and compliance functions

Type B = A flat tympanogram, which indicates there is fluid in the middle ear

Type C = Retracted tympanic membranes with a shift to the negative side; may be indicative of otitis media or blockage of the eustachian tube

Type A_S = A shallow tympanogram which may indicate otosclerosis or tympanosclerosis

Type A_D = A deep tympanogram, which could be indicative of a flaccid tympanic membrane or ossicular chain discontinuity

Speech Audiometry

Speech audiometry is the evaluation of a client's ability to hear and understand speech, and, when appropriate, to determine the effects of amplification. The client wears headphones through which words are spoken or delivered by a tape through the audiometer. Adults are instructed to either repeat or write down the target words. Children may point to pictures of the target words. The two findings of speech audiometry are the Speech Reception Threshold (SRT) and Speech Recognition scores. Speech Reception Thresholds may also be referred to as Spondee Thresholds (ST). A Spondee Threshold is the lowest decibel level at which a client can correctly identify a series of two-syllable words 50% of the time. These two-syllable words contain syllables that are equally stressed, and are called spondees. Table 17–3 contains a list of commonly used spondees.

TABLE 17-3 Commonly used spondaic words			
baseball	airplane	birthday	grandson
railroad	hotdog	armchair	hothouse
toothbrush	cowboy	schoolboy	workshop
outside	playground	duckpond	pancake

"The main function of the ST is to confirm the pure tone thresholds; in addition, it serves as a reference for the level at which word discrimination testing is performed" (Roeser & Downs, 1988).

A pure tone average is the average of pure tone thresholds at 500 Hz, 1000 Hz, and 2000 Hz. An SRT is considered to be within normal limits when it is within ± 6 dB from the pure tone average (Shipley & McAfee, 1998).

Word discrimination scores reveal the client's ability to recognize words. The audiologist selects a comfortable decibel level that is above the speech reception threshold. The client then repeats a series of words presented by the audiologist. These words may be single words, or they can involve choosing the correct word from similar sounding pairs of words (Shipley & McAfee, 1998). A normal score is 90–100% correct, and a score of 50–60% is considered to be poor discrimination (Roeser, 1988).

Behavioral Observation Audiometry (BOA), Conditioned Orientation Reflex Audiometry (COR), and Visual Reinforcement Audiometry (VRA)

BOA, COR, and VRA are all audiometric tests that can be used with infants and/or difficult-to-test children. All three tests involve placing the child in the sound-treated room. In BOA, stimuli are presented in sound field through calibrated speakers. The child is observed for reactions, such as looking for the source of the sound, awakening from a light sleep, ceasing ongoing activity, changing his facial expression, or vocalizing. The lack of a response is not necessarily considered significant, but the presence of a response is of considerable significance (Martin, 1994). Also of significance could be the child's reaction to the cessation of an ongoing sound.

Depending on the technique used, the child can be reinforced for his responses. In 1961, Suzuki and Ogiba developed a procedure known as conditioned orientation reflex (COR). In COR, the child is placed between and in front of two speakers through which the tone is introduced. When the child looks toward the source of the sound, he is rewarded by an illuminated doll on the appropriate speaker. Initially, the light and the tone are presented simultaneously to condition the child to look toward the speaker that is the source of the sound. Once the response is conditioned, there is a delay between the sound and the light so that the light becomes a reinforcer after the child looks at the sound source.

Visual reinforcement audiometry (VRA) is based on the same principles as COR. However, VRA may be used with the child hearing the tone through earphones as well as in sound field, and speech is used in addition to pure tones (Martin, 1994).

Central Auditory Processing Disorders

A central auditory processing disorder can be defined as "a difficulty in processing the acoustic speech signal that interferes with accurate and efficient perception of speech" (Sloan, 1991, p. 35). A team approach should be used in diagnosing central auditory processing disorders, with the team members including an audiologist, a speech-language pathologist, the classroom teacher, and the parents of the child being assessed. The role of the speech-language pathologist should be to determine why the child is having academic difficulties, using tests based on information processing, task analysis, and multimodality comparisons of information processing. The role of the audiologist is to determine the site of the lesion within the auditory pathway and to assess the child's ability to understand speech in a variety of conditions (Wallach & Butler, 1994).

According to Keith (1988), there are three assumptions that underlie testing for central auditory processing deficits:

1. A conglomeration of tests that assess auditory memory, auditory closure, auditory discrimination, auditory figure-ground perception is necessary.

2. The auditory system is redundant. "Therefore, it is necessary to reduce and manipulate the redundancies by filtering, alternating between the right and left ears, compressing the message, lowering the signal-to-noise ratio, and presenting competing noise in the opposite or same ear" (Vinson, 1999, p. 186).

3. It is difficult to determine whether the central auditory processing disorder contributes to the language disorder, or whether the language disorder causes the central auditory processing disorder. Thus, diagnostic information should be interpreted very carefully when labeling a child and determining eligibility for services (Northern & Downs, 1991).

Musiek, Geurkink, and Kietel (1984) listed seven tests that could be used to assess central auditory processing. These are outlined in Table 17–4.

TABLE 17–4 Tests used to assess central auditory processing

Test	Explanation
Rapid Alternating Speech Perception (RASP)	The listener repeats simple sentences that alternate every 300 ms between the right and left ears.
Binaural Fusion	The listener repeats spondees presented binaurally but filtered such that the low frequencies are presented to one ear and the high frequencies to the other ear.
Low Pass Filtered Speech (LPFS)	The listener repeats monosyllabic CVC words passed through a filter that rejects energy above 500 Hz. The words are presented monaurally.
Staggered Spondaic Word Test (SSW)	The listener repeats spondees whose onsets are staggered between the two ears such that the last half of the first word and the first part of the second word are dichotic while remaining portions are presented in isolation to opposite ears.
Competing Sentences	Two different sentences are presented simultaneously, one to each ear. The target sentence is at 35 dB SL while the competing sentence is at 50 dB SL.
Dichotic Digits	Two different digits are presented simultaneously, one to each ear (dichotically).
Frequency Patterns	The listener detects which of three tones presented in succession is a different frequency.

TREATMENT

Digital Hearing Aids

A digital hearing aid is defined by Martin (2000) as "an amplification system in which the input signal is stored, as by a computer, as sets of binary digits that represent the frequency, intensity, and temporal patterns of the input acoustical signal" (Martin, 2000, p. 416).

There are two types of digital hearing aids: the Digital Signal Processing (DSP) hearing aid that was originally marketed in the 1980s, and the Digitally Controlled Analog (DCA) hearing aid. Analog means "that the signal is processed in a manner that is continually varying over time" (Stach, 1998, p. 490). This differs from digital in that digital refers to representation of a signal as "discrete numeric values as discrete moments in time" (Stach, 1998, p. 490). The original DSP hearing aid did not gain widespread acceptance due to battery consumption, the size of the device, and other technological constraints (Stach, 1998).

DCA hearing aids were introduced about the same time but were more accepted than the DSP hearing aids. The main advantage to DCA hearing aids is that they have enhanced flexibility because they are programmable. This permits remote "fine tuning" of the hearing aid using an "interface that communicates with a personal computer or dedicated hearing aid programmer" (Stach, 1998, p. 492). Another advantage is that the hearing aid has a greater range of output. This is because the DCA hearing aid contains a variety of matrices that can be programmed for use by the hearing aid. This is in contrast to a conventional hearing aid that contains only a single amplifier matrix. Flexibility is also increased in that DCA hearing aids have a greater number of controls than does a conventional hearing aid. For example, a conventional hearing aid may have only one or two controls, whereas the DCA hearing aid has "separate controls for on-off, gain control, frequency response, compression parameters, output limiting, and other characteristics" (Stach, 1998, p. 492).

In a DSP hearing aid, the "analog signals from the microphone are converted into digital form by an analog-to-digital converter. Once in digital form, the signals are manipulated by sophisticated processing algorithms and then converted back to analog form by digital-to-analog conversion" (Stach, 1998, p. 492). DSP hearing aids have an advantage over more traditional models in that they provide "more precise and flexible frequency shaping, better acoustic feedback reduction, more sophisticated compression algorithms, and enhanced noise reduction" (Stach, 1998, p. 493).

Conventional Hearing Aids

The four most common styles of conventional hearing aids include the behind the ear (BTE), in-the-ear (ITE), in the canal (ITC), and completely in the canal (CIC) models. BTE hearing aids are used for mild to severe hearing losses. Canal hearing aids are typically used for milder hearing losses but can also be used for hearing losses ranging from mild to moderately severe (Stach, 1998; Martin, 2000).

Another style is the body-type hearing aid. The body-type hearing aid contains a microphone, an amplifier, circuit modifiers, and a battery compartment within a case. The case can be clipped to the client's clothing or worn in a pocket or special pouch. Advantages of the body-type hearing aids are that the controls are easy to adjust because they are larger than those in the smaller hearing aids, and the batteries last longer. Also, because of the separation of the microphone and the receiver, there is less acoustic feedback. Disadvantages include the cosmetic aspect and frequent breakage of the cords. Also, when worn under clothing, the rubbing of the clothes against the microphone results in a competing noise. Because of advances in hearing aids worn over and in the ear, very few people choose to use body-type aids (Martin, 2000).

The BTE hearing aid hangs behind the ear by a plastic hook that fits over the top of the ear. The BTE consists of a microphone, amplifier, and receiver. A microphone/telephone off (MTO) switch and volume control are typically mounted on the back side of the hearing aid, with other controls being concealed behind a removable plate that is on the underside of the casing. The tubing that holds the hearing aid in place also serves as a conduit between the hearing aid receiver and the earmold. The earmold is custom designed to fit into the auricle and serves to conduct sounds from the earhook and tubing into the external auditory meatus. Frequency gain characteristics can be altered through modifications to the earmold and tubing (Stach, 1998).

ITE hearing aids are custom-made to fit into the concha of the auricle. This hearing aid also contains a microphone, amplifier, and receiver. "The microphone port is located on the hearing aid faceplate. This provides an advantage over BTE hearing aids in that the microphone is located in a more natural position on an ITE. This advantage increases with ITC and CIC devices" (Stach, 1998, p. 496). The MTO switch and volume control switch are located on the faceplate of the ITE. If it is a DCA or DSP hearing aid, the interface connection is also on the faceplate. Other controls typically are located on the inside surface of the casing or in the battery compartment (Stach, 1998).

ITC hearing aids are similar to the ITE hearing aid, but smaller. The ITC hearing aid fits into the canal and extends into the concha only minimally (Stach, 1998).

CIC hearing aids are barely visible because they do not extend into the external auditory meatus. The lateral end of the hearing aid fits 1–2 mm inside the opening of the ear canal, and it ends near the tympanic membrane. The microphone port and other controls for a CIC hearing aid are on the faceplate. There is also typically a small filament that protrudes from the faceplate and is used to remove the hearing aid from the canal. In some models, the filament is attached to the volume control to allow easier manipulation of the volume by the client (Stach, 1998).

Choosing between the different types of hearing aids is a cosmetic decision for some clients. However, there are several other factors that govern which hearing aid a client selects. Some of these factors are summarized in Table 17–5.

Cochlear Implants

A cochlear implant is not a hearing aid because it does not amplify sound. Instead, the cochlear implant bypasses the damage to the cochlea and directly stimulates the auditory nerve. The cochlear implant is surgically implanted in patients with profound sensorineural hearing loss. Specifically, adults with postlingual hearing loss and children with either a congenital or postlingual hearing loss can benefit from a cochlear implant. A profound hearing loss is the result of a loss of hair cell functions in the cochlea. The hair cell dysfunction

TABLE 17-5	Factors in hearing aid style selection
Factor	*Explanation*
Acoustic feedback	When amplified sound from a loudspeaker is rerouted back into the microphone, feedback (whistling) occurs. Thus, the greater the separation between the microphone and the loudspeaker, the less the feedback.
Venting	Two problems typically occur with canal hearing aids. One is that normal aeration of the canal is reduced and can lead to problems with external otitis. The other problem is that the insertion of the hearing aid into the canal results in further hearing loss. To resolve these problems, a bore, or vent, is made in the earmold or the hearing aid so that sound and air can be transmitted through the canal.
Device size	More and larger electronic components can be placed in larger hearing aids. Thus, there is enhanced flexibility in the use of the hearing aid the larger the aid. However, with DSP technology, this is no longer an issue.
Durability	Canal hearing aids are less durable due to the effects of perspiration and cerumen on the components of the hearing aid.
Deep insertion	CIC hearing aids present more acoustic advantages because their use does not interfere with the influences of the auricle and concha, and because they are closer to the tympanic membrane. This is particularly important in the transmission of high-frequency sounds. There is also less wind noise, and it is easier to use the telephone.

Adapted from *Clinical Audiology: An Introduction* (pp. 498–501), by B. A. Stach, 1998, San Diego, CA: Singular Publishing Group. Copyright 1998 by Singular Publishing Group. Adapted with permission.

leads to a lack of generation of neural impulses so that electrical activity of the auditory nerve is not initiated. Thus, the purpose of the cochlear implant is to stimulate the auditory nerve (Stach, 1998).

A cochlear implant consists of an internal part and an external device. The internal part is made up of a receiver and a wire electrode (Ross, Brackett, & Maxon, 1991). The internal receiver, consisting of a tiny coil and wire electrodes, is placed under the skin in the mastoid process behind the pinna. "Active electrodes are placed 22 to 24 mm into the scala tympani within the cochlea. Ground electrodes are placed outside the bony labyrinth, often in the temporalis muscle" (Martin, 1994, p. 441). The external portion consists of a small microphone that is attached to an earhook and worn behind the ear, a signal processor that is worn on the body, and a stimulator that fits over the receiver (Ross, Brackett, & Maxon, 1991). Electrical impulses are fed from the microphone to a speech processor. The speech processor then codes the speech information to be transmitted to the electrode array. The auditory signal goes from the processor to a transmitter, and the transmitter converts the signal to magnetic impulses. The magnetic impulses are then sent to the electrodes. "An electrical signal is induced from the magnetic field in the cochlea and flows on to stimulate the auditory nerve" (Martin, 1994, p. 441).

There are two types of cochlear implants: single channel systems and multichannel systems. In the multichannel system, "22 active electrodes rest in the inner ear, and the processor is individually tuned to provide the most salient signal in all 22 channels" (Ross, Brackett, & Maxon, 1991, p. 207).

Cochlear implants have advantages over hearing aids because they have "better high-frequency hearing, enhanced dynamic range, better speech recognition, and no feedback-related problems" (Stach, 1998, p. 508).

Assistive Listening Devices (ALDs)

ALDs usually are "not used as general purpose amplification devices; rather, they are used as need-specific amplification in a particular environment or listening situation" (Stach, 1998, p. 501). Examples of ALDs include telephone amplifiers, television listeners, FM systems, and personal amplifiers. Like hearing aids, ALDs consist of a microphone, an amplifier, and a receiver. However, the microphone is separated from the amplifier and receiver. This helps to narrow the gap between the listener and the signal source (Stach, 1998).

Some clients may use ALDs to supplement their hearing aids, particularly individuals with a severe hearing loss. Other clients may use ALDs instead of a hearing aid if their hearing problems are limited to specific situations such as listening in church or when watching television. A third category of individuals who use ALDs are those whose hearing problems are related to processing instead of acuity. In other words, the hearing problem is associated with a central nervous system disorder (central auditory processing disorder). For these individuals, "enhancement of signal-to-noise ratio is more appropriate than amplification from a conventional hearing aid" (Stach, 1998, p. 502).

Personal FM Systems

Personal FM systems consist of two parts: a microphone-transmitter and an amplifier-receiver. The microphone-transmitter is worn by the speaker, and the amplifier-receiver and headphones are worn by the listener. Via FM radio waves, the signals are sent from the transmitter to the receiver. The personal FM system provides enhancement of the signal-to-noise ratio, bridging the gap between the speaker and the listener. Detaching the microphone from the receiver provides an advantage in settings such as church, classrooms, restaurants, theaters, and parties.

Personal Amplifiers

According to Stach (1998), a personal amplifier "consists of a microphone that is connected to an amplifier box, usually by a cord. The microphone is held by the person who is talking. The signal is then routed to a small case, which is often about the size of a deck of cards. The box contains the battery, amplifier electronics, and volume control. The loudspeaker is typically a set of lightweight headphones or an ear-bud transducer" (pp. 505–507). As with the FM system, the microphone is separated from the amplifier, which enhances the signal-to-noise ratio. Personal amplifiers are typically used as a substitute for a conventional hearing aid when the individual does not have access to his hearing aid or when the client is in an acute listening situation (Stach, 1998).

Other ALDs

Closed captioning and text telephones are among the most popular ALDs. Text telephones allow the message to be sent by typing. Other ALDs include alarm clocks, fire alarms, and doorbells that either flash a light or vibrate a bed when they are activated. Telephone amplifiers of assorted types are also heavily used ALDs (Stach, 1998).

Intervention in Central Auditory Processing Disorders

The treatment of central auditory processing disorders requires a team approach with the involvement of the child's teacher, the audiologist, a speech-language pathologist, and the child's family. A team approach is particularly critical since some children with central auditory processing disorders present with the same symptomatology as children with attention deficit disorder (ADD), attention deficit disorder with hyperactivity (ADDH), language-based learning disabilities, or dyslexia. Therefore, some of the therapy techniques used for each of these disorders may also be used in the treatment of central auditory processing disorders (CAPD). The team needs to work together to make a definite and precise diagnosis and to recommend the appropriate intervention.

Procedures to strengthen environmental localization, sound sequencing, memory tasks, sound blending, and discrimination of speech in the presence of background noise are some specific targets that have been developed for children with CAPD. Some of these same tasks are used in children with language-based learning disabilities and ADD.

The Auditory Discrimination in Depth program was developed by Lindamood and Lindamood in 1969 and still is in use. According to Willeford and Burleigh, the Lindamoods' program was devised "for developing the function of the ear in monitoring correspondence between the contrasts, sequences, and shifts of our spoken language and the sets of graphic symbols which represent them" (Willeford & Burleigh, 1985, p. 123). The Auditory Discrimination in Depth program has four levels of activities:

1. Gross level: includes activities that focus on problem-solving techniques and gross discrimination of sounds;

2. Oral-aural level: focuses on auditory discrimination of sounds, consonant/vowel changes in syllable patterns, and changes in syllable combinations;

3. Sound-symbol level: geared toward the orthographic representation of the phonemes;

4. Coding level: includes activities focusing on the coding of nonsense syllables into graphic and oral patterns and generalization into words (Willeford & Burleigh, 1985).

In addition to the Lindamood program, there are several programs available for treating central auditory processing disorders. Most of them have in common the teaching of auditory discrimination of speech-sound contrasts in phonetic sequences of increasing difficulty (Sloan, 1991).

Use of FM Systems

An FM system for classroom use consists of a receiver that the child wears and a microphone that is worn by the teacher. The system provides amplification of the teacher's voice without amplifying the ambient noise in the classroom.

Other Suggestions for Classroom Modification

Other suggestions for modifying the classroom to accommodate children with CAPD include the following:

1. Provide the child with preferential seating so that he is in the optimal auditory and visual location in the classroom.

2. The teacher should use visual aids, particularly when teaching a new concept.

3. Rephrase any information the child does not appear to be comprehending.

4. Instruct the teacher to speak clearly and use gestures if they are not distracting to the child.

5. Instruct the teacher to ask short, simple questions and to have the child repeat the question before providing the answer.

6. Isolate key words to help the child focus on the information or question being presented.

7. Teach reading using a phonics approach.

8. Include auditory activities in the curriculum that emphasize memory, sequencing, rhythm, and discrimination (Barr, 1972).

CHAPTER EIGHTEEN
Language Disorders in Children

DEFINITION/DESCRIPTION

When discussing language functioning in children, one must distinguish between a language delay, a language disorder, and a language difference. A language delay means that the acquisition of normal language competencies occurs at a slower rate than would be expected given the child's level of functioning and chronologic age. A language disorder refers to a disruption in the learning of language behaviors and skills. A language disorder typically encompasses the use of language constructs that would not be considered a normal part of developing linguistic skills. Language differences refer to "language behaviors that are not in concert with those of the person's primary speech community or native language" (Vinson, 1999, p. 4).

Language delays and disorders can be described based on the features of language (semantics, morphology, phonology, pragmatics, syntax) or based on etiology (specific syndromes, mental retardation, autism, etc.). Those based on etiology are described elsewhere in this book. The assessment and treatment of language disorders based on the features of language are described in this chapter.

DSM-IV DIAGNOSTIC CRITERIA FOR 315.31 EXPRESSIVE LANGUAGE DISORDER

A. The scores obtained from standardized individually administered measures of expressive language development are substantially below those obtained from standardized measures of both nonverbal intellectual capacity and receptive language development. The disturbance may be manifest clinically by symptoms that include having a markedly limited vocabulary, making errors in tense, or having difficulty recalling words or producing sentences with developmentally appropriate length or complexity.

B. The difficulties with expressive language interfere with academic or occupational achievement or with social communication.

C. Criteria are not met for Mixed Receptive-Expressive Language Disorder or a Pervasive Developmental Disorder.

D. If Mental Retardation, a speech-motor or sensory deficit, or environmental deprivation is present, the language difficulties are in excess of those usually associated with these problems.

Coding note: If a speech-motor or sensory deficit or a neurological condition is present, code the condition on Axis III.

DSM-IV DIAGNOSTIC CRITERIA FOR 315.32 MIXED RECEPTIVE-EXPRESSIVE LANGUAGE DISORDER

A. The scores obtained from a battery of standardized individually administered measures of both receptive and expressive language development are substantially below those obtained from standardized measures of nonverbal intellectual capacity. Symptoms include those for Expressive Language Disorder as well as difficulty understanding words, sentences, or specific types of words, such as spatial terms.

B. The difficulties with receptive and expressive language significantly interfere with academic or occupational achievement or with social communication.

C. If Mental Retardation, a speech-motor or sensory deficit, or environmental deprivation is present, the language difficulties are in excess of those usually associated with these problems.

Coding note: If a speech-motor or sensory deficit or a neurological condition is present, code the condition on Axis III.

ASSESSMENT

The lack of universal screening measures for speech and language development in preschoolers is an ongoing problem that delays the identification of many children until they achieve school age. However, there are numerous measures available for the assessment of children beginning at birth. The purpose of this chapter is to address the assessment and treatment of speech and language disorders in children.

Lund and Duchan (1998) list five major objectives of the assessment process in Table 18–1.

The assessment process can be defined as the process of interviewing, observing, and testing an individual to determine the nature, extent, and severity of his or her language disorder,

TABLE 18–1   Five major objectives of the assessment process
1. Determine whether or not the child has a language disorder, a language delay, or a language difference
2. Identify etiological factors
3. Identify weaknesses in the child's use of language
4. Describe the strengths in the child's language behaviors
5. Make the appropriate recommendations for the child

Adapted from *Assessing Children's Language in Naturalistic Contexts*, by N. Lund and J. Duchan, 1988, Englewood Cliffs, NJ: Prentice-Hall, as cited in *An Introduction to Children with Language Disorders* (p. 417), by V. Reed, 1994, Boston: Allyn and Bacon. Copyright 1994 by Allyn and Bacon.

TABLE 18-2	Diagnostic process based on the scientific model
Scientific Model	*Diagnostic Process*
Definition and delineation of the problem	**Constituent analysis** a. **Definition/delineation of the clinical problem** b. **History** c. **Normal vs. abnormal**
Develop hypothesis to test	**Clinical hypothesis: Derivation of cause and/or effect relationships**
Research design: Develop procedures to test hypothesis	**Clinical design: Planning the diagnostic session; measurable plan to systematically observe and measure behaviors**
Collection of data	**Clinical testing** a. **Is tool appropriate?** b. **Control stimuli presentation** c. **Control responses** d. **Rapport** e. **Efficient data collection**
Analysis of data	**Clinical data analysis: Objective categorization of data in relationship to cause-effect hypothesis**
Interpretation of data to support or reject the hypothesis	**Clinical interpretation to:** a. **Determine the meaning and significance of the results** b. **Support/reject the hypothesis** c. **Vital for referral** d. **Look at whole picture** e. **Logical interpretation**
Conclusions: Generalize data	**Conclusions: Patient management**

Based on information from *Diagnosis of Speech and Language Disorders* (2nd ed.) (pp. 55–62), by J. E. Nation and D. M. Aram, 1984, San Diego, CA: College-Hill Press. Copyright 1984 by College-Hill Press.

delay, or difference (Vinson, 1999, p. 51). Nation and Aram (1984) have developed a model for diagnosis of communication disorders based on the scientific model of research. The steps of this model are outlined in Table 18–2.

The first step encompasses the case history and initial interview with the caregivers of the child. The first and most critical questions to be addressed are, "Why are you here?" and "What do you expect me to answer as a result of this session today?" Both of these questions provide a baseline from which the clinician can approach the diagnostic process. The first question, "Why are you here?" gives the clinician a good reading as to the family's understanding of the possible language deficit. The second question, "What do you expect me to answer as a result of this session today?" lets the clinician know the primary concern of the family. Also, the family is more likely to feel like the evaluation session was worthwhile and productive if the clinician is sure to answer the primary questions the family has. Another function of these two questions is to empower the family to be a part of the assessment process. "No matter how much knowledge a clinician has, it is important to remember that the clinician's knowledge relates to the disorder and the academic aspects of the process. Just as important is the fund of knowledge the family has about their child" (Vinson, 1999, p. 55).

TABLE 18-3 Questions to determine the communication environment and status of a child

1. What are the child's communication abilities at this time?

2. For what purposes does the child communicate at this time?

3. What are the demands and expectations in the child's daily environment?

4. How does the child interact with his or her environments?

5. Is there any difference in how the child communicates in one environment as opposed to other environments?

From *Language Disorders across the Lifespan* (p. 56), by B. P. Vinson, 1999, San Diego, CA: Singular Publishing Group. Copyright 1999 by Singular Publishing Group. Reprinted by permission.

A third critical question in the history-gathering phase of the assessment process is, "How does the child communicate now?" The answer to this question can improve the effectiveness of the communication exchanges between the child and the clinician. It is also important to assess the communication environment of the child in answering this question. The questions outlined in Table 18–3 can help determine the communication environment and status of the child.

The development of a clinical hypothesis constitutes the second step of the diagnostic process. Based on the history, what does the clinician believe to be the problem? Is the speech and/or language problem a delay, a disorder, or a difference? What may be at the root of the speech and/or language deficit?

Third, the clinician must plan the diagnostic process. The driving question at this stage of the assessment process is "What tests and procedures will be used to determine the nature and extent of the child's language deficiencies?" (Vinson, 1999, p. 57). If the wrong tools for assessment are chosen, the clinical hypothesis will remain untested, and the diagnostic questions unanswered. Questions to guide test selection are listed in Table 18–4.

Step four of the assessment process is the actual testing and observing of the child—collecting the data. This aspect of the process may involve screening of speech and language prior to a complete assessment. A screening is "the administration of short tests in order to determine if a child's language is within normal limits or if he or she needs to be referred for a complete diagnostic process" (Vinson, 1999, p. 63). A screening test at the beginning of an assessment procedure may help the clinician decide what additional tests to administer.

TABLE 18-4 Questions preceding test selection

1. What is the purpose of the test?

2. Has the test been validated for this purpose?

3. What is the standardization group?

4. Are the characteristics of the patient similar to those of the sample group?

5. Are there any data or experiences to support differing performances across cultural groups (age, sex, socioeconomic status, geographic location)?

6. Would different values, experiences, behaviors, or other factors affect any of the responses?

From *Language Disorders across the Lifespan* (p. 58), by B. P. Vinson, 1999, San Diego, CA: Singular Publishing Group. Copyright 1999 by Singular Publishing Group. Reprinted by permission.

Table 18–5 Types of receptive tasks		
Type	*Used For*	*Potential Limiting Factors*
Identification tasks (child selects a picture in response to the examiner's questions)	Lexicon Morphology	Child can use guessing or use a process of elimination; may be more a test of recognition than comprehension
Acting out using schemes, role play, and scripts; child manipulates toys and objects in response to the examiner's directions	Semantics Morphology Pragmatics Syntax Comprehension	Have to be careful that the child is truly responding to the examiner's questions, and not performing tasks that he knows due to real-world familiarity with the item (the monster scared the boy; the boy scared the monster)
Judgment tasks: child makes formal judgment of the suitability of a word word or sentence—examiner makes a statement, and the child responds if the statement is wrong or right, silly or OK, and so forth	Semantics Syntax Lexicon Morphology	Very difficult for children under 4 years as it requires processing of the word or sentence's form independent of the meaning (requires metalinguistic skills)

From *Language Disorders across the Lifespan* (p. 63), by B. P. Vinson, 1999, San Diego, CA: Singular Publishing Group. Copyright 1999 by Singular Publishing Group. Reprinted by permission.

For example, a screening test may help the clinician decide whether to focus more on receptive language or expressive language.

There are different types of expressive and receptive language tests. These are outlined in Tables 18–5 and 18–6. Receptive tests assess linguistic knowledge; that is, what does the child know?

Expressive tasks test linguistic performance, or how well the child uses his linguistic knowledge. Standardized and nonstandardized tests can be used to assess the child's language. The decision as to which to use may be dictated by the child's level of expressive language as explained in the next section of this chapter.

The fifth step of the diagnostic process is to analyze the data. Standardized tests will yield standard scores, percentile levels, age scores, and/or grade scores that can be used to compare the child's performance to that of his age-level peers. However, just as important (if not more important) is an analysis of the items the child missed. The question that begs to be asked is, "Why did the child miss or pass this item?" There could be numerous explanations for why a child misses (or gets) a particular test item. The results of this type of analysis can be summed up in a four-box system (Table 18–7) to interpret the findings from the diagnostic tests and procedures.

Regardless of whether the information is gained through standardized tests, criterion-referenced tests, observation, or interview, the information can be entered into the four-box system. The strengths can then be easily amassed and applied to improving the weaknesses.

Step six involves the interpretation of the assessment data. At this point, the clinician is testing the clinical hypothesis and determining whether there are any cause-and-effect statements that can be made regarding the child's speech and language skills. Interpretation addresses the question, "Now that the data are gathered and analyzed, what do they mean?" Careful interpretation of the data will form the foundation of the recommendations.

TABLE 18-6 Types of expressive tasks		
Type	*Used For*	*Potential Limiting Factors*
Elicited imitation tasks; examiner says a sentence, and the child repeats it	Semantics Syntax Morphology Rule out auditory memory problems	Works on the assumption that if a child does not use a particular construction in his or her speech, he or she will omit it in imitation
Delayed imitation tasks: show child 2 pictures and say, "The man sees the boy; the man sees the boys. Which one is this?"	Semantics Syntax Morphology	Works on the assumption that if a child does not use a particular construction in his or her speech, he or she will omit it in imitation
Carrier phrase task: Child completes incomplete sentences spoken by the clinician	Semantics Morphology Lexicon	Child can fail if there is an auditory memory deficit
Parallel sentence production tasks: place 2 pictures in front of child. Examiner describes first one, and child describes second one using a similar format	Semantics Syntax Lexicon Morphology	Works on the assumption that if a child does not use a particular construction in his or her speech, he or she will omit it in imitation
Analysis of spontaneous language sample: child and clinician engage in spontaneous conversation which is recorded mechanically and later analyzed by the clinician	Semantics Syntax Lexicon Morphology	Getting a sample with an adequate number of utterances

From *Language Disorders across the Lifespan* (p. 64), by B. P. Vinson, 1999, San Diego, CA: Singular Publishing Group. Copyright 1999 by Singular Publishing Group. Reprinted by permission.

TABLE 18-7 A four-box system to interpret findings from diagnostic tests and procedures		
	Non-communicative	Communicative
Strengths		
Weaknesses		

From *Language Disorders across the Lifespan* (p. 71), by B. P. Vinson, 1999, San Diego, CA: Singular Publishing Group. Copyright 1999 by Singular Publishing Group. Reprinted by permission.

Making conclusions and recommendations constitutes the seventh step of the assessment process. The clinician should share the information obtained from the tests with the family of the child. Even if the test has not yet been scored, information on the types of items missed and passed should be shared with the family. It is also helpful to ask whether that information is an accurate reflection of the child's typical abilities based on their own observations. A helpful question at this stage is, "What do you need to know from me at this point?" The answer to this question will guide the clinician as to how much information the family members are willing and able to receive. Also, remember that in the preassessment interview the family was empowered to be part of the diagnostic team. At this point in the process, the clinician and family should decide together the appropriate recommendations.

Another part of the concluding phase is the writing of the diagnostic report. This is further discussed in the Documentation section under Professional Issues. However, it bears repeating at this point that the diagnostic report may be all that a referral source knows about the referring clinician. In other words, if the clinician decides to refer the child to another professional, the report should precede the child's visit to that professional. In many instances, the clinician and the professional to whom the child is being referred may not know each other personally. Thus, the clinician is known by that professional only by the quality of the referring report. Thus, it is of utmost importance that the report be written in a succinct manner with no grammatical or spelling errors.

Assessment for Children at the Nonverbal, Single-Word, and Early Multi-Word Level

Nonverbal Children

McCathren, Warren, and Yoder (1998) "identify four proven predictors of later language development in prelinguistic children: (1) use of babbling, (2) development of pragmatic functions, (3) vocabulary comprehension, and (4) the development of combinatorial/symbolic play skills" (Haynes & Pindzola, 1998, p. 89). Two tests that address these specific variables are the *Communication and Symbolic Behavior Scales* (Wetherby & Prizant, 1993) and *Assessing Prelinguistic and Early Linguistic Behaviors in Developmentally Young Children* (Olswang, Stoel-Gammon, Coggins, & Carpenter, 1987).

With nonverbal children, the clinician will be unable to use most standardized testing instruments. Thus, it may be necessary to rely on observational checklists, parental interview, case history forms, and informal assessment procedures.

First, the clinician should determine the child's developmental level. Does the child use gestures or any other nonverbal means to control his environment? What is the level of the child's play skills? Is the child at the presymbolic or symbolic level?

Second, the clinician should determine (often by ruling out) that the child has the biological substrates necessary for language development. Specifically, the clinician should delineate the child's medical history, social history, neurological status, and audiometric capabilities.

Third, the clinician should observe the child interacting with his caretakers. As part of this observation, the clinician should create an inventory of the child's communicative intents. Does he show negation, and, if so, what types and how often? Does he initiate interactions? Is he a passive or an active communicator? Does he show objects and wait for comments?

A vocalization analysis should also be done. A phonemic inventory should be taken of the sounds the child is able to produce (as in babbling or jargon). If the child is using any sound combinations, they should be documented and analyzed for the syllable shape (CV, VC, CVC).

Cognitive analysis can be done using play, observational checklists, and screening tasks. Examples of observational checklists include the *Uzgiris and Hunt Infant Scales of Psychological Development* (Uzgiris & Hunt, 1975) and the *Early Communication Checklist* (Lombardino, Stapell, & Gerhardt, 1987). The Early Communication Checklist is included in Appendix 18–B of this chapter.

Finally, the clinician should assess the child's lexical comprehension by simple tasks such as selection of pictures and/or objects from an array of at least three items, having the child follow directions, and asking the parents for information they have regarding their child's ability to understand what they say (Haynes & Pindzola, 1998).

Single-Word Level

This level of development is also difficult to assess using standardized measures. Basically, the evaluation should follow the same format as that for a nonverbal child. However, in addition to those tasks, a phonological analysis of the child's lexicon and transitional elements should be done.

Typically, a child develops a vocabulary of approximately 50 words prior to beginning to combine words. This allows an adequate sample of words to determine the child's phonological processes using tests such as the *Khan-Lewis Phonological Analysis* (Khan & Lewis, 1986) of the *Goldman-Fristoe Test of Articulation* (Goldman & Fristoe, 1986) or the *Assessment of Phonological Processes–Revised* (APP-R) (Hodson, 1986).

An analysis of the child's lexicon should be done, reflecting the number of words the child uses and the different grammatical types of words the child uses. A form/function analysis would also be beneficial in determining the functions that are served through the child's lexicon. Finally, an analysis of the transition elements the child is using in preparation for the use of multi-word combinations should be done (Haynes & Pindzola, 1998).

Early Multi-Word Combinations

All the analyses and testing mentioned previously should be done in addition to an analysis of the word combinations used by the child in terms of their syntax and their functions. A child at this level should be able to participate in some standardized testing such as that listed in Appendix 18–A.

Speech/Language Samples

A speech/language sample should contain a minimum of 100 utterances, with up to 200 being recommended by some clinicians (Lahey, 1988). It is suggested that the first 25 and the last 25 statements be eliminated, with those in the middle serving as the sample.

Obtaining a language sample can sometimes be an arduous task. Shipley and McAfee (1992) suggest these facilitating techniques:

- Strive for a long sample.
- Vary the subject matter of the sample.

- Seek out multiple environments (e.g., clinic, playground, home, workplace, etc.).
- Alter the contexts (e.g., conversation, narratives, responses to pictures, etc.).
- Request other people to record samples for you (e.g., spouse, parent, teacher, etc.).

It is helpful to avoid yes-no questions and short-answer questions. Instead, use "how" and "tell me about . . . " statements to elicit complete thoughts and sentences.

Analysis of language should include an evaluation of the child's lexicon, semantics, syntax, pragmatics, and morphology. Two useful systems for analyzing a language sample are the Systematic Analysis of Language Transcripts and the Fey and Damico analysis.

The child's articulation, phonology, voice, and fluency should also be analyzed. Assess intelligibility in connected speech. Shipley and McAfee (1992) recommend focusing on the following aspects in the analysis of a speech sample:

> Number of errors; error types; consistency of errors between the speech sample and the articulation test, within the same speech sample, and between different speech samples; correctly produced sounds; intelligibility; speech rate; prosody. (pp. 133–134)

Shipley and McAfee (1992) also suggest the following guidelines for transcribing a language sample based on the work of Bloom and Lahey (1978), Hubbell (1988), Owens (1995), and Retherford (1993):

- transcribe the entire sample;
- indicate the speaker for all utterances;
- use phonetic symbols to transcribe unintelligible or partially intelligible utterances;
- use a dash (—) to indicate unintelligible words;
- capitalize only proper nouns and I;
- minimize punctuation;
- number the client's utterances.

Calculating the Mean Length of Utterance (MLU)

In addition to the transcription of the speech/language sample, the child's MLU should be calculated. For comparison purposes, Brown's (1973) developmental stages are as follows:

Stage	Age (years)	MLU
I	1 to 2:2	1.0–2.0
II	2:3 to 2:6	2.0–2.5
III	2:7 to 2:10	2.5–3.0
IV	2:11 to 3:4	3.0–3.75
V	3:5 to 3:10	3.75–4.5
	3:11+	4.5+

Based on the work of Lund and Duchan, Shipley and McAfee (1992) make the following suggestions with regard to calculating the mean length of utterance (MLU):

Exclude from your count:

1. *Imitations* which immediately follow the model utterance and which give the impression that the child would not have said the utterance spontaneously.

2. *Elliptical answers* to questions which give the impression that the utterance would have been more complete if there had been no eliciting question (e.g., "Do you want this?" "Yes." "What do you have?" "My dolls").

3. *Partial utterances* which are interrupted by outside events or shifts in the child's focus (e.g., "That's my—oops").

4. *Unintelligible utterances* that contain unintelligible segments. If a major portion of a child's sample is unintelligible, a syllable count by utterance can be substituted for morpheme count.

5. *Rote passages* such as nursery rhymes, songs, or prose passages which have been memorized and which may not be processed linguistically by the child.

6. *False starts and reformulations* within utterances which may either be self-repetitions or changes in the original formulation (e.g., "I have one [just like] almost like that"; [We] we can't").

7. *Noises* unless they are integrated into meaningful verbal material such as "He went xx."

8. *Discourse markers* such as *um, oh, you know* not integrated into the meaning of the utterance (e.g., [Well] it was [you know] [like] a party or something").

9. *Identical utterances* that the child says anywhere in the sample. Only one occurrence of each utterance is counted. If there is even a minor change, however, the second utterance is also counted.

10. *Counting or other sequences of enumeration* (e.g., "blue, green, yellow, red, purple").

11. Single words or phrases such as "hi," "thank you," "here," "know what?"

Count as one morpheme:

1. Uninflected lexical morphemes (e.g., *run, fall*) and grammatical morphemes that are whole words (articles, auxiliary verbs, prepositions).

2. Contractions when individual segments do not occur elsewhere in the sample apart from the contraction. If either of the constituent parts of the contraction are found elsewhere, the contraction is counted as two rather than one morpheme (e.g., *I'll, it's, can't*).

3. Catentatives such as *wanna, gonna, hafta* and the infinitive models that have the same meanings (e.g., *going* to go). This eliminates the problem of judging a morpheme count on the basis of the child's pronunciation. Thus "am gonna" is counted as two morphemes.

4. Phrases, compound words, diminutives, reduplicated words which occur as inseparable linguistic units for the child or represent single items (e.g., *oh boy; all right; once upon a time; a lot of; let's; big wheel; horsie*).

5. Irregular past tense. The convention is to count these as single morphemes because children's first meanings for them seem to be distinct from the present tense counterparts (e.g., *did, was*).

6. Plurals which do not occur in singular form (e.g., *pants; clothes*), including plural pronouns (*us; them*).

7. Gerunds and participles that are not part of the verb phrase (*Swimming* is fun; He was *tired;* That is the *cooking* place).

Count as more than one morpheme:

1. Inflected forms: regular and irregular plural nouns; possessive nouns; third person singular verb; present participle and past participle when part of the verb phrase; regular past tense verb; reflexive pronoun; comparative and superlative adverbs and adjectives.

2. Contractions when one or both of the individual segments occur separately anywhere in the child's sample (e.g., *It's* if *it* or *is* occurs elsewhere).

The MLU is calculated by dividing the number of morphemes by the number of utterances. Some clinicians calculate the MLU by dividing the number of words by the number of utterances. Either one gives the clinician a fairly accurate estimation of the child's grammatical development up to four to five morphemes.

Calculating the Type-Token Ratio

The Type-Token Ratio (TTR) can also be calculated to measure functional vocabulary skills. To calculate the TTR, the clinician divides the number of different words by the number of total words in the sample. For comparison purposes, Templin (1957) calculated the TTRs of normally developing children between the 3 and 8 years of age as being 0.45–0.50. A variation of the TTR is presented by Retherford (1993), who tallies the different types of words used by the child. The words are counted in each of the following categories: nouns, verbs, adjectives, adverbs, prepositions, pronouns, conjunctions, affirmatives, negatives, articles, and wh- words.

The calculation of the TTR is done by dividing the number of words in a category by the total number of words in the utterance. This can give you a Type-Token Ratio for semantic skills.

TREATMENT

The treatment sequence consists of two major portions: the evaluative-planning process and the clinical process. The initial assessment of the child and the determination of therapeutic goals comprise the evaluative-planning process. The process of establishing and habituating new skills, then generalizing the skills to the client's natural environment constitute the clinical process (Leith, 1984). Regardless of whether the child has a language delay or a language disorder, the treatment principles are generally the same.

Sensory Integration

Sensory integration is defined as the organization and interpretation of input from the various sensory systems of the body (Vinson, 1999, p. 91). Sensory integration is a key component in structuring a child's environment to facilitate communication. A key question in this structuring is, "How much sensory stimulation can the child tolerate?" The clinician should pay attention to the child's distraction level and monitor the amount of visual, auditory, and tactile feedback the child can handle. A child who is distracted will not get maximum benefit from therapy.

A second key factor in the treatment of language delays and language disorders in children is to procure the family's cooperation to facilitate generalization and maintenance of the child's language skills. Recall that during the assessment portion of the treatment sequence, the clinician empowered the family to be part of the process. This empowerment extends into the intervention phase of the assessment process. The parents should be instructed to use a level of language that is equal to or slightly above the child's current level.

A third major consideration in designing therapeutic intervention for language is to ascertain whether the child is at the presymbolic or symbolic level of communication. Symbolic communication occurs when the "individual understands the relationships among words and objects and events" (Vinson, 1999, p. 92). Language and cognition parameters such as means-end, causality, object permanence, turn taking, joint attention, use of gestures, requesting, behavior regulation, play schemes, and imitation skills serve as the foundation for language intervention. As expressed by Dunst (1980),

> the description of the child's sensorimotor performance in qualitative terms represents the critical and most important step in the overall clinical-educational process. Procedures used to describe a child's performance in qualitative terms permit an assessment of the extent to which a child is delayed in development, whether or not a child's pattern of development is typical or atypical, a determination of a child's strengths and weaknesses, and an identification of appropriate interventions designed to remediate or ameliorate any delays and/or deficits found. (Dunst, 1980, p. vii)

The Social Stages of Development

Bates, Camaioni, and Volterra (1975) described three social stages of communication development. The first stage, the perlocutionary stage, occurs between birth and 8 months of age. In the perlocutionary stage, the child is interactive but uses nonverbal and unintentional communication. During this stage, the adult assigns meaning to the behaviors of the child.

The second stage is the illocutionary stage of development. This stage develops around 10 months of age. In the illocutionary stage, communication is still primarily nonverbal, but it is intentional. "The infant may use eye gaze, conventional gestures (e.g., waving good-bye and pointing), and vocalizations to convey a message in an organized and coordinated manner. During this stage the use of jargon is noted as the child uses proto-words. Proto-words are words the child invents that may or may not sound like standard English words" (Vinson, 1999, p. 95).

The locutionary stage is the third social stage of development. This stage begins around 12 months of age when the child begins to use intentional linguistic communication, and speech consists primarily of nouns and labels. By 18 months of age, most children begin to combine words and have an expressive vocabulary of approximately 50 words.

These stages can provide a framework from which the clinician can judge if a child is developing a deficit in expressive language skills. If a child is not using single words by 18 months of age and is not combining words by 30 months of age, there may be reason to be concerned about the child's development of language.

Therapy Procedures Based on a Behavioral Paradigm

The behavioral approach to therapy relies on a stimulus-response relationship. Sometimes it is necessary to provide prompting to attain the desired response. Prompting can consist of physical assistance, modeling and imitation, visual assistance, and verbal assistance.

Physical assistance consists of physically guiding the child through making the correct response. This may include assisting the child in making a target gesture or physically manipulating the articulators to demonstrate how a particular sound is produced.

Modeling and imitation is the next level of assistance. In this case, the clinician demonstrates the target behavior in an effort to prompt an imitative response. "Imitation is a powerful teaching tool and forms the foundation for the development of many different skills in normal development" (Vinson, 1999, p. 109). Children with severe and profound retardation frequently do not have an imitative response, so the use of physical assistance to teach imitation could be a therapy goal and procedure for these children. Another problem is that some behaviors are difficult to model. This is typically more problematic in speech therapy than in language therapy. Regardless, research principles support the use of modeling and imitation as a teaching tool.

Shaping is rarely used in its purest form. Shaping is defined as the differential reinforcement of successive approximations to a specified target to create a new behavior (Leith, 1984). In true shaping, the clinician does not offer a model, and he/she does not tell the client why he is being reinforced. Thus, shaping can be a very slow process unless combined with other therapy strategies, such as modeling and imitation. Shaping requires that the clinician have a good understanding of task analysis, since the goals must be broken down into discrete steps. It is important that the steps not be too small because therapy will be inefficient; it is also important that the steps not be too large because reinforcement will not be sufficient enough to keep the child on task. In shaping, the clinician determines where the child is on the ladder of achieving the desired skill and begins therapy at that point.

Prompting with visual assistance and prompting with verbal assistance are two more therapy techniques. A prompt is also referred to as a supplementary antecedent because it is added to the original stimulus in hopes of increasing the probability of getting the desired response. It is important to always use the weakest prompt possible and to fade the prompts as quickly as possible.

Chaining is a therapeutic procedure used to teach skills that consist of many different components. A chain is a sequence of behaviors, all of which must be done to produce the desired response. There are three types of chaining: forward chaining, in which the first steps of a sequence are taught first; backward chaining, in which the last steps of the sequence are taught first; and total task presentation, in which the entire series of sequential skills must be completed in order to master the skill and receive reinforcement. Academic skills are typically taught using forward chaining, while self-help skills are usually taught using backward chaining. Total task presentation can be used when the child can do each individual component of the sequence but does not perform them in the proper sequence.

Finally, fading refers to the gradual removal of all prompts and reinforcers so that the client is responding independently to the stimuli. This is a critical component of generalization and maintenance of the new skills.

Models of Intervention

The traditional model of intervention in the schools has been the "pull-out" model in which the clinician takes a child out of his classroom to a designated area in which therapy is provided. In this model, the clinician must rely on the teacher to provide feedback as to how well the child is generalizing his therapy skills to the classroom.

A much more productive model that is currently in vogue is the collaborative model. This is also known as classroom-based, or curriculum-based, therapy. The intervention focuses on learning strategies and using them in materials related to the child's academic curriculum. The collaborative model implies a cooperative partnership between the clinician and the teacher. The principle that underlies the collaborative model is that "language learning is intrinsic to literary development" (Naremore, Densmore, & Harman, 1995). In 1995, ASHA supported the collaborative model of intervention, claiming it to be the most efficient and effective model of intervention for children with language-based learning disabilities in public schools.

The consultative model is a third model of intervention. The consultative model is a service delivery model in which the speech-language pathologist provides indirect therapy through inservice and input to classroom teachers on appropriate methods for encouraging effective speech and language skills. Other indirect models of therapy include counseling, tutoring, and adapting education materials to address communication and language in the classroom curriculum.

Selecting Intervention Targets

Hegde (1996) makes several recommendations regarding the selection of intervention targets.

Select language intervention targets that:

- are child-specific and ethnoculturally appropriate

- are useful in natural settings

- can make an immediate and socially significant difference in the child's communicative skills

- help meet the academic and social demands the child faces

- help expand communication skills into conversational speech in natural settings

- are within the child's reach as judged by current performance (words, phrases, sentences, conversational speech) (Hegde, 1996, p. 144)

The clinician should then design a sequence of treatment and prepare the stimulus materials.

Therapy Techniques

Activity-based therapy: With young children, activity-based therapy utilizing naturalized settings provides the best opportunities for learning a skill, generalizing the skill, and maintaining the skill beyond the therapy setting. A comprehensive approach, activity-based therapy can address lexicon, semantics, syntax, morphology, phonology, and pragmatics. In this type of approach, therapy activities are grounded around themes, or schemes, to facilitate the use of language in "real-world" settings. For example, the clinician might set up a cooking scheme and develop language related to that scheme. Within the scheme, foundations such as turn taking, maintaining a topic, joint attention, causality, and means-end can be addressed.

If a child does not readily interact with the clinician when acting out a scheme, the clinician can engage in parallel talk and parallel play in which he/she plays beside the child without actively seeking out an interaction. For example, in a cooking scheme, the clinician could feed a baby doll at the same time that the child feeds another baby doll. The clinician could model expressive language at a level appropriate for the child and expand any utterances the child makes.

Reversed imitation: Using reversed imitation, the clinician imitates what the child says. This can be used as one way to teach a child who does not imitate to do so.

Conversational repair: Conversational repair is a technique to teach children to make requests, ask for clarification, and maintain a topic. Thus, it addresses pragmatics of language. Situations can be set up in which the clinician requires the child to ask for clarification or to make other requests. For example, the clinician could have an array of toys and ask the child, "Will you please give me a toy?" If the child does not ask for clarification ("Which toy?"), the clinician then models the behavior and repeats the request. If the child still does not ask for clarification, the clinician can progress through the prompting hierarchy outlined previously in this chapter.

APPENDIX 18-A: SAMPLE OF PUBLISHED TESTS FOR ARTICULATION AND LANGUAGE

Test	Author(s)	Ages
Peabody Picture Vocabulary Test – III	Dunn & Dunn	2–6 thru 90+
Carrow Elicited Language Inventory	Carrow-Woolfolk	3–0 thru 7–11
Test for Auditory Comprehension of Language – 3	Carrow-Woolfolk	3–0 thru 9–11
Test of Early Language Development – 3	Hresko, Reid, Hammill	3–0 thru 7–11
Preschool Language Scale – 3	Zimmerman, Steinen Pond	Birth thru 6–11
Expressive Vocabulary Test	Williams	2–6 thru 90+
Birth to Three Assessment and Intervention System—2nd ed.	Ammer & Bangs	Birth–3
Early Language Milestone Scale—2nd ed.	Coplan	Birth–3
Fluharty Preschool Speech and Language Screening Test	Fluharty	2–6
Token Test for Children	DiSimoni	3–12
Sequenced Inventory of Communication Development	Hedrick, Prather, & Tobin	4 mo–4 years
Receptive One-Word Picture Vocabulary Test	Gardner	2–0 thru 11–11
Preschool Language Assessment Instrument	Blank, Rose, & Berlin	3–0 thru 5–11
Photo Articulation Test (3rd ed.)	Lippke, Dickey, Selmar, Soer	3–0 thru 8–11
Bankson-Bernthal Test of Phonology	Bankson & Bernthal	3–0 thru 9–0
Quick Screen of Phonology	Bankson & Bernthal	3–0 thru 7–11
Arizona Articulation Proficiency Scale, 2nd ed.	Fudala & Reynolds	1–5 thru 13 years
Reynell Developmental Language Scales	Reyness & Gruber	1–6 years
Receptive-Expressive Emergent Language Test (REEL – 2)	Bzoch & League	Birth–3 years
Kaufman Survey of Early Academic and Language Skills	Kaufman & Kaufman	3–0 thru 6–11

APPENDIX 18-B: EARLY COMMUNICATION CHECKLIST *+

Linda J. Lombardino, Ph.D., Jamie B. Stapell, M. A., and Kenneth J. Gerhardt, Ph.D.

Child's Name _____   Date of Birth _____

Examiner _____   Test Date _____

Reactive Primitive Behaviors (1–3 months)
(Early perlocutionary)

_____ Arouses from sleep by sudden noises

_____ Startles to unexpected loud noises

_____ Looks to/fixates on adult's face

_____ Looks to/fixates on inanimate objects

_____ Responds to adults' facial expressions and vocalizations (cooing sounds)

_____ Smiles during face-to-face interactions

_____ Responds differentially to familiar vs unfamiliar, angry vs happy, male vs female voices

Purposeful Primitive Behaviors (4–7 months)
(Late perlocutionary)

_____ Begins to make rudimentary head turns toward sound source

_____ Searches for sound sources that are out-of-sight

_____ Demonstrates a listening attitude

_____ Reaches for an object held out to child or close by

_____ Pushes away (or turns body away from) undesired object or event

_____ Uses global body movements (vocal/gestural/eye contact) as a means to reinstate a desired activity

_____ Responds to familiar phrases to reinstate a desired activity

_____ Produces syllable repetitions

Transitional/Instrumental Communicative Behaviors (8–11 months)
(Transition from perlocutionary to illocutionary)

_____ Turns to out-of-sight sound sources in the lateral plane

_____ Enjoys shaking rattle or noise maker

_____ Participates in social games such as pat-a-cake and peek-a-boo

_____ Gives an object in response to adult's outstretched hand

_____ Uses adult's hand to recreate a spectacle (does not look to adult's face as if to bid for help)

_____ Reaches for objects at a distance (does not look back at adult)

_____ Engages in "showing off" behaviors

_____ Extends arms to be picked up

_____ Waves "hi" or "bye" (with prompting from parent)

_____ Responds to own name

_____ Responds to "no," and a few single words

_____ Uses ma-ma or da-da (void of any real meaning)

Intentional/Conventional Communicative Behaviors (11–14 months)
(Illocutionary)

_____ Alerts to telephone ring

_____ Looks to the television when certain programs or commercials come on

_____ Initiates routine games

_____ Spontaneously waves hi or bye

_____ Spontaneously gives objects to adult

_____ Spontaneously shows objects to adults

_____ Spontaneously points to request objects from adult

_____ Spontaneously points to request assistance

_____ Shakes head "no" to indicate rejection

_____ Uses a few words as performatives (proto-words)

_____ Responds to a number of single words (names of family members, names of pets, labels for games or social routines, food-related items)

First Words (14–16 months)

(Locutionary)

_____ Localizes to sounds in all planes (left, right, down, up, diagonal)

_____ Responds to name when called from another room

_____ Uses gestures, varying intonation patterns, and/or words to express a number of communicative functions

     _____ Draws attention to self

     _____ Draws attention to objects

     _____ Requests objects

     _____ Requests actions or social routines

     _____ Expresses dislikes or protests

     _____ Expresses pleasure or surprise

     _____ Greets

     _____ Answers

_____ Uses a few words to refer to objects, events, actions, attributes, and locations

_____ Responds to several words in addition to questions such as "Where's daddy?" "Where's your nose?"

---

*Indicate whether behavior was directly observed (D) or reported by parent (P)

+From "Evaluating Early Communication Behaviors in Infancy," by L. J. Lombardino, J. B. Stapell, and K. J. Gerhardt, 1987, _Journal of Pediatric Health Care_, 1(5), pp. 240–246. Reprinted with permission.

CHAPTER NINETEEN
Laryngectomy

DEFINITION/DESCRIPTION

Patients who face the diagnosis of laryngeal cancer express many concerns and fears that need to be addressed by the patient, his family, and the medical team involved in his care. These fears and concerns are much the same as those facing anyone with any type of cancer—recurrence of the cancer, the possibility of death, the ability to continue with work, and the ability to maintain his current lifestyle. However, in addition to these concerns, the individual with laryngeal cancer faces the possibility of losing oral communication and, thus, the ability to control his environment (Cassisi, Sapienza, & Vinson, 1996).

The term "laryngectomy" refers to the surgical removal of all or part of the larynx. A partial laryngectomy is the removal of less than the whole structure. A hemilaryngectomy is removal of one-half of the larynx, and a supraglottic laryngectomy is the removal of the laryngeal structures above the true vocal folds (Casper & Colton, 1998). "A partial laryngectomy conserves sufficient laryngeal structure and function to permit audible voice production utilizing pulmonary airflow. The voice quality may be hoarse, breathy, and altered in fundamental frequency and other acoustic parameters" (Casper & Colton, 1998, p. 2).

Etiological Factors

The most prevalent cause of laryngeal cancer is the smoking of cigarettes, pipes, and/or cigars. However, it should be noted that abstention from the use of tobacco for 5 years results in a decline in tobacco-related cancers of the alimentary and respiratory tracts, and after 10 years of nonuse, the risk approaches that of nonsmokers (Wynder, 1978). Smoking of more than 10 marijuana cigarettes also appears to lead to an increase of laryngeal cancers. In spite of preoperative counseling regarding the role of smoking in laryngeal cancer, the relationship is not acknowledged by many male patients and their wives. In a study by Kommers, Sullivan, and Yonkers (1977), 98% of the male patients with laryngeal cancer smoked at least one pack of cigarettes per day, and 36% smoked two or more packs per day. Nonetheless, 42% of their wives denied that smoking was related to their husband's laryngeal cancer.

Alcohol abuse, and particularly when alcohol and smoking are combined, is another etiological factor in cancer of the larynx. In fact, persons who combine the consumption of alcohol and smoking are 15.5% more likely to develop malignancies of the larynx than is the general population. (McKenna, Fornataro-Clerici, McMeamin, & Leonard, 1991).

Occupational exposure to chemicals and other substances can also lead to laryngeal cancer. Finally, diet is also believed to play a role in the occurrence of cancer of the larynx (Casper & Colton, 1998).

Onset and Course of the Disorder

Anatomically, the larynx is divided into the supraglottic, glottic, and subglottic larynx. The symptoms and course of the disease will vary according to which anatomic site is affected by the cancer.

Supraglottic Cancer

The supraglottic larynx consists of the epiglottis, the false vocal cords, the ventricles, the aryepiglottic folds, and the arytenoids. Therefore, unless the lesion becomes quite large, hoarseness is not a prominent symptom of supraglottic cancer. Patients typically will complain of mild and persistent pain when swallowing, with this pain being the initial symptom. In addition, patients may complain of a globus sensation, otherwise known as a "lump in the throat." Referred pain to the ear (by way of Arnold's nerve) may occur in lesions of the epiglottis. An asymptomatic neck mass may be the first sign of a supraglottic cancer, with later symptoms including dysphagia and weight loss (Cassisi, Sapienza, & Vinson, 1996).

Glottic Cancer

A carcinoma of the true vocal cords typically has hoarseness as the initial symptom. The patient may exhibit inspiratory and expiratory stridor caused by airway obstruction. Pain and coughing may occur also (Casper & Colton, 1993). Tumors of the true vocal cords range in size and shape. However, 95% of the tumors are localized to the mid-membranous portion of the true vocal cord and are whitish in color (Aronson, 1990).

Subglottic Cancer

Frequently, patients with early lesions in the subglottic area are asymptomatic. Hoarseness is the most common symptom, followed by obstruction of the airway.

ASSESSMENT

The first portion of the assessment process is typically to have the patient complete a history form that includes questions related to the psychological and physiological factors the patient is experiencing. The examiner should glean information related to the onset of the disorder, related illnesses, previous treatments, social and occupational considerations, and overall functionality of the patient in daily living (Case, 1991).

An audio recording of the patient's voice should be analyzed to obtain objective measures regarding the acoustic and aerodynamic characteristics of the voice. The acoustic measures include frequency, intensity, and duration. The aerodynamic measures encompass quantification of the airflow and air pressure during phonation. In addition, perceptual measures (which are less objective) should be done as part of the voice evaluation.

A visual examination of the larynx is a critical component of the evaluation for laryngeal cancer. Initially, this may be a mirror exam, but it should be complemented with fiberoptic examination. This can be done with either a transnasal fiberoptic endoscopic procedure or through indirect examination via a rigid or flexible scope.

Lesions of the epiglottis should be described in terms of their relationship to the hyoid. Thus, they should be designated as either infrahyoid or suprahyoid. Lesions of the true vocal cords should be described in terms of the extent of the lesion. This includes noting whether or not the opposite cord is involved and/or whether the arytenoids are affected. The mobility of the cords should be addressed prior to direct laryngoscopy and biopsy.

The clinical workup of lesions of the larynx should include indirect laryngoscopy, CT scanning with contrast, MRI in selected cases, chest X-ray, and direct laryngoscopy with biopsy. In addition, the vibratory characteristics of the vocal folds should be assessed using video-stroboscopy. All imaging should be done prior to direct laryngoscopy and biopsy (Cassisi, Sapienza, & Vinson, 1996).

Staging

A classification system that stages cancer of the larynx was developed by the American Joint Committee on Cancer (AJCC). Its staging is based on three factors: tumor, node, and metastasis (TNM) (McKenna et al., 1991). This staging is outlined in Table 19–1.

TABLE 19–1 American Joint Commission on Cancer staging of laryngeal lesions

I. Tumor (T)

  A. Supraglottis

    T1 Tumor limited to one subsite of supraglottis with normal vocal fold mobility.

    T2 Tumor invades more than one subsite of supraglottis or glottis with normal vocal fold mobility.

    T3 Tumor limited to larynx with vocal fold fixation and/or invades postcricoid area, medial wall of pyriform sinus or pre-epiglottic tissues.

    T4 Tumor invades through thyroid cartilage and/or extends to other tissues beyond the larynx (e.g., to the oropharynx, soft tissues of the neck).

  B. Glottis

    T1 Tumor limited to vocal folds (may involve anterior or posterior commissure with normal mobility).

    T1a Tumor limited to one vocal fold.

    T1b Tumor invades both vocal folds.

    T2 Tumor extends to supraglottis and/or subglottis with impaired vocal fold mobility.

    T3 Tumor limited to the larynx with vocal fold fixation.

    T4 Tumor invades through thyroid cartilage and/or extends to other tissues beyond the larynx (e.g., oropharynx, soft tissues of the neck).

  C. Subglottis

    T1 Tumor limited to the subglottis.

    T2 Tumor extends to vocal folds with normal or impaired mobility.

    T3 Tumor limited to larynx with vocal fold fixation.

    T4 Tumor invades through cricoid or thyroid cartilage and/or extends to other tissues beyond the larynx (e.g., oropharynx and soft tissues of neck).

II. Regional Lymph Nodes (N)

  NX Regional lymph nodes cannot be assessed.

  N0 No regional lymph node metastasis.

  N1 Metastasis in a single ipsilateral lymph node, 3 cm or less in greatest dimension.

continued

TABLE 19–1	continued

N2 Metastasis in a single ipsilateral lymph node, more than 3 cm but not more than 6 cm in greatest dimension, or in multiple ipsilateral lymph nodes, none more than 6 cm in greatest dimension, or in bilateral or contralateral lymph nodes, none more than 6 cm in greatest dimension.

N2a Metastasis in a single ipsilateral lymph node more than 3 cm but not more than 6 cm in greatest dimension.

N2b Metastasis in multiple ipsilateral lymph nodes, none more than 6 cm in greatest dimension.

N2c Metastasis in bilateral or contralateral lymph nodes, none more than 6 cm in greatest dimension.

N3 Metastasis in a lymph node more than 6 cm in greatest dimension.

III. **Distant Metastasis (M)**

MX Presence of distant metastasis cannot be assessed.

M0 No distant metastasis.

M1 Distant metastasis.

IV. **Stage Grouping**

Stage 0	Tis	N0	M0
Stage I	T1	N0	M0
Stage II	T2	N0	M0
Stage III	T3	N0	M0
	T1	N1	M0
	T2	N1	M0
	T3	N1	M0
Stage IV	T4	N0, N1	M0
	Any T	N2, N3	M0
	Any T	Any N	M1

Used with the permission of the American Joint Committee on Cancer (AJCC®), Chicago, Illinois. The original source for this material is the *AJCC® Cancer Staging Manual, 3rd Edition* (1988) published by Lippincott-Raven Publishers, Philadelphia, Pennsylvania.

The Voice Examination

During the information gathering interview with the patient and/or his family, the examiners learn specific information about the disorder such as the onset of the symptoms, a description of the symptoms, related illnesses, previous treatments, social and occupational considerations, and overall functionality of the patient with regard to daily living (Case, 1991). A sample case history form is found in Appendix 19–A. Based on the case history information, the speech-language pathologist and other team members have an array of factors that may be related to the patient's symptoms and can plan the steps of the assessment process.

One important component of the assessment is the voice evaluation. Perceptual ratings may be done to assess the degree of hoarseness and the pitch and loudness level of the voice. However, as Baken (1987) points out, perceptual ratings can be unreliable. Therefore, a combination of perceptual judgments and objective indices are recommended in the voice evaluation.

Objective measures are helpful in that they provide a means of numerically documenting the status of the patient's voice prior to intervention. Gould (1988) presents an overview of the instrumentation often used in the clinical voice laboratory. These measures are typically divided into two categories: aerodynamic and acoustic. Aerodynamic measures quantify the amount of airflow and air pressure during phonation. Acoustic measures evaluate the frequency, intensity, and duration of the voice.

Aerodynamics

"Aerodynamics refer to the average air pressures, airflows, and air volumes that are produced as part of the peripheral mechanics of the respiratory, laryngeal, and supralaryngeal airways" (Bless & Hicks, 1996, p. 145). In other words, laryngeal valving efficiency and respiratory support can be evaluated through clinical measures of air pressure, airflow, and air volume (Bless, 1988; Hirano, 1981). Aerodynamic measures are indirect measures of voice production changes that occur as a result of respiratory support. They should be supplemented by acoustic, glottal kinematic, and other measures of vocal function. As with acoustic measures, aerodynamic measures of voice usually follow a dichotomy between fine and gross characteristics (Scherer, 1990).

The major reasons for measuring laryngeal aerodynamics are to monitor change in the voice, evaluate degrees of dysphonia, and differentiate between respiratory and laryngeal problems (Bless & Hicks, 1996). The most frequently used measures, according to Hirano (1981), are mean airflow rate and the maximum phonation time.

Acoustics

With regard to acoustical measures of the voice, standards have been suggested by the National Center for Voice and Speech (1995). These standards are reflected in Table 19–2.

Bless and Hicks (1996) describe the Voice Range Profile (VRP) as a recording of frequency versus intensity. The VRP

> circumscribes the maximum range a person can produce and as such can be used to establish the boundaries for further testing. Low, medium and high pitch are defined as a percentage of the fundamental frequency range (e.g., 10%, 50%, and 80%), and soft, medium, and loud as a percentage of intensity range. Strategic vowels are elicited at specific locations within the range to determine stability. A series of pitch, loudness, adduction, and register glides are elicited to determine the range, speed, accuracy, and stability of phonation within the VRP. (Bless & Hicks, 1996, p. 148)

In summation of assessment, one must take a multipronged approach to the evaluation of the patient with cancer of the larynx. A careful case history must be gathered prior to proceeding with any other evaluation. Evaluation should consist of a visual examination, laryngoscopy, and a complete voice evaluation. Attention should also be paid to the psychological state of the patient and his caregivers.

TABLE 19-2 Test utterances recommended by the National Center for Voice and Speech acoustics standards meeting participants in 1995 for clinical recording and analysis of acoustic signals

NONSPEECH

Voice Range Profile defines test frequencies and intensities (low = 10% of F range, medium = 45% of F range, high = 80% of F range; soft = 10% of intensity range, medium = 50% of intensity range, loud = 80% of intensity range)

Sustained [ ], [i], [u] Vowels

1. low, soft, 2s
2. low, loud, 2s
3. high, soft, 2s
4. high, loud, 2s
5. medium high, medium loud, 2s
6. comfortable pitch and loudness, 2s
7. comfortable pitch and loudness, maximum duration

Sustained [s] Consonant

comfortable pitch and loudness, maximum duration

Sustained [z] Consonant

comfortable pitch and loudness, maximum duration

Pitch Glides

1. low-high-low, one octave, 0.25 Hz
2. low-high-low, one octave, 1.0 Hz
3. low-high-low, one octave, maximum rate

Loudness Glides

1. soft-loud-soft, 0.25 Hz
2. soft-loud-soft, 1.0 Hz
3. soft-loud-soft, maximum rate

Adductory Glides [ɑ] and [hɑ]

1. onset-pressed-offset, 0.1 Hz
2. onset-pressed-offset, 2.0 Hz
3. onset-pressed-offset, maximum rate

Register Glides

1. modal-pulse-modal, 0.1 Hz
2. modal-falsetto-modal, 0.1 Hz
3. modal-falsetto-modal, maximum rate, as in yodeling

SPEECH

Counting from 1 to 100, comfortable pitch and loudness

All voice sentence, "Where are you going?", soft, medium, loud

Sentence with frequent voice onset and offset "The blue spot is on the key again," soft, medium, loud

Oral reading of "Rainbow Passage"

Descriptive speech, "Cookie Theft" picture

Parent-child speech, "Goldilocks and The Three Bears"

Dramatic speech involving deep emotions (fear, anger, sadness, happiness, disgust)

Singing part of "Happy Birthday to You," modal and falsetto register

TREATMENT

Because of the complex effects of laryngectomy on an individual and his family, it is highly recommended that the treatment team include the surgeon, a speech-language pathologist, social workers, psychologists, and nurses. Casper and Colton (1998) recommend a three-pronged approach to therapy: psychosocial, swallowing, and speech.

Surgical Treatment

Treatment for vocal fold carcinoma depends largely on whether the treatment occurs in the early or late stage of the disease. Treatment in the early stages of the disease often results in some sort of voice-sparing treatment. However, in the late stages, the treatment is typically a total laryngectomy. However, a trial period of radiation is an option (Million, Cassisi, & Mancuso, 1994).

In the early stages, at most centers, irradiation is the initial form of treatment. If irradiation fails, some viable surgical alternatives are a hemilaryngectomy, a cordectomy, and laser incision. However, the voice is likely to be better following radiation treatment than it will be following surgical intervention. When comparing voice quality pre- and postintervention, the voice may actually be better following radiation treatments. However, following a hemilaryngectomy, the voice typically remains hoarse, or it may be worse with breathiness and a loss of vocal loudness often occurring.

Moderately advanced vocal fold carcinomas typically include lesions that cause vocal fold fixation. These lesions are classified as favorable or unfavorable, with the latter usually having extensive bilateral disease and a compromised airway. A favorable T3 lesion will be limited to one side of the larynx, with the maintenance of a good airway. Historically, the majority of persons with a T3 lesion underwent a total laryngectomy. However, patients are now offered an option of radiation therapy and surgical salvage if the radiation therapy fails. There is approximately a 5–10% reduction in the 5-year survival rate of those who do not undergo a total laryngectomy.

> Using this philosophic approach for these moderately advanced vocal fold cancers, the local control rate with voice preservation is 50–70%. Of the ones that fail, 50–70% are cured with surgical salvage. The major problem with this approach is that, with more advanced lesions, it is sometimes difficult to distinguish between radiation edema and local recurrence. Often the recurrence is submucosal, and deep biopsies are required to diagnose the recurrence. (Cassisi, Sapienza, & Vinson, 1996)

Total laryngectomy and neck dissection are the treatments of choice for advanced vocal fold carcinoma. In addition, postoperative radiation is often recommended. The tracheal stoma, cervical lymph nodes, and base of the tongue are the most common sites of failure.

Treatment for supraglottic laryngeal carcinoma can readily be treated with external beam irradiation or subtotal supraglottic laryngectomy. The subtotal supraglottic laryngectomy is the treatment of choice "if the lesion is bulky and infiltrative and if the patient has good pulmonary reserve" (Cassisi, Sapienza, & Vinson, 1996). For early lesions, radiation therapy is often recommended. However, it is preferable to use only one modality of treatment for early lesions. Therefore, some type of neck dissection on the most involved side of the lesion is usually done.

Psychosocial

Patients and their families need the support of the medical team in accepting the diagnosis, understanding the implications of the surgery, and becoming educated about the various options available postoperatively. Depression among patients who are undergoing a laryngectomy is a predominant emotion. However, it needs to be addressed because depression "can compromise the patient's recovery, retard physical healing, and be a hindrance to initiating alaryngeal communication training" (Casper & Colton, 1998, p. 5).

Other emotions that are frequently found in patients undergoing laryngectomy are anxiety, nervousness, denial, isolationism, irritability, and difficulty adjusting to the physical changes that have been incurred (Blood, Luther, & Stemple, 1992). Blood, Simpson, Dineen, Kauffman, and Raimondi (1994) found that 30% of the spouses of laryngectomees expressed that the period of postoperative adjustment following a laryngectomy was more difficult than they had anticipated. However, according to Gardner (1961), "success or failure in rehabilitation often depends on the attitude of the spouse toward the laryngectomee's handicap and his/her effort to talk."

The patient with a laryngectomy and his family may go through a grief process in working toward acceptance of the changes in their lives. Many times, the patient becomes "self-focused, even selfish, as he or she passes through the stages of grief. While focusing on his or her own needs, the laryngectomee becomes less able to recognize the anxieties felt by family members, and is frequently unavailable to them as they work through their own set of worries and concerns" (Cassisi, Sapienza, & Vinson, 1996). This points out the need for support groups for the laryngectomees, as well as separate support groups for the spouses and family members of laryngectomees.

Swallowing

Swallowing problems can occur at the oral, pharyngeal, and/or esophageal stages of the swallow. Patients who have lost a portion of their tongue, or for whom there is restricted mobility of the tongue, may have difficulty with the oral phase of swallowing in that forming a bolus and positioning it to be swallowed may be problematic. Patients who undergo a supraglottic laryngectomy may have difficulty swallowing without aspirating. This problem needs immediate intervention given the possible life-threatening aspects of aspiration. If there has been extensive esophageal or pharyngeal reconstruction, the patient may experience constrictions that interfere with the passage of food through the esophagus. These patients will need to be taught modified swallowing and eating habits (Casper & Colton, 1998).

Speech

As soon as the patient is diagnosed, the clinician should begin to provide information about the use of alaryngeal speech following the surgery. The loss of ability to speak can contribute to a feeling of being powerless and exacerbate any sense of isolation and depression the patient may be experiencing. Thus, in addition to providing instruction on alaryngeal methods of speech, the speech-language pathologist may be involved in some rudimentary counseling as well.

Internal Methods of Speech

Internal methods of speech for laryngectomees include esophageal speech and tracheoesophageal fistulization/puncture (TEF/TEP). The support for esophageal speech comes from driving air into the upper esophagus. The PE segment, which is located approximately between the cervical vertebrae C3–C6, is the source of vibration. The PE segment is formed by the inferior pharyngeal constrictor muscle and the cricopharyngeous muscles (lower portion of the inferior constrictor muscle). During vocalization, the PE segment is narrowed. When constricted, air can be driven out of the esophagus under pressure to produce a vibratory air source.

One advantage of esophageal speech is that it can be produced naturally without the use of external devices. Another advantage is that it does not require additional surgery to produce vocalization as does the TEP procedure. Disadvantages include short duration of speech since air must be replenished frequently. Other disadvantages include a lack of success with esophageal speech due to poor vibratory characteristics of the PE segment, or poor motivational and compliance factors.

There are two main techniques for supplying air to vibrate the PE segment: injection and inhalation. In the injection method, air is injected from the mouth into the esophagus using coordinated movements of the tongue and pharynx. The first phase is the glottal press in which air is trapped behind the tongue and moved backward into the oral cavity. The second phase includes tongue movement back toward the pharyngeal wall to drive the air down into the esophagus. The inhalation method is based on driving air from the lungs. Air is inhaled into the lungs. "If the PE segment can be relaxed, the air pressure within the esophagus will become substantially lower than atmospheric pressure, creating a force that pulls the air from the mouth and pharynx into the esophagus" (Cassisi, Sapienza, & Vinson, 1996).

The tracheoesophageal fistulization (TEF) and tracheoesophageal puncture (TEP) procedures require surgical intervention. A primary TEF/TEP is one done at the time the laryngectomy is performed; a secondary TEF/TEP is done later. A prosthesis is placed into a fistula of the trachea, thereby providing a pathway for the pulmonary air to be directed into the esophagus. The airflow then travels through the PE segment in the same manner as for esophageal speech. It is modified by the resonating cavities of the upper vocal tract to produce speech sounds. In general, TEF/TEP speech has been found to have advantages over esophageal speech and speech associated with mechanical devices. One reason is that duration of speech is longer since a greater amount of air capacity is available. Second, loudness and pitch can be controlled to some extent.

A comparison of alaryngeal speech modes can be found in Table 19–3.

Table 19-3 Comparison of alaryngeal speech modes

Type of Speech	Advantages	Disadvantages
Pneumatic speech aid	"Natural," nonelectric sound Easy to learn Intelligible speech Inexpensive initial cost Inexpensive operating costs (no batteries)	Bulky size Requires access to stoma Sometimes difficult to maintain seal at stoma
Electronic speech aid (Neck type)	Easy to learn to use Fits in pocket or purse Volume and pitch controls for individual preference Adequate volume to be heard in noisy places Intelligible speech when used well	Noisy electronic sound Cannot be used with heavily scarred or erythematous neck Moderate initial cost Occasional extra cost for repair Requires very clear articulation skills
Electronic speech aid (Oral type)	Easy to learn to use Fits in pocket or purse, but may be larger than neck type Volume and pitch controls for individual preference May be less noisy than neck types (with or without oral adapter) Can be used soon after surgery even in presence of much scar tissue Intelligible when used well	Electronic sound very obvious to all observers "Clumsy" feeling initially to talk with tube in mouth Moderate initial purchase cost Occasional additional cost for repairs Requires excellent articulation skills for easy intelligibility
Esophageal speech	"Natural" nonelectronic sound Requires no dependence on mechanical instrument or other device Sound of the voice does not call attention to itself (may be perceived as having a cold)	A period of therapy required for most people May be difficult for one third or more patients to learn well enough to be easily intelligible Difficult to hear in noisy environments Requires excellent articulation skills May exacerbate symptoms of gastroesophageal reflux
Tracheoesophageal speech	"Natural" nonelectronic sound Requires short learning period Smooth, fluent speech using long sentences because of availability of pulmonary air Flexibility of loudness and pitch variations Sound of the voice does not call attention to itself Extended wear prosthesis types obviate need for frequent removal	If not done as primary procedure, requires another surgical procedure Requires manual dexterity, visual acuity, and level of alertness to care for Requires use of finger to occlude stoma or daily affixing of valve to peristomal area Buildup of candida deposits requiring frequent cleaning

From *Clinical Manual for Laryngectomy and Head/Neck Cancer Rehabilitation* (2nd ed.) (pp. 56–57), by J. K. Casper and R. H. Colton, 1998, San Diego, CA: Singular Publishing Group. Copyright 1998 by Singular Publishing Group. Reprinted with permission.

External Methods of Speech

There are two types of external speech methods: the pneumatic devices and the electro-laryngeal devices. Pneumatic speech aids

> usually consist of a piece that fits over the stoma, a small unit with a reed inside to provide the sound, and tubing that carries the sound to the mouth. The patient places the tube in the corner of his or her mouth as exhalatory air from the lungs drives the reed to produce sound that is resonated in the usual way in the patient's oral cavity and shaped into words by the action of the articulators. (Casper & Colton, 1998, pp. 55–57)

Specific types include the DSP8 Speech Aid, the Tokyo Speech Aid, and the ToneAire Artificial Larynx.

Electronic speech aids use electric power to drive a vibrator that provides the sound source. There are three types of electronic devices:

1. A handheld vibrator that is placed against the neck. Sound is delivered through the skin;

2. A tube attached to an electrically driven vibrator that functions much the same as the pneumatic devices; and

3. A device contained in a dental plate that is activated by a handheld unit (Casper & Colton, 1998).

Specific types of electronic speech aids include the following: the Cooper Rand Electronic Speech Aid; Servox Inton; Romet Speech Aid; SPKR; Denrick Speech Aid; TruTone Electronic Speech Aid; Nu-Vois Artificial Larynx; P.O.Vox; UltraVoice; the SolaTone; and Optivox Electrolarynx. Ordering information for electronic aids is listed in the book's Appendix B.

Counseling

It is necessary for the speech-language pathologist to offer pre- and post-surgery counseling, with an ultimate goal of helping the patient to achieve "a functional level of intelligibility" (Golper, 1998, p. 5). During this time, the clinician should also instruct the patient on health and safety concerns, where he can buy supplies such as an electrolarynx and shower shields, and on use and care of the prosthesis (Golper, 1998).

For patients using non-vocal means of communication and for those who have tracheo-stomas, the instruction from the clinician should include information on Passey-Muir (speaking) valves. For these patients, information should also be provided regarding alter-native and augmentative communication devices for patients who cannot phonate because of severe motor speech deficits or the presence of an endotracheal tube (Golper, 1998).

The speech-language pathologist should also be involved in interdisciplinary team confer-ences, staff education, research, continuing education, reimbursements (terminology and protocols), risk management, program reviews, cost containment, and program monitoring (Golper, 1998).

APPENDIX 19-A: LARYNGECTOMEE CASE HISTORY AND ASSESSMENT FORM

Syracuse Voice Center
SUNY Health Science Center, Syracuse, NY

Name: _____ DOB: _____

Evaluation date: _____

Address: _____

Phone: ( ) _____ Referred by: _____

Medical History

Primary site of tumor: _____ ICD9: _____ Surgery date: _____

Staging: T: _____ N: _____ M: _____ Surgeon: _____

Prelaryngectomy Rx: ☐ none ☐ radiation ☐ chemotx ☐ prior surgery

(specify procedure and date) _____

Extent of surgery: ☐ partial laryngectomy ☐ total laryngectomy ☐ myotomy
☐ pharyngectomy ☐ esophagectomy ☐ partial anterior glossectomy
☐ partial lateral glossectomy ☐ <50% ☐ >50%
☐ neck dissection: ☐ unilateral ☐ bilateral ☐ standard ☐ modified

Closure/reconstruction: ☐ primary ☐ free flap ☐ jejunal ☐ gastric pullup

☐ other (describe) _____

Complications: (describe) _____

TEP: ☐ primary ☐ secondary (date: _____)

Postop radiotx: #treatments _____ #rads _____ Date completed: _____

General health: (other conditions, other surgeries): _____

_____

Medications: _____

Social/Occupational History:

Occupation:_____

Do you plan to return to work? ☐ same job ☐ different job ☐ no

With whom do you live? _____

Family/friends adjustment? _____

Current Status:

Hearing: ☐ unaided ☐ aided ☐ untested;   self-appraisal: ☐ OK ☐ problem

Vision: ☐ glasses ☐ no glasses;   self-appraisal: ☐ OK w/glasses ☐ problem

Dental: ☐ edentulous ☐ full dentures ☐ other (describe)_____

Swallowing: (describe any difficulties) _____

_____

Chewing: _____ Taste: _____ Smell: _____

Tongue: range of motion: _____

Reconstruction or prosthesis: _____

Cognitive status: _____ Emotional status: _____

Prior voice/speech rehab: (describe) _____

Primary communication: ☐ writing ☐ artificial larynx (type) _____

                          ☐ TEP ☐ esophageal ☐ other _____

Secondary communication: ☐ writing ☐ artificial larynx (type) _____

                          ☐ TEP ☐ esophageal ☐ other _____

For TE prosthesis users only: style and size of prosthesis _____

Date fitted: _____ Date placed: _____ Tracheostoma valve ☐ yes ☐ no

Prognosis for Acquisition of:

Electronic/mechanical speech: _____

Esophageal speech: _____

Tracheoesophageal speech: _____

Independent prosthesis management skills: _____

Recommendations:

Clinician: _____

CHAPTER TWENTY
Multicultural Issues in Speech-Language Pathology

Understanding multicultural issues goes beyond speaking a second language or dialect and being familiar with a culture's holiday celebrations, art, music, and food. Rather, one must learn about interaction patterns, beliefs, and value systems to understand a culture different from one's own (Westby, 1994). Also, one should remember that speakers of another dialect can come from across the town, not just across major geographic borders.

One of the most underserved populations of persons with communicative disorders comes from the rural populations of the United States. The prevalence of adults aged 65 and over in rural communities is increasing when compared to other segments of rural society. This is, in part, caused by the younger adults leaving the rural areas to pursue employment in more urban communities (Stewart-Gonzalez, 2000). However, there are still close to 5 million children attending school in rural areas that, according to the American Speech-Language-Hearing Association, are underserved (ASHA, 1985a, 1985b). They further point out that "the content of most standardized tests typically reflects formal language used in white middle-class school settings. Obviously, this precludes accurate assessment of many segments of our community" (Wilson, Wilson, & Coleman, 2000, p. 105). The rural culture is a non-dominant culture in mainstream America.

To successfully diagnose a language or speech disorder in a person from a non-dominant culture, one must have an understanding of the following:

1. The development of communication in different cultures;

2. The causes and effects of communication disorders in various racial/ethnic populations;

3. The effects of culture and second language acquisition on the process of testing and test interpretation;

4. Dialect differences versus speech-language disorders; and

5. Alternative assessment approaches for culturally/linguistically different clients. (Westby, 1994, p. 31)

Wilson, Wilson, and Coleman (2000) reference Losardo and Coleman (1996) in pointing out that "normative samples frequently do not include various racial/ethnic/cultural groups. When representatives of these groups are included, it is usually not in proportion to the groups' representation in the general population" (Wilson, Wilson, & Coleman in Coleman, 2000).

Testing is affected in both verbal and nonverbal aspects. Time is one of the nonverbal aspects that merits some consideration. Americans typically are bound by time and achieving goals within a set time period (e.g., completing an evaluation in 2 hours). People from some other cultures may not feel the need to complete a task quickly. Also, in the United States, we traditionally teach with words, whereas in other cultures, many children learn by observing others, with little or no verbal information being provided. This has implications for standardized testing because the client may want the clinician to show him how to do a task, and this may be prohibited by the testing protocol.

Another difference involves individual versus group orientation. In the United States, much value is put on individual achievement. However, in many cultures, one is encouraged to work toward group potential and goals, with little value being placed on individual accomplishments. Thus, the client may be hesitant to participate in testing that identifies his individual skills as separate from the group. In addition, in such cultures, children expect to be helped in accomplishing a new task, so they may be hesitant to participate in the testing situation without help from their peers.

Verbal aspects of testing can also be affected by different cultural backgrounds. For example, Americans use many "pseudoquestions" when educating their children. As a parent reads a picture book to a child, he will point to a picture and say, "What is this?" even though, clearly, the adult knows the answer to the question. Native American children are likely not to answer such a question because it would be considered an insult to the elder, as it suggests that the adult does not know the answer. Thus, on identification tasks, Native American children may not respond even if they know the answers.

In other cultures, questioning of an individual usually means that person is in trouble. This is true in the Carolina Piedmont culture. Because questioning is a critical component of most language testing, the clinician should know the implications of questions in the culture of the person being tested.

Another problem is the reliance on context to understand what is being asked or said. Because many test questions are decontextualized, this may also be problematic with regard to standardized testing. Standardized tests often do not take into account contextual language or behavioral and cultural influences on the measurement of language (Coleman, 2000).

A third problem, with regard to verbal aspects of testing, lies in the type of organizational structure of conversations in the testing atmosphere. Normally, there is a give-and-take of information between two persons. However, in the testing situation, one person asks questions and the other person answers. Persons with neurological impairments may have difficulty keeping the topic and the individual statements in mind at the same time. Similarly, persons from a different linguistic background may never have been involved in this type of discourse so that their testing indicates disorganized language not unlike that of a client with a language-based learning disability. It is critical to identify the language and learning needs of the client in different situations and observe how quickly they learn what is taught in these varied settings and situations. Otherwise, they may be assumed to have a language-based learning disability when, in actuality, they do not know how to structure the language in the asymmetrical style of testing.

Depending on the timing of the testing, a child may be losing his first language while learning a second language. Thus, if one were to test a child at this point in his development, he may test as having a language delay in each language, which, in fact, is not the case. Language proficiency needs to be evaluated in everyday situations, not just in the testing environment (Westby, 1994).

TABLE 20-1 Framework for language assessment	
Cognitively Demanding	*Context-Embedded*
Converses with familiar person	Participates in games
Follows spoken directions with concrete props	Describes content of school lessons
	Follows spoken directions without concrete props
Relates a personal experience	*Context-Reduced*
Follows simple pictorial or written directions	Tells or writes imaginary stories
	Tells or writes explanations and persuasive essays

From "Multicultural Issues," by C. Westby, 1999, in *Diagnosis in Speech-Language Pathology* (2nd ed.) (p. 52), by J. B. Tomblin, H. L. Morris, and D. C. Spriestersbach, San Diego, CA: Singular Publishing Group. Copyright 1999 by Singular Publishing Group. Reprinted with permission.

Westby proposes a framework for language assessment as outlined in Table 20–1. She divides common assessment tasks into cognitively demanding, context-embedded, and context-reduced aspects.

PROBLEMS WITH COMMON SUGGESTIONS FOR EVALUATION OF NON-DOMINANT LANGUAGE PERSONS

Westby points out several problems with the frequently cited suggestions for improving tests used in the evaluation of persons speaking a minority language or dialect.

The first suggestion is to translate the test. This is problematic because there is not always a one-to-one correspondence between a word in English and a word or concept in another language. In addition, concepts are often learned at different rates and in different orders than in standard English. Furthermore, morphology in standard English does not always have a counterpart in other languages.

Second, people often suggest standardizing existing tests using people from minority populations. According to Westby (1994), "standardized tests are based on mainstream culture. Consequently, nonmainstream individuals who are unfamiliar with the concepts on the test will usually score lower than mainstream individuals. There is a tendency to assume that lower test scores are indicative of lower innate potential" (p. 43).

Modifying existing tests to make them appropriate for clients from other cultures is also a suggestion that has problems. It is essential that the complexity of the content be maintained on a modified test. However, it is difficult to do that. Westby (1994) warns us that we must have knowledge of the culture for which the modifications are made to ensure the possibility of equal credit.

Others have suggested using a language sample, criterion-referenced tests, and other observations to assess the speech and language of those from another culture. Again, adequate knowledge about the culture of the minority client must be maintained by the assessing clinician. In most instances, we have inadequate norms and developmental information to make a meaningful analysis of a minority language.

If using a language sample, according to James (1989), as cited by van Keulen, Weddington, and DeBose (1989), two aspects of pragmatics can be determined from the language sample: "communication intentions and conversational ability. Intention refers to the ability to use the language to perform various communicative acts, such as describing, arguing, and responding. Conversational ability refers to the process of communicating with a partner and includes turn taking, topic maintenance, and relevance" (van Keulen, Weddington, and DeBose, 1998, p. 129).

Van Keulen, Weddington, and DeBose (1998, p. 124) make the following suggestions regarding modification of response requirements:

> Allowing more time than recommended by the test
>
> Accepting responses that are different from allowable responses, but appropriate for the language or culture
>
> Allowing the client to change responses
>
> Allowing the client to clarify responses or ask questions
>
> Allowing the client to respond using sign or foreign language or gesture.

Of course, if any of these modifications are made, the test cannot be counted as being administered in the standardized format. The test can be used to gather information about the client's language, but it cannot be scored based on the test's norms. The use of criterion-referenced testing may be a good alternative to using standardized tests. By using criterion-referenced testing, the clinician can test a skill in a variety of formats and be better able to compare the client's language to that of his peers.

Alternative Assessment Approaches

One alternative assessment approach is to use ethnographic interviews. "Ethnographic interviews have the goal of helping the interviewer understand the social situations in which the clients live and how the clients and their families perceive, feel about, and understand situations" (Westby, 1994, p. 44). Through such interviews, clinicians can gather information about the client's strengths, weaknesses, and needs from the perspective of the client and/or his family. One way to gather the information is to ask the client or family member to describe a typical day. From this information, the clinician can gather information as to what is important to the family, the daily communication needs, what they like or do not like, and an idea of the activities in which the client and/or his family participates.

Westby delineates several types of information that would be helpful to the clinician assessing a pediatric client from another culture:

> the language skills expected of children at different ages; who talks to children and who children talk with; how people talk with children; the topics of conversation for boys, girls, men, women; the beliefs about how children learn to talk; reasons for talking (giving directions, asking questions, telling stories, joking, etc.); roles of boys, girls, men, women in the culture; and how the culture defines and views a handicap. (Westby, 1994, p. 44)

For school-aged children, the child should be observed in his classroom, and his teacher should be interviewed to assess his/her concerns about the child. Information such as how the child is doing in different aspects of the curriculum is critical. It is also helpful to know the child's ability to relate the events of a story and to understand elements of stories such as the problems and solutions and the characters' personalities and feelings. The child's ability to comprehend complex sentences and assigned texts should also be evaluated. Writing samples are a good adjunct to a verbal language assessment that is gathered in the child's natural environment.

Feuernstein (1979) introduced the concept of dynamic assessment. Traditional assessment focuses on *what* has been learned; dynamic assessment focuses on *how* the client learns. This is a more appropriate assessment model for the evaluation of persons from minority cultures because the assessor has a better understanding of what needs to be done to improve the learning of the individual.

Interpreting Assessment Information

The client and/or his family should be told that they can bring anyone they choose to the interpretative meeting to hear the results of the assessment. In some cultures, the parents are not the decision makers, so whoever the decision makers are (grandparents, tribal elders, etc.) should attend the meeting.

The clinician should be aware that miscommunications may arise because of cultural interplay. In some cultures, men may be reluctant to accept information from a woman. Different rates of speaking could convey different meanings. Turn-taking patterns may also differ. Thus, the pragmatic differences between the clinician's dominant language and the client's minority language may affect how the results of the assessment are interpreted by the client and/or his family. It is important that the clinician explain why the questions that are asked are important because they may be viewed as rude or too personal to answer by members of a different culture.

Clinicians should also be aware of gender and racial biases that may exist based on previous experiences and/or the client and his family.

The African-American Child

It is important to remember that members of a minority culture do not necessarily embrace that culture if they are living in America. Thus, the clinician should be careful about identifying a patient's linguistic patterns as typical of, for example, Black English.

After reviewing eight research studies addressing the acquisition of African-American language, Stockman (1986) concluded that the features typically associated with African-American English are not prominent in children under 3 years of age. However, as the child becomes older, the presence of the features increases.

SUMMARY

In summary, there are many considerations in the area of multicultural issues with regard to assessment and treatment. It is difficult to give most standardized tests to members of non-dominant cultures without modifying the format, which results in a nonstandardized administration. However, the information gained from the testing can be used as part of the foundation to set up appropriate intervention goals. Awareness of different customs and linguistic aspects of minority languages is critical when interviewing, assessing, and treating persons from those minority areas.

CHAPTER TWENTY-ONE
Pediatric Feeding Problems

DEFINITION/DESCRIPTION

There are many different causes of pediatric feeding and swallowing disorders. A delineation of neurological conditions of childhood that are associated with dysphagia is in Table 21–1.

TABLE 21–1 Neurologic conditions of childhood associated with dysphagia

Dysfunction of Cortex or Basal Ganglia

Static encephalopathy (e.g., in utero intoxications, chromosomal defects, CNS infection, cerebrovascular accidents, trauma)

Progressive encephalopathy (e.g., Wilson's disease, HIV, multiple sclerosis, drug-induced movement disorders)

Brainstem

Congenital CNS anomalies

Tumors of brainstem or posterior fossa

Trauma

Brainstem encephalitis

Cranial Nerves

Trauma (basilar skull fracture)

Motor neuron disease (poliomyelitis, progressive bulbar paralysis of childhood, spinal muscular atrophy)

Tumors (schwannoma, neurofibromatosis)

Toxins (diphtheria, heavy metals)

Neuromuscular Junction

Myasthenia gravis

Drugs/intoxications (e.g., tetanus, streptomycin, bacitracin, beta blocker, phenothiazines)

Muscle

Congenital (e.g., muscular dystrophy)

Errors of metabolism

Endocrine (e.g., hyperthyroidism, hypothyroidism)

Esophageal Motility

Associated with CNS dysfunction

Induced by reflux esophagitis

Drug induced (e.g., beta adrenergics, muscle relaxants associated with myopathies)

From *Diagnosis and Evaluation in Speech Pathology* (5th ed.) (p. 312), by W. O. Haynes and R. H. Pindzola, 1998, Boston: Allyn and Bacon. Copyright 1998 by Allyn and Bacon. Reprinted with permission.

One of the most frequent causes of swallowing disorders in children is cerebral palsy. Typically, the oral stage of the swallow is the most affected, with the degree of involvement varying widely from child to child.

> Children may exhibit inappropriate oral reflexive behaviors; inability to hold material in a cohesive bolus, especially if the material is being masticated; and/or disorganized lingual movements that do not contribute to a smooth peristaltic action of the tongue in moving the material posteriorly. (Logemann, 1998, p. 324)

In some children, there may be oral residue following the swallow, or pieces of food may break off and lodge in the oral cavity prior to the oral swallow. Rarely does this result in aspiration, possibly because the pharyngeal swallow is not triggered when these small particles fall into the airway. However, children with severe oral motor problems, pharyngeal delay, and neuromuscular problems associated with the pharyngeal swallow typically do have oral and pharyngeal residue that can lead to aspiration (Logemann, 1998).

The development of coordinated movements of the oral musculature in children involves sensory, tactile, cognitive, respiratory, and oral motor skills. Disruptions in any of these skills can result in feeding and/or swallowing deviations in the pediatric population. These problems can lead to malnourishment and its associated sequelae.

The relationship between oral motor skills for eating and oral motor skills for speech is unclear. As Pinder and Faherty (1999) express, "although some children exhibit adequate eating skills, their speech is unintelligible. In our clinical experience and in our professional reading, we know of no children whose speech is clear but who are unable to chew their food due to lack of oral motor skill development" (Pinder & Faherty, 1999, p. 281). Many researchers and practicing clinicians have noted that many children who experience problems in developing their oral motor skills for feeding also have difficulty developing intelligible speech (Evans-Morris & Klein, 1987; Fogel & Thelen, 1987; Mueller, 1974; Pinder & Faherty, 1999). Pinder and Faherty (1999) go on to note that "as the sensitivity decreased and the child's practice with textures increased, the oral structures (lips, cheeks, tongue, and jaw) became more mobile both in range and coordination . . . (and) as the oral movements and oral feeding continued to improve, the child typically vocalized more with increasing variety of consonant-vowel combinations as well as increasingly accurate vocal imitation skills. Increased clarity of speech also followed, sometimes with startling rapidity" (Pinder & Faherty, 1999, pp. 281–282).

The implied improvement of speech following improvement of oral motor skills makes an oral motor approach to therapy for children with feeding and/or swallowing disorders a critical concern. However, the improvement of speech is secondary to improving the nutrition and physical health of the children. This is particularly true in children with cerebral palsy, apraxia, dysarthria, structural defects, failure to thrive, Möebius Syndrome, Pierre Robin syndrome, Down syndrome, and/or other motor speech disorders. In addition, early feeding problems may be the initial indicator of a neuromuscular or neuromotor disorder. Therefore, they should be treated with all due consideration.

DSM DIAGNOSTIC CRITERIA FOR 307.59 FEEDING DISORDER OF INFANCY OR EARLY CHILDHOOD

A. Feeding disturbance as manifested by persistent failure to eat adequately with significant failure to gain weight or significant loss of weight over at least 1 month.

B. The disturbance is not due to an associated gastrointestinal or other general medical condition (e.g., esophageal reflux).

C. The disturbance is not better accounted for by another mental disorder (e.g., Rumination Disorder) or by lack of available food.

D. The onset is before age 6 years. (DSM, 1994, p. 99–100)

ASSESSMENT

Feeding disorders in the pediatric population is an important topic because of the nutritional impact on brain development in the first few months of life. Usually, dysphagia in children is part of a more pervasive problem, such as gastrointestinal difficulties, neurologic and airway problems, and disruption of the caregiver-child relationship. It is also important because it is known that children with physiologically based feeding problems often develop behavioral complications.

It is important that the clinician has a good understanding of the anatomical differences between children and adults. Comprehension of the interrelationships of physiologic systems and their effects on swallowing and feeding, as well as the impact of the caregiver-child relationship, is critical as well (Arvedson & Rogers, 1998).

One anatomical difference between adults and children is the presence of sucking pads in the masseter muscles. These facilitate the baby's sucking patterns that are critical to acquiring adequate nutrition. Also, the baby's tongue essentially fills the oral cavity, and it rests in a more anterior position in the child than it does in the adult. Relatively speaking, the child's mandible is smaller. The larynx is suspended higher in the neck than it is in adults. This elevated position, combined with the close proximity of the tongue, the soft palate, and the pharynx, helps to facilitate nasal breathing during the first 3–4 months of life (Arvedson, Rogers, & Brodsky, 1993).

As in adult therapy, a team approach for assessment and treatment is critical. Typically, the members of a pediatric swallowing team include developmental physicians (including those knowledgeable in otorhinolaryngology, neurology, respiratory, and upper gastrointestinal problems), a speech-language pathologist (to address the oral motor and swallowing issues), and an occupational therapist (responsible for sensory development and self-feeding). Physical therapists, radiologists, nutritionists, social workers, nurses, and parents are also critical members of the team (Arvedson & Rogers, 1998).

Table 21-2 When to assess a child for feeding problems
Child is gagging more than two times per meal
Child is unable to keep fluid/food in his mouth
Child does not swallow
Child exhibits primitive or pathological reflexes
Child does not tolerate solids
Child is abnormally postured at mealtime
Child has abnormal muscle tone
Child exhibits tongue thrust beyond 6 months of age
Child bites down hard on the spoon
Parent reports mealtime difficulties
Child is nutritionally at risk

Children who are slow feeders (mealtimes typically longer than 30–40 minutes), who exhibit signs of aspiration, or who exhibit the symptoms of oral motor dysfunction should be evaluated for feeding and/or swallowing difficulties. Other criteria are listed in Table 21–2.

The decision about which children to assess would include children who demonstrate a new feeding problem, or a change in feeding patterns, including increased drooling and nasopharyngeal reflux. Signs of aspiration include "breathing interruptions or apnea during oral feeding, 'gurgly' vocal quality before and after swallows, incoordination of sucking and swallowing in infants, oral motor inefficiencies that delay movement of the bolus over the back of the tongue, and history of recurrent pneumonia and feeding difficulty" (Arvedson & Rogers, 1998, p. 49).

In addition, there may be behavioral symptoms that indicate the possibility of gastroesophageal reflux disease (GERD). These include behavior problems and/or irritability during meals, unexplained food refusal, failure to thrive, lethargy, and decreased arousal during feedings. Failure to gain weight over a period of 2–3 months, and a diagnosis of any disorder associated with failure to thrive or dysphagia are also reasons for referral. Finally, signs of delayed development such as not spoon feeding by 9 months of age, not chewing table foods by 18 months of age, and/or not drinking from a cup by age 24 months should also signal the need for an evaluation of feeding and/or swallowing disorders (Arvedson & Rogers, 1998).

A feeding observation form is found in Appendix 21–A, and an Oral Motor and Feeding Evaluation form comprises Appendix 21–B. Either of these can be used to guide the observation and assessment of children with feeding disorders.

Initially, children should be observed being fed by their primary feeder, using the equipment, food textures, and food amounts typically used when feeding. This enables the assessor to determine whether there are mechanical changes that can be made in the physical approach to feeding that will facilitate better eating on the part of the child. Once this observation is complete, the assessor can make modifications in the child's position, equipment, food texture, and/or food amount to see whether they have any effect on the child's eating. Food and liquid should be presented by spoon using about one-third of a teaspoon, initially using the texture that is best handled by the child. If chewables are used, it is recommended that graham crackers or plain sugar cookies be used because these form a bolus with a minimal amount of chewing or munching. Foods that should be avoided include the following: foods that flake apart (saltine crackers, pretzels, potato chips); foods with skins or shells (peas, hot dogs, corn); foods that are small and/or have hard textures (M & M's, hard candy, peanuts) (Arvedson, 1993).

Muscle Tone

Speech-language pathologists, occupational therapists, and physical therapists should jointly assess muscle tone, postural tone, and movement patterns to determine their effects on feeding and eating. The child should be assessed in a variety of positions, including supine, prone, and sitting. The clinician should observe symmetry of the muscles in the upper extremities, the lower extremities, the trunk, and the neck at rest and in movement. The clinician should pay particular attention to hyperextension because it is frequently accompanied by abnormal movements of the oral musculature. The child's ability to extend and flex into and against gravity should be assessed, as well as his ability to pull to a sit. When pulling to a sit, note whether the child's head follows along with the body without dropping back from the neck. In other words, the child's head should remain in flexion when the child is being pulled to a sit.

When the child is sitting, notice whether the child exhibits a pelvic tilt. Also, make note of the child's use of his abdominal muscles to maintain a sitting position. The clinician should notice whether there is any neck hyperextension used to maintain a sitting balance, as well as taking note of the child's mouth position in the sitting position. For example, the child may have hyperextension with the shoulders retracted. In this case, the child will probably exhibit lip and tongue retraction as part of a generalized abnormal movement and posturing pattern.

Other aspects of movement that should be assessed include the following:

- Does the child have enough dissociation to roll over?
- Does the child have lateral movement?
- Is the child able to shift his weight without losing his balance?
- Does the child have protective righting responses?

Hand-eye and hand-to-mouth coordination should also be assessed because they will have a significant impact on the child's ability to self-feed.

Abnormal muscle tone is a primary factor in pediatric feeding problems. If the tone is abnormal, it can lead to problems with tactile and proprioceptive feedback and sensations, which possibly will interfere with muscle coordination. The clinician should determine whether the child is hypotonic or hypertonic. A list of characteristics of hypotonia is in Table 21–3, and characteristics of hypertonia are in Table 21–4.

Jaw Movement

When feeding the child, the clinician should observe jaw movement to determine whether there is an up-down movement and a rotary component. Both are necessary for efficient chewing. Some children may have difficulty grading the opening of the jaw, either not

TABLE 21-3 Characteristics of hypotonia

Affects entire body

Floppy

No righting or protective response

Shallow, rapid breathing

Poor head control

Chest deformities

Paucity of phonation

Poor basis for movement; must "fix" abnormally for stability

TABLE 21-4 Characteristics of hypertonia

Affects all or part of body

Stiff and rigid

Influenced by limb positions in relation to body and by body position in relation to gravity

Extensor pattern characterized by jaw thrust, tongue thrust, legs close and/or scissored, spine extended, arms pulled back at shoulders, and elbows stuck in flexion or extension

Flexor pattern characterized by legs flexed, knees apart, spine and arms flexed, hands fisted, head pulled down, and a bite reflex

A neck and shoulder retraction pattern often accompanied by retraction of the lips, jaw, and tongue

Abnormal increase in resistance to passive movement

opening the jaw wide enough to accommodate a spoon, or opening the jaw too widely. Opening the jaw too widely is often accompanied by a reflexive bite in which the child clamps down on the spoon because he cannot grade the closing of the jaw. This "clamping down" is known as a tonic bite, and the child may have difficulty releasing the bite when it occurs. In some children, such as those with athetosis, this bite may be an attempt to stabilize the head by biting on the spoon. The bite can be released by applying firm pressure on the temporomandibular joint. Pulling on the spoon will only result in a stronger bite. The tonic bite also contributes to sensitization problems in the mouth. Children with a tonic bite will clamp down on their own fingers, resulting in a negative experience that is not likely to be repeated. Thus, the child does not actively engage in exploration of the environment using the oral sensations, resulting in a lack of sensitization of the oral cavity (Arvedson, 1993).

Lip Closure

Some children, particularly those with spasticity, may have habitually retracted lips. When the lips are retracted, the child cannot achieve lip closure. Thus, this interferes with getting food off of a spoon, sucking liquids through a nipple or a straw, and achieving cup drinking. Lip retraction may also lead to increased oral defensiveness.

Lip retraction is often accompanied by shoulder retraction and/or neck extension. Both of these interfere with proper positioning for feeding and other activities. Thus, it may be necessary to normalize a generalized body posture before proceeding with additional therapy.

Tongue Movement

Tongue movement should also be assessed. The child may have difficulty using controlled tongue movements such as retraction, elevation, and protrusion. The child may exhibit tongue thrust and tongue retraction. Tongue thrust will interfere "with placement of food in the mouth, as well as the child's ability to suck, chew, and swallow" (Arvedson, 1993, p. 276). In fact, the thrust may push the food out of the mouth before the lips can close. Thus, tongue thrust interferes with the ability of the child to chew the food, form a bolus, and position the food for swallowing.

Observations that should result in a referral of a child for the evaluation of feeding and/or swallowing problems include the following: prolonged feeding times (longer than 30–40 minutes); presence of neuromotor deficits; cleft palate; weak or breathy cry; hoarseness; gurgly vocal quality; increased rate of respirations during feeding; increased respiratory effort; incoordination of respirations and sucking and/or swallowing; unexplained weight loss (Arvedson & Rogers, 1998: Pinder & Faherty, 1999).

A bedside and clinical assessment protocol for children is delineated in Table 21–5.

Videofluoroscopic Swallowing Studies (VFSS), also known as the modified barium swallow, are the most frequently used method of evaluating the oral and pharyngeal phases of the swallowing process. Specifically, the following observations can be made:

- Extent of lip closure on the nipple, cup, or spoon
- Initiation of sucking response following nipple placement
- Tongue shaping, elevation, and movement during bolus manipulation
- Variance of bolus control in sucking, drinking, or chewing different textures
- Pooling of the bolus on the floor of the mouth, in the buccal cavities, or sticking to the hard palate
- Gradation of tongue and jaw movements
- Oral hypersensitivity (e.g., gagging, tongue retraction, etc.)
- Delayed oral transit time. (Pinder & Faherty, 1999, p. 298)

Another advantage of VFSS is that therapeutic management can be attempted and the results of the various procedures evaluated for their effectiveness (see Table 21–6).

The modifications suggested in Table 21–6 are expanded upon in Table 21–7.

Other diagnostic measures include technetium scans, 24-hour pH probes, and upper gastrointestinal radiographic series to assess the function of the esophagus and to determine the presence of gastroesophageal reflux. These procedures are described in the chapter on dysphagia in adults.

> In summary, the diagnostic workup for children with feeding and swallowing problems must be comprehensive (1) to establish etiology, (2) to describe the structures and function in all aspects of feeding and swallowing, (3) to clarify oral, pharyngeal, and esophageal phase physiology and the risk for aspiration with oral feeding, and (4) to delineate nutrition status and risks. (Arvedson & Rogers in Johnson & Jacobson, 1998, p. 55)

TABLE 21-5 A bedside and clinical assessment protocol for children

Test	*Measurements*
Observations	Parent-child interaction
	Positioning during feeding
	General postural tone
	Respiratory status
	Level of alertness
	Temperament
	Ability to self-calm and self-regulate
	Speech and sound production (variety, frequency, volume, and quality)
Oral motor exam	Lip and jaw position/symmetry at rest
	Lip and jaw position/symmetry with movement
	Presence (and awareness) of drooling
	Tongue position and symmetry at rest
	Tongue position and symmetry during movement
	Shape and height of palate
	Presence and absence of oral reflexes (rooting, bite, suck-swallow, gag, cough)
	Laryngeal function
	Nonnutritive sucking in infants
Feeding observation	Self-feeding (drinking, hand-to-mouth with fingers and utensils, maintenance of good oral motor patterns when self-feeding)
	Presence of munching and/or chewing
	Bolus formation
	Timing of oral phase of swallowing
	Timing of pharyngeal phase of swallowing
	Number of active swallows per bolus
	Progression through various textures
	Signs of hypersensitivity or hyposensitivity (tactile, taste, temperature, auditory, visual, movement)
	Positioning (head, neck, and shoulder stability, postural control)
	Observe a minimum of 15–20 minutes to observe for fatigue and increasing disorganization
Flexible endoscopy	Congenital anomalies
	Stenosis
	Compression from vascular rings or masses
	Laryngotracheal malacia or other structural airway problems
	Examination of upper airways (laryngoscopy)
	Examination of lower airways (bronchosopy)
	Airway protection (nasopharyngoscopy)

Based on information from "Dysphagia in Children," by J. C. Arvedson and B. T. Rogers, 1998, in *Medical Speech-Language Pathology: A Practitioner's Guide* by A. F. Johnson and B. H. Jacobson, New York: Thieme Medical Publishers. Copyright 1998 by Thieme Medical Publishers; and "Issues in Pediatric Feeding and Swallowing," by G. L. Pinder and A. S. Faherty, 1999, in *Clinical Management of Motor Speech Disorders in Children,* by A. J. Caruso and E. A. Strand, New York: Thieme Medical Publishers. Copyright 1999 by Thieme Medical Publishers.

TABLE 21–6 On-line therapeutic modifications to be assessed during the VFSS based on witnessed dysphagia symptoms

Modification Attempted	Dysphagia Symptom Witnessed
Feeding Delivery Method Changes	• Oral phase difficulties • Suck-swallow-breathe incoordination • Piecemeal deglutition
Thermal Stimulation (e.g., chilled liquid/food)	• Swallow reflex delay • Aspiration before the swallow
Textural Modifications	• Oral phase difficulties • Piecemeal deglutition • Swallow reflex delay • Nasal reflux • Aspiration before, during, or after the swallow • Residue after the swallow
Increased Liquid Viscosity	• Nasal reflux • Reduced speed of laryngeal elevation with frequent supraglottal penetration • Aspiration during the swallow
Positioning/Postural Changes	• Oral phase difficulties • Limited laryngeal elevation • Asymmetrical dysfunction

From "Issues in Pediatric Feeding and Swallowing," by G. L. Pinder and A. S. Faherty, 1999, in *Clinical Management of Motor Speech Disorders in Children* (p. 298), by A. J. Caruso and E. A. Strand (Eds.), New York: Thieme Medical Publishers. Copyright 1999 by Thieme Medical Publishers. Reprinted with permission.

TABLE 21–7 Additional therapeutic modifications to be assessed during the VFSS based on witnessed dysphagia symptoms

Analysis of the Effectiveness of a Specific Intervention	Situation
Palatal Lift	Dysphagia symptoms witnessed that might suggest use of a palatal lift: Oral phase difficulties, particularly obstruction of liquid flow by flaccid soft palate Suck-swallow-breath incoordination Significant nasal reflux Nasal and pharyngeal residue after the swallow Aspiration after the swallow
Medication Change	Aspiration before, during, or after the swallow, on a child previously orally fed, following the introduction of a new drug or a new dosage increase in a previous drug
Oral Motor Treatment	Objective analysis of changes in symptoms can be conducted in serial VFSS procedures to verify that the treatment has had an impact, and therefore, to advance oral diet

From "Issues in Pediatric Feeding and Swallowing," by G. L. Pinder and A. S. Faherty, 1999, in *Clinical Management of Motor Speech Disorders in Children* (p. 299), by A. J. Caruso and E. A. Strand (Eds.), New York: Thieme Medical Publishers. Copyright 1999 by Thieme Medical Publishers. Reprinted with permission.

TREATMENT

In the pediatric population, frequently the primary goal of therapy is adequate nutrition. For children with neuromotor disorders, such as cerebral palsy, one of the first goals is adequate positioning to facilitate the feeding and swallowing processes. Central alignment as described by Arvedson and Rogers (1998) is outlined in Table 21–8.

Desensitization

It should be remembered that children normally explore their world through use of all their senses, including taste. Thus, developmentally, one would encourage mouthing of toys as part of a desensitization and exploratory process. One of the primary goals is to develop "coordinated movements of the mouth, respiratory, and phonatory systems for communication as well as for oral feeding" (Arvedson & Rogers, 1998, p. 57). Toothbrushing without toothpaste can also be used to desensitize the oral cavity and facilitate exploring different temperatures and textures of foods. Desensitization of the oral cavity will also result in a decrease in the gag reflex.

Normalizing the Gag Reflex

The gag reflex is a normal survival mechanism for protecting the trachea from foreign bodies. However, in some children, the gag is hyperactive or hypoactive. In these cases, the gag reflex must be normalized. The gag reflex can be normalized through the use of a sensory stimulation program.

One way to normalize sensation is to use a plastic swizzle stick or a tongue blade (the child must not have a tonic bite) to "walk" back on the tongue. In the case of a hyperactive gag, the goal is to increase the distance between the front of the mouth and the faucial pillars that the clinician can move the stick without eliciting the gag reflex. In the case of a hypoactive gag, the goal is to decrease the amount of space between the front of the mouth and the point at which the gag reflex is elicited. Other methods of desensitization/sensitization can also be used, including having the child do oral play (mouthing toys and other objects).

TABLE 21–8 Central alignment
Neutral head flexion (symmetry, midline, stability) with a balance between flexion and extension
Neck elongated
Shoulder girdle stable and depressed
Trunk elongated
Pelvis stable and symmetrical and in neutral position
Hips at 90°, with neutral base of abduction and rotation
Feet in neutral with slight dorsiflexion and never plantarflexed

From "Dysphagia in Children," by J. C. Arvedson and B. T. Rogers, 1998, in *Medical Speech-Language Pathology: A Practitioner's Guide* (p. 57), by A. F. Johnson and B. H. Jacobson (Eds.), New York: Thieme Medical Publishers. Copyright 1998 by Thieme Medical Publishers. Used with permission.

Normalizing the Suck-Swallow Reflex

In the early stages of moving from liquids to solids, children prefer to suck their food (as opposed to chew) because it softens the food prior to its being swallowed. However, this normalizes around 6–9 months with the development of munching and chewing behaviors. Children who continue to use a suck-swallow pattern to swallow their food may have deficits in sensory processing, oral motor difficulties, or problems with swallowing (Murphy & Caretto, 1999).

Again, a sensory stimulation program may be of benefit to children with a persistent suck-swallow reflex. The goal of sensory stimulation programs is to normalize sensitivity in the oral area.

Sensory Stimulation Programs

There are certain guidelines that should be followed when implementing a sensory stimulation program. The first is to move from distal to proximal. Even when working on sensitization in the oral area, stimulation should begin distally (with the hands, arms, and trunk), moving gradually toward the face, then to the mouth in particular. It is not unusual for a child who is hypersensitive in the oral area also to be hypersensitive on his hands. Thus, normalizing sensation should begin on the hands; this also prepares the child for self-feeding (Murphy & Caretto, 1999).

A second premise is to use deep, firm pressure. Light touch arouses the central nervous system and serves as an "alert" that an "invasion" is about to occur. A small amount of deep pressure that is provided symmetrically does not result in a strong "alert" response.

Third, the stimulation should be smooth and continuous. In Table 21–9, Murphy and Caretto (1999) delineate what types of contact should be provided.

When providing sensory stimulation in the oral area, the clinician should always wear protective gloves. However, the clinician should be sure the child is not latex-sensitive, and the clinician should not use powdered gloves. If the child does not tolerate the sensation created by the gloves, the clinician can wrap his/her hand or finger in a washcloth or other soft fabric that is better tolerated. The materials should be dry because the cold sensation of wet cloth may trigger a negative reaction (Murphy & Caretto, 1999).

If a child reacts negatively toward being approached in the facial area, the clinician can create distractions in the environment to minimize the negative reaction. For example, the

TABLE 21–9 Types of sensory input

Area	Type of Sensory Input
Cheeks	Use palm instead of fingertips.
Lips	Use sides of fingers instead of fingertips.
Cheeks	If muscle tone is decreased, use quick strokes. If muscle tone is increased, use slow strokes.

From "Sensory Aspects of Feeding," by S. M. Murphy and V. Caretto, 1999, in *The Educator's Guide to Feeding Children with Disabilities* (Chpt. 6), by D. K. Lowman and S. M. Murphy (Eds.), Baltimore, MD: Paul H. Brookes Publishing Co. Copyright 1999 by Paul H. Brooks Publ. Co.

clinician could place a small towel on the child's head and play peek-a-boo as the towel is moved across the child's face. Songs can be sung, music can be played, or soothing talking can be used to minimize the implied threat (Murphy & Caretto, 1999).

Sensory stimulation can involve touch, icing, brushing, and vibration. Because of the complex nature of the sensory system, icing, brushing, and vibration should be done only by those who are trained specifically in the use of those techniques.

When working on the musculature of the lips and cheeks, it is important to work toward the mouth. Murphy and Caretto (1999, p. 118) recommend the following method of facial stimulation:

- Stroke downward on the cheeks toward the corners of the lips.
- Stroke downward from the nose toward the upper lip with the side of one finger.
- Stroke upward from the chin to the bottom lip with the side of one finger.
- Stroke around the lips in a circular motion with a finger pad to stimulate the 'pucker' muscle.

Facial stimulation provided prior to meals can help facilitate preparation of the muscles for the movements required for eating. Specifically, the stimulation can have significant effects on the sensory awareness of the facial musculature, the muscle activity, and the muscle length.

Oral stimulation is more invasive than stimulation of the face, because it involves stimulation to the gums, the tongue, and the internal cheek muscles. Care should be taken when working with a child who has a tonic bite reflex or who has a hyperactive gag reflex. One method of oral stimulation is to rub a beginner's toothbrush over the teeth and gums. The Nuk toothbrush is a knobby rubber device that provides excellent stimulation for the gums. When toothbrushes are used, they should be used without toothpaste. If the child does not have a tonic bite reflex, digital stimulation can be provided by the clinician. Even if the child does have a tonic bite reflex, the clinician can stimulate the gums between the teeth and the cheeks, and the inside of the cheeks as long as care is taken to avoid the teeth.

Visual stimuli (e.g., a spoon of food) should be presented slightly below the child's line of vision if he were facing straight ahead. If the stimulus is presented too high, it may lead to hyperextension. Similarly, if it is presented too low, it will encourage the child to go into a flexion pattern. If the stimulus is presented slightly below the child's line of vision, it will encourage a slight chin tuck, which will facilitate oral posturing for feeding.

Facilitating Head and Trunk Stability

Etiological factors in poor head and trunk stability include distractibility, poor sitting balance, absence of head and/or trunk control, spasticity, athetosis, poor sensory integration, structural deformities, static positioning, and compensatory or habitual movements/fixations. Associated problems related to feeding include lack of oral control and the development of postural blocks at the level of the neck, shoulders, and/or pelvis. Activities to facilitate maintenance and carryover of good head and trunk stability include feeding the child in a non-distracting environment, positioning the child properly (see Table 21–8), use of oral control as needed, and movement to counteract tone problems. The physical therapist can be a tremendous asset to the team in developing appropriate movement and posturing patterns. Expected results of these manipulations are a decrease in the bite reflex, decreased reflexive sucking (and the use of a more mature sucking pattern), facilitation of lip closure, stimulation of chewing, and stimulation of swallowing.

Facilitating Jaw Stability

Etiological factors in jaw instability include many of those associated with poor head and trunk control. In addition, a tongue thrust pattern, persistence of a suck-swallow pattern, innervation problems, and/or ataxia can contribute to jaw instability. Normally, a child should be able to keep his jaw in a midline, stable position with the mouth closed for eating. Individuals with cerebral palsy frequently cannot control the jaw movement, so others must provide stability until the muscles are trained to do so on their own. As a result, lip closure, chewing, sucking, and control for speech production will be adversely affected. Any child with poor muscle tone and/or innervation problems in the oral and/or facial area will have problems with jaw stability. Associated feeding problems include poor lip closure, poor sucking patterns, and problems with chewing. Jaw instability is a major problem for children with cerebral palsy. A child with jaw instability gets no lateral jaw movement; the jaw only moves up and down. This prevents the development of the rotary component that is critical to a mature chewing pattern. Children with cerebral palsy are often mouth breathers, with the mouth typically being open at rest. Thus, these children frequently have problems with drooling.

External jaw control can be offered by the clinician if the child will tolerate touch in the oral and facial area. External jaw control is provided by the following positioning of the clinician's hand on the child's face:

> The clinician's thumb should rest firmly on the child's chin; the index finger should be extended and provide pressure on the temporomandibular joint (TMJ), thus providing side-to-side stability; the remaining fingers should be crooked below the chin, with the side of the third finger providing upward pressure on the base of the tongue. The thumb and index finger help to provide stability of the head, and the third finger presses up on the base of the tongue to help stimulate a swallow if necessary.

> If a child has very poor head control, it may be necessary to modify the external jaw stability. One method that may be helpful is to stand behind the child with the clinician's forearms providing head control, with regard to preventing lateral movement of the head. The clinician's thumb should be placed on the TMJ, the index finger across the upper lip, the middle finger on the lower lip, and the other two fingers under the chin. Regardless of which method of external jaw stability is used, the provision of stability helps to inhibit the bite reflex and the suck-swallow reflex and assists in facilitating lip closure and correct chewing and swallowing patterns.

> If a child resists external jaw control, a sensory stimulation program to normalize the child's tolerance of touch should be implemented.

Facilitating Sucking Ability

Etiological factors associated with poor sucking ability include hypertonicity, hypotonicity, ataxia, jaw instability and/or asymmetry, compensatory or habitual movements, innervation problems, dental malocclusion, improper positioning, lack of lip closure/lip seal, hypersensitive skin over the orbicularis oris and/or masseters, and a hyperactive gag reflex. Associated feeding problems include difficulty removing food from the spoon, difficulty drinking through a nipple or a straw, and difficulty swallowing.

Facilitation techniques include positioning the child correctly and providing external jaw stability. Lightly stroke the cheeks going down in an arc from the ears to the lips. Lightly stroke the area around the mouth. Encouragement of straw drinking is also effective. The clinician can trap a small amount of liquid in the straw by placing his/her finger over the opposite end of the straw. The straw is then placed in the child's mouth, and when he approximates a sucking movement, the finger can be removed and the liquid will be released into the child's mouth. Sucking can be shaped using this procedure. If the child will tolerate cold items, popsicles can be provided for sucking. Pacifiers can be used to establish a non-nutritive sucking pattern. Puckering can be stimulated with blowing exercises. Use a tongue depressor or flat-bowled spoon to put food on the middle of the tongue. Applying a slight downward pressure will cause the upper lip to approximate the lower lip, thus facilitating lip closure and a sucking movement of the tongue.

Facilitating Chewing

Chewing problems can be attributed to any of the etiological problems associated with sucking difficulties. However, poor tongue control and, in particular, the inability to make lateral movements with the tongue, are the most influential factors. Inability to chew may also be associated with a strong bite reflex.

Chewing is an extremely complex process involving balanced, coordinated movements of the cheeks, the mandible, the lips, and the tongue. Chewing involves an up-down motion of the jaw, a rotary movement of the jaw, and tongue lateralization. Some children may exhibit only the up-down motion of the jaw; this is called munching, and it is normal when a child is first learning to chew. However, the rotary component of jaw movement and lateralization of the tongue are necessary to transfer food throughout the oral cavity and to assist in preparing and positioning the food to be swallowed.

As a rule, the most frequently encountered chewing difficulties are as follows:

1. Inability to transfer food from the front of the mouth to the molars

2. Inability to keep food between the molars for grinding

3. Difficulty in transferring food from one side of the mouth to the other

Remediation techniques for chewing include a wide variety of activities. It should be noted that therapy for chewing should not begin until the bite reflex has been eliminated and the suck-swallow and gag reflexes normalized. Initially, a bite must be elicited by placing a food bit between the molars, pulling downward on the child's jaw, and pressing on the temporomandibular joint of the jaw. If this fails, push upward on the jaw until a bite is obtained. Food should be placed in the mouth when it is open to a normal width. If food does not stay between the molars, use an applicator stick or a tongue blade to hold the food in place. If the child does not move the food from side to side on his own, the applicator stick can also be used to do this. One technique that is particularly successful is to wrap a cube of sugarless bubble gum securely in a piece of gauze. Leave about a 6- to 8-inch tail of gauze, which the clinician can use to hold onto the gum. Place the gum between the molars, and after a few chews, transfer it to the opposite side. Continue this process until the child moves the gum back and forth using his own tongue.

Jaw stability may need to be provided to facilitate chewing. If so, it may be helpful to gently massage the masseters with the thumb, unless this action stimulates a bite reflex. Constant firm pressure under the chin is the best stimulus for chewing.

It should be stressed that in children without handicapping conditions, chewing movements start to become mature and voluntarily initiated around 7 months of age. If the child in therapy is functioning below an age level of 6–8 months, he is not developmentally ready to begin a chewing program. Also, since chewing motions do not completely mature until age 12 months, a child who functions below 12 months of age may have difficulty learning to chew.

Facilitating Swallowing

Swallowing problems may be due to hypertonicity, hypotonicity, ataxia, insufficient tongue control, a habitually open mouth, poor or absent sucking ability, a hyperactive gag, and faulty compensatory or habitual movement patterns. One should suspect swallowing problems if the child drools, holds food in his mouth for a longer-than-average time, or chokes frequently. If the child has a hyperactive gag reflex, it must be normalized before working on the swallowing skills. Associated feeding problems include choking and/or gagging, drooling, and dehydration.

The child should be positioned properly, and external jaw stability should be provided. It is very important that the clinician not let the head tilt backward. This opens the airway and makes the child susceptible to aspiration. Also, gravity forces the swallow, and the child does not develop an active swallowing response. Lip closure should be facilitated, and manual pressure should be applied under the chin. It may be helpful to stroke the neck in a downward motion and to gently pinch the laryngeal protuberance. These manipulations will result in a relaxation of the oral musculature, decreased tongue thrust, and improved tongue control. Improved tongue control will result in better formation and positioning of the bolus for swallowing. Slight upward pressure on the base of the tongue will trigger the swallow reflex to propel the food from the oral cavity into the pharynx.

A delineation of the signs and symptoms of swallowing problems and treatment options is found in Table 21–10.

In summary, the child's eating and drinking skills should be assessed as outlined previously to determine whether the child has the prerequisite skills to benefit from oral motor therapy. It should be remembered that nutrition, not oral feeding, is a primary goal in children, not oral feeding. Oral feeding may occur as a byproduct of therapy. "A systematic developmental approach focuses on heightening sensory awareness, perception, and discrimination within the mouth" (Arvedson & Rogers, 1998, p. 57).

TABLE 21-10 Signs and symptoms of swallowing problems in the oral preparatory, oral, and pharyngeal phases with treatment options

Phase of Swallow	Sign or Symptom	Treatment to Improve
Oral preparatory	Food falls out of mouth	Lip closure
	Pooling in anterior sulci	Jaw elevation and lip closure
	Lack of tongue action to form bolus	Tongue exercises
	Lack of chewing	Rotary tongue and jaw action
Oral	Pooling in lateral sulci	Lip closure and buccal tension
	Food pushed out of mouth	Tongue exercises to reduce thrusting
	Slow bolus formation	Tongue manipulation
	Piecemeal deglutition	Lateral tongue and jaw action and rotary jaw action
	Delayed swallow	Initiate tongue action quickly
Pharyngeal	Pooling in vallecula and pyriform sinuses	Improve timing of swallow production
	Residue in pharyngeal recesses after swallow	Multiple swallow per bite; alternate textures
	Gurgly voice quality	Improve vocal fold closure with voice therapy
	Aspiration on liquids, safe for thicker textures	Thicken liquids
	Aspiration on paste, safe with liquids	Make food thinner texture
	Choking on mixed textures in the same bite	Make each bite of a consistent texture; alternate per bite
	Swallow delayed > 10 seconds for best texture	Non-oral feedings
	Aspiration for all textures (frequent)	Non-oral feedings; oral stimulation without food except for taste

From "Oral-Motor and Feeding Assessment," by J. Arvedson, 1993, Chapter 8 in *Pediatric Swallowing and Feeding: Assessment and Management* (p. 277), by J. C. Arvedson and L. Brodsky (Eds.), San Diego, CA: Singular Publishing Group. Copyright 1993 by Singular Publishing Group. Reprinted with permission.

APPENDIX 21-A: HOLISTIC FEEDING OBSERVATION FORM

Child's Name: _____ Age: _____

Date(s) Observed: _____ Time: _____

Environment(s) Observed: _____ Observer(s): _____
Reason for Referral:

I. Collaboration with the Family
Sample Questions
- What is the feeding routine at home? What is the feeding routine in school?
- How is the child fed? What equipment is used?
- What are the feeding issues identified by the family?
- What is pleasurable specific to the feeding interaction?
- What is difficult specific to the feeding interaction?
- What cultural implications are important to consider?
- Are there medical or nutritional issues that must be addressed?

Observations:

II. Respiratory Issues
Sample Questions
- Is the gag reflex present and effective (i.e., not over- or underresponsive)?
- Is the swallow reflex present and effective (i.e., not inhibited or delayed; no paralysis)?
- Is the feeding pace determined by the child (i.e., not the feeder)?
- Is swallowing relaxed and without gagging, coughing, or aspiration?
- If a respiratory infection is present, is enough extra time allowed for coordination of breathing and swallowing?
- Is the coordination of breathing, swallowing, and talking difficult?

Observations:

III. Oral Motor Development

Sample Questions

- Has overall muscle tone been determined (e.g., low, normal, high)?
- Have muscle tone issues specific to the face and mouth been determined?
- Have needs for oral motor treatment been identified?

Observations:

IV. Physical Development/Positioning

Sample Questions

- Is 90°-90°-90° position achievable?
- Are feet and arms supported by a flat surface (i.e., not dangling)?
- Are knees at a comfortable 90° angle?
- Are hips resting symmetrically against a supportive surface?
- Is trunk upright and symmetrical?
- Is a neutral head position ensured for most effective swallow and eye contact?

Observations:

V. Sensory Development

Sample Questions

- Are any limitations of the sensory modalities present (e.g., visual, auditory, tactile, gustatory, olfactory, proprioceptive)?
- Which textures are most easily tolerated?
- Which tastes are most easily tolerated (likes versus dislikes)?
- Which temperatures are most easily tolerated? (Note preferences.)
- Which type(s) of touch are most easily tolerated (arousing versus calming)?

Observations:

VI. Communication, Behavioral, and Socialization Skills

Sample Questions

- Does the child have the maximum control possible?
- How does the child indicate hunger with food present?
- How does the child indicate hunger when food is not present?
- How does the child indicate his or her need for a change of pace/pause in feeding?
- How does the child indicate a choice of food or liquid?
- How does the child indicate readiness for more food?
- How does the child indicate that he or she is finished eating?
- How does the child indicate a desire for social closeness/distance?

Observations:

VII. Feeding Process and Implementation Plan

Sample Questions

- Have the family, all feeders, and needed specialists participated in the development of this plan?

- Has needed medical information (including physician orders and nutrition requirements) been received and factored into this feeding plan?

- Has needed feeding equipment been identified and obtained?

- Has the most effective sequence (i.e., the best order of feeding) been determined?

Observations:

From *The Educator's Guide to Feeding Children with Disabilities* (pp. 231–233), by D. K. Lowman and S. M. Murphy, 1999, Baltimore: Paul H. Brookes. Copyright 1999 by Paul H. Brookes. Reprinted with permission.

APPENDIX 21–B: ORAL MOTOR AND FEEDING EVALUATION

Name _____ Chart Number _____

Date of Evaluation _____ Referral _____

Date of Birth _____ Diagnosis _____

C.A. _____ Adjusted Age _____ Clinician _____

Summary _____

_____

Put a √ to indicate presence of any factor; describe briefly. NA = not applicable.

History

I. **Family and Social History**

_____ Primary caregivers: ☐ parent ☐ babysitter ☐ foster parent

_____ Other _____

_____ Other persons in the home _____

_____ Neurologic problems _____

_____ Cleft palate or other craniofacial anomalies _____

_____ Feeding problems in family _____

_____ Respiratory/breathing problems
(asthma, allergies) _____

_____ Environmental factors (smoking, pets) _____

II. **Prenatal History**

_____ Medications _____

_____ Substance abuse (smoking, alcohol, other drugs)

_____ Mother _____

_____ Father _____

_____ Maternal infection _____

_____ Radiation _____

_____ Toxemia _____

_____ Bleeding _____

_____ Thyroid disease _____

_____ Polyhydramnios _____

_____ Other _____

III. Birth History

_____ Birth weight _____ Gestational age

_____ Trauma _____

_____ Apgar scores _____

_____ Intubation

_____ Prolonged hypoxia or anoxia/respiratory distress _____

_____ Surfactant therapy _____

_____ Cardiac problems _____

_____ Other complications _____

IV. Neonatal period (first 28 days)

_____ Alert _____ Lethargic, difficult to rouse _____

_____ Respiratory problems

_____ Supplemental ventilation _____

_____ Pneumonia/bronchitis _____

_____ Chronic upper respiratory infection _____

_____ Allergies and/or asthma _____

_____ Sleep problems _____

    _____ Lengthy night waking times _____

    _____ Snoring _____

_____ Rooting reflex intact _____ Absent _____ Inconsistent

_____ Drooling _____ Intermittent _____ Frequent _____ Excessive

_____ Medication _____

_____ Weak or dysrhythmic non-nutritive suck (pacifier or finger)

_____

V. Feeding History — Describe each factor

Position: _____ Cradles in arms _____ Upright in arms _____ Upright in chair

Duration: _____ 20 minutes _____ 30–40 minutes _____ More than 45 minutes

Intervals: _____ 2 hours _____ 3 hours _____ 4 hours _____ Other

Tube feedings: _____ If yes, type _____

    How long: _____ weeks _____ months

Sucking: _____ Breast _____ Bottle (_____ nipple type _____ formula)

    Lip seal: _____ No liquid loss _____ Liquid loss at corners of mouth

        _____ Excessive vertical jaw action _____ Hard to burp

Textures in diet: _____ Liquid only _____ Liquid and pureed

        _____ Liquid, pureed, and solid _____ Pureed and solid

Diet (per 24-hour day)

    Quantity of food _____

    Quantity of liquid (oz/cc) _____

    Vitamin/mineral supplement _____

Appetite: ____ Good ____ Inconsistent ____ Poor

Food allergies or intolerance _____

Gagging or emesis: ____ During feed ____ After feed (at least 30 minutes)

Preferred food temperature: ____ Warm ____ Cold

Preferred liquid temperature: ____ Warm ____ Cold

Location for feeding: ____ One place ____ Several locations

Utensils: ____ Bottle and nipple ____ Cup ____ Straw

____ Spoon ____ Fingers

Respiratory status

____ Supplemental ventilation

____ Aspiration or pneumonia

____ Bronchitis or chronic upper respiratory infection

____ Allergies or asthma

____ Noisy breathing: ____ With feeds ____ After feeds

____ Gurgly voice quality: ____ During feeds ____ After feeds

____ Coughing or choking: ____ During feeds ____ After feeds

____ Trouble breathing during feeds

Other signs of distress

____ Fussing during feeding

____ Head turning to avoid feeding

____ Falling asleep during feeding

____ Postural changes: ____ Stiffening ____ Hyperextending

VI. Other Factors

Past medical/surgical history

_____ Upper GI or Scintiscan _____

_____ Videofluoroscopic modified barium swallow study: _____

_____ Surgical procedures — describe: _____

Sleep

_____ Waking in night

_____ Snoring

_____ Mouth breathing

Communication

_____ Nonverbal

_____ Verbal: _____ Intelligible (more than 50%)   _____ Unintelligible

Miscellaneous comments: _____

_____

Physical Examination

I. Prefeeding Observations

A. Position at rest

_____ Prone   _____ Supine   _____ Sidelying

_____ Independent sitting   _____ Supported sitting

_____ Flexion   _____ Hyperextension

_____ Trunk asymmetry   _____ Limb asymmetry

_____ Variable: _____

B. Level of arousal and alertness

_____ Sustained for at least 10 minutes

_____ Intermittent and fluctuating

_____ Falls asleep within 4–5 minutes

C. Muscle tone and movement patterns

_____ Tone normal   _____ Hypertonicity   _____ Hypotonicity   _____ Variable

_____ Proximal stability: _____ Adequate   _____ Deficient

_____ Distal stability: _____ Adequate   _____ Deficient

D. Irritability (state)

_____ Usually quiet   _____ Infrequent and calms easily

_____ Frequent, but calms with holding   _____ Frequent, difficult to quiet

E. Airway status

_____ No problem   _____ Stridor

_____ Dusky spells: _____ with feeding   _____ apart from feeding

_____ Oxygen dependent

_____ Tracheotomy: _____ size   _____ type

_____ Ventilator dependent

F. Communication

_____ Nonverbal

_____ Verbal: _____ Intelligible   _____ Breathy   _____ Shrill

_____ Hypernasal   _____ Gurgly   _____ Weak

_____ Hyponasal

_____ Vocal quality normal   _____ Abnormal

_____ Pitch normal   _____ High   _____ Low

_____ Volume normal   _____ Weak   _____ Overloud

G. Face and mouth — structure and function

_____ Facial symmetry _____ Facial asymmetry

_____ Mandible normal _____ Small

_____ Cheek tone normal _____ Reduced

_____ Tongue symmetrical _____ Tongue asymmetrical

_____ Tongue protrusion midline _____ Tongue protrudes to one side

_____ Tongue soft (hypotonic) _____ Tongue contracted (hypertonic)

_____ Hard palate symmetrical _____ High arch _____ Narrow _____ Cleft

_____ Soft palate normal _____ Cleft

_____ Jaw stability normal _____ Jaw instability

_____ Gag reflex

_____ Rooting reflex

_____ Bite reflex

_____ Non-nutritive suck/swallow coordinated _____ Uncoordinated

H. Drooling

_____ Seldom _____ Variable _____ Frequent _____ Constant

_____ Minimal _____ Moderate _____ Severe _____ Profuse

_____ To lip _____ To chin _____ To clothes _____ To table

_____ Bib or clothing changes each day: How many _____

_____ Awareness high _____ Occasional _____ Never

II. Non-nutritive Sucking

_____ Responsive to stroking around mouth: _____ Eager _____ Inconsistent

_____ Rooting when stroked near corners of mouth:

_____ Always _____ Inconsistent _____ Never

_____ Sucking on little finger: _____ Rhythmic _____ Dysrhythmic

III. Oral Motor Function and Feeding Assessment

A. Movement of oral structures (check if present)

_____ Lips _____ Retraction _____ Pursing

_____ Tongue elevation _____ Protrusion

_____ Lateralization _____ Rapid movement

_____ Soft palate elevation during phonation

_____ Mandible vertical movement _____ Rotary movement

B. Protective mechanisms — upon command, no food

_____ Swallow _____ Cough _____ Gag

C. Primary feeder with infant — describe:

Communication/interaction _____

Positioning _____

Utensils _____

Amount per meal _____

Length of meal (minutes) _____

Avoidance/refusal _____

D. Feeding Assessment

_____ Suck/swallow/respiratory sequence normal _____ Uncoordinated

_____ Sucking bursts with appropriate pauses _____ Not pause

_____ Suck/swallow/respiratory sequence normal _____ Uncoordinated

_____ Flow rate normal (bubbles with each suck) _____ Poor

_____ Lip closure normal _____ Open mouth

_____ Loss of liquid: _____ Minimal _____ Moderate

_____ Tongue normal _____ Lateral movement _____ Thrusting

_____ Laryngeal elevation noted during swallow _____ Absent

_____ Pocketing of food/liquid: _____ Cheeks _____ Front of mouth

_____ Nasopharyngeal reflux: _____ Liquid only _____ Food

_____ Changes in respiratory functioning

    _____ Noisy breathing

    _____ Chest retractions

    _____ Inconsistent rate of breathing or dysrhythmia

    _____ Nasal obstruction

    _____ Bradycardia _____ Apnea _____ Cyanosis

    _____ Desaturation (usually measured by pulse oximetry)

_____ Alert for entire feed _____ Lethargy noted

_____ Coughing _____ Choking _____ Gagging _____ Spitting

_____ Emesis (vomiting)

_____ Spoon feeding: _____ Sucks food off spoon

    _____ Closes lips _____ Upper lip active _____ Upper lip no movement

_____ Chewing: _____ Suck-swallow _____ Munching

    _____ Rotary jaw _____ Lateral tongue _____ Abnormal

_____ Straw drinking: _____ Anticipates

    _____ Lip seal _____ Successful _____ Unsuccessful

_____ Associated movements

    _____ Arching back, neck, or head

    _____ Squirming or withdrawing

    _____ Falling asleep

    _____ Feeding time less than 30 minutes _____ More than 30 minutes

E. Changes made during assessment with positive outcome _____

_____

_____

_____

F. Changes made during assessment with negative outcome _____

_____

_____

_____

CHAPTER TWENTY-TWO
Reading and Spelling Disorders

DEFINITION/DESCRIPTION

Dyslexia is a developmental reading disability. Typically, dyslexia is caused by an individual's difficulty with phoneme-grapheme association. That is, people with dyslexia have difficulty associating the sound a letter or letter combination makes with its written representation. Usually, they are also poor spellers, although not all poor spellers are dyslexic. Dyslexia is not related to intelligence, but the individual with dyslexia may have other language-based learning disabilities (Guilmette, 1997). Johnson and Myklebust (1967) described children with dyslexia as having "problems perceiving the similarities in the initial and final sounds in words. These children also had problems breaking words into syllables and phonemes, retrieving the names of letters and words, remembering verbal information, and pronouncing phonologically complex words in speech" (Catts & Kamhi, 1999, p. 53).

Difficulties with phonemic awareness seem to be at the base of most reading and spelling problems. Torgesen (1999) defines phonemic awareness as follows:

> It involves a more or less explicit understanding that words are composed of segments of sound smaller than a syllable, as well as knowledge, or awareness of the distinctive features of individual phonemes themselves. It is this latter knowledge of the identity of individual phonemes themselves that continues to increase after an initial understanding of the phonemic structure of words is acquired. (p. 129)

Normal Reading

Developmental dyslexia is a deficit of auditory processing both in decoding and encoding. It is the most prevalent learning disability, accounting for 75–80% of all learning disabilities (Livesay, 1995). Reading has phonetic, syntactic, semantic, and memory components, all of which must be integrated if a person is to be a successful reader. Therefore, to determine a child's status with regard to reading, it is necessary to assess his or her visual and auditory modalities in order to determine whether there is a problem, and, if so, where the problem lies. Auditorily, an emphasis should be placed on phonics, phonetics, and linguistic information. The child must be able to decode letters to form an accurate phonological image of each word, then retrieve the definition of each word from memory. He or she must then combine syntactic and semantic information from the definitions into proper representation of a sentence. Finally, the child must combine the representations of individual sentences to comprehend the passage.

TABLE 22-1	Stages of reading	
Stage	*Ages*	*Primary Development*
0	Birth to 5–6 years	Accumulation of knowledge about letters, words, and books
1	5–7 years	Initial reading or decoding
2	7–9 years	Decoding becomes more automatic; beginning of reading for comprehension
3	9–14 years	Reading to learn; decoding skills become fully automatic
4	14–18 years	Multiple viewpoints due to increased cognitive skills, which enable abstract thinking
5	18+ years	Construction and reconstruction in critical reading; development of hypothetical-deductive reasoning

Adapted from *Stages of Reading Development*, by J. Chall, 1983, New York: McGraw-Hill. Copyright 1983 by McGraw-Hill.

These skills are all taught in the first three years of elementary school, with the expectation that the child will integrate the knowledge and be a successful reader by third grade. In kindergarten through second grade, the emphasis is on perceptual-cognitive skills and preoperational skills. In the third and fourth grades, the emphasis shifts to require a child to exercise his or her linguistic and symbolic language skills. The content of all subject areas requires the child to abstract, analyze, and synthesize the information with the expectation that the child can read for content and no longer needs to focus on decoding each word because word recognition and understanding have become a internalized operations. Furthermore, the child is faced with a higher level of vocabulary, more complex sentence structure, and more abstract concepts.

Chall (1983) sums up this academic progression in reading by dividing the development of reading into six stages (see Table 22–1).

Stage 0 is the longest stage and the one with the most changes. During this period, children accumulate knowledge about letters, words, and books. They learn to produce syntactically correct utterances and develop early metalinguistic skills. These early metalinguistic skills involve "the awareness that language consists of discrete phonemes, words, phrases, and sentences" (Kamhi & Catts, 1989, p. 26). At this point, the children do not understand letter order and phoneme-grapheme correspondences. However, they do show interest in initial sounds and word shapes.

In Stage 1, children who are 5 to 7 years old learn about phoneme-grapheme correspondences and learn to decode words. The children decode to read, and then read for comprehension once they are beyond the single-word level in their reading. During Stage 2, decoding becomes more automatic so they can begin to focus on meaning. They also use their knowledge of scripts and story structure to assist in reading for meaning as they develop reading fluency. Decoding skills become fully automatic by Stage 3, which covers ages 9 to 14 years. Finally, in Stages 4 and 5, children become mature readers. They also develop cognitive skills that enable them to become critical readers (Chall, 1983).

Problem Areas with Readers in Trouble

According to Wiig and Semel (1984), readers in trouble experience difficulty with many skills as outlined in Table 22–2.

TABLE 22–2	Trouble areas for poor readers

Visually decoding the printed, graphic words

Integrating auditory-visual inputs

Associating printed words, phrases, concepts, and relations with their underlying meaning

Processing the surface structure of the printed sentences and relating it to the underlying meaning

Difficulty integrating grapho-phonemic, syntactic, and semantic information

Generating a tentative, anticipatory hypothesis about subsequent printed messages

Verifying, rejecting, or revising the anticipatory hypothesis with reference to the actual printed, graphic representation

Trouble with developmental sensitivity to grammar in written language

Adapted from *Language Assessment and Intervention for the Learning Disabled* (p. 596), by E. H. Wiig and E. Semel, 1984, New York: Merrill. Copyright 1984 by Merrill Publishers.

Children who experience reading difficulties frequently will have trouble encoding the information, retrieving it from memory, and using phonological memory codes to decode the words (Kamhi & Catts, 1989). It is also important to analyze the child's visual and auditory skills because successful reading requires a high level of integration of both sets of skills. The integration of these skills is critical for the child to associate written language with underlying meanings and structures.

Another major problem area for poor readers is grammar. Children having difficulty in reading will have problems correcting incorrect grammar. Regular and irregular morphemes are particularly problematic for these children. It is also known that poor readers typically have poor short-term memory for various sentence structures, which increases the problems they have because they have difficulty processing complex sentences.

Dyslexia

Originally referred to more than 65 years ago as "congenital word blindness," dyslexia is a developmental reading disorder. Hynd (1991) defines dyslexia as a rare but definable and diagnosable form of primary reading retardation with some form of central nervous system dysfunction. Dyslexia runs in families and is more common in boys than in girls (Leonard, 1998). Children with dyslexia have unexpected reading failures that often are accompanied by tendencies toward atypical spelling and handwriting. In addition, evidence exists to support the concept that the difficulties with phonologic awareness originate in "the phonologic component of the larger specialization for language" (Shaywitz et al., 1998).

With regard to the IQ discrepancy in the ICD-10 codes, questions have been raised as to whether or not IQ-reading discrepancies are a valid measure to determine the presence of dyslexia (Siegel, 1992; Stanovich, 1991). Historically, a discrepancy between IQ scores on neuropsychological tests and reading achievement scores on reading tasks has been used to determine or confirm the presence of dyslexia. However, this discrepancy is now seen as an inappropriate and invalid marker. Recent research studies do not support the use of a discrepancy-based definition of developmental dyslexia. In fact, when looking at the reading-impaired population, minimal differences are observed between reading-disabled children who meet discrepancy criteria and reading-disabled children who do not show a wide IQ-reading achievement gap (often referred to as "garden variety" poor readers).

Actually, measures of phonological awareness provide the most robust difference in performance between normal and impaired readers, making phonological awareness, not IQ-reading discrepancies, a better tool for diagnosing reading problems such as dyslexia.

Neurological Factors in Dyslexia

Most reading literature supports the belief that the brain abnormalities observed in people with dyslexia are atypical of development, just as if one extremity were larger than the other. That is to say, the brain abnormalities are structural anomalies, not physiological. Dyslexia is not believed to be part of a disease process that would involve progressive weakness or deterioration of brain structures and functions. Also, some disorders that appear to be developmental may in fact result from acquired lesions in early stages of development, with possible accompanying central nervous system dysfunction. Furthermore, significant deficits in social skills are sometimes reported in children with reading disorders. This may relate to the difficulty with increasing complexity of sentences and the general language difficulties experienced by some children who have language-based learning disabilities.

As the field of brain pathophysiology advances, we will have better answers to the questions on the identification of structural abnormalities in the brains of individuals with dyslexia. Galaburda (1989) reported abnormalities in brain structures and symmetries postmortem. Recent advances in the use of neuroimaging techniques such as functional magnetic resonance imaging (MRI) have contributed significantly to our knowledge of the morphology of the brain (Hynd, Semrud-Clikeman, Novey, & Eliopulos, 1990; Leonard, 1998).

Most recently, Shaywitz et al. (1998) used functional MRI techniques to study brain activation patterns in people with dyslexia. They designed a set of tasks that required their subjects to decide whether two stimuli presented simultaneously were the same or different. Their subjects included 29 dyslexic readers and 32 non-impaired readers, all completing the tasks as outlined in Table 22–3.

They found that the reading performance of the subjects with dyslexia was significantly impaired compared with that of the non-impaired readers. The biggest discrepancies were on the single-letter rhyme and non-word rhyme tasks, both of which require phonological processing. Using functional MRI, Shaywitz et al. (1998) studied those areas of the brain that were "activated" when the subjects were performing the various tasks. They found that the portions of the brain responsible for segmenting words into their phonological components functioned imperfectly in the subjects with dyslexia. Thus, the cognitive and behavioral deficits commonly associated with dyslexia were linked to problematic activation patterns in posterior and anterior language regions of the brain.

Table 22–3 Tasks performed by subjects in the study by Shaywitz et al. (1998)

Task	Example	Adds the Demand of
Line orientation	Do [\\V] and [\\v] match?	Visual-spatial processing
Letter case	Do [bbBb] and [bbBb] match?	Orthographic processing
Single-letter rhyme	Do the letters [T] and [V] rhyme?	Phonologic processing
Non-word rhyme	Do [leat] and [jete] rhyme?	Difficult phonological processing
Semantic category	Are [corn] and [rice] in the same category?	Retrieval from lexicon

Although MRI had been used extensively to study brain morphology in individuals with dyslexia, it had not been used to study brain morphology in children with specific language impairment (SLI). Using the MRI scans, Gauger, Lombardino, and Leonard (1997) studied brain morphology in 11 children with SLI. They found that "(a) pars triangularis was significantly smaller in the left hemisphere of children with SLI, and (b) children with SLI were more likely to have rightward asymmetry of language structures" (Gauger, Lombardino et al., 1997, p. 1272).

The Role of the Speech-Language Pathologist in Diagnosing and Treating Developmental Dyslexia

Children with dyslexia need intervention that includes speaking, listening, reading, and writing because reciprocity appears to occur in oral-written language. Dyslexia is a specific deficit in the processing of phonological information, an area about which most speech-language pathologists are well versed with regard to assessment and remediation. The primary role of the speech-language pathologist should be early identification. A test battery (see Table 22–4) that is designed to evaluate language production and processing (including phonology, semantics, and syntax) should be administered to children who are at risk for problems in reading (Lombardino et al., 1997). In addition, all children in kindergarten and first grade should be given tests of phonological awareness that predict reading disabilities. Because of the interplay between auditory and visual processing, it also makes sense that a speech-language pathologist would be involved in the remediation because many children with developmental dyslexia show deficits in their oral language. Similarly, many of the same strategies that the speech-language pathologist uses to treat auditory processing disorders can be used to treat developmental dyslexia. With the understanding of phoneme-grapheme information possessed by the speech-language pathologist, it is only logical that he or she be involved in the early identification and treatment of developmental dyslexia. There is no doubt that the speech-language pathologist should work collaboratively with classroom teachers and specialists in reading or learning disabilities in modifying the curriculum to facilitate optimal academic success for children with developmental dyslexia.

DSM-IV DIAGNOSTIC CRITERIA FOR 315.00 READING DISORDER

A. Reading achievement, as measured by individually administered standardized tests of reading accuracy or comprehension, is substantially below that expected given the person's chronological age, measured intelligence, and age-appropriate education.

B. The disturbance in Criterion A significantly interferes with academic achievement or activities of daily living that require reading skills.

C. If a sensory deficit is present, the reading difficulties are in excess of those usually associated with it.

Coding note: If a general medical (e.g., neurological) condition or sensory deficit is present, code the condition on Axis III.

ASSESSMENT

At the University of Florida Speech and Hearing Clinic, a battery of tests has been assembled to test the reading, writing, and spelling skills of children with suspected reading and spelling disorders. It is particularly important to assess the student's knowledge of sound-letter correspondences. This battery is outlined in Table 22–4.

Catts, Wilcox, Wood-Jackson, Larrivee, and Scott (1997) identified more than 20 tasks that have been used in research to measure phoneme awareness in words. They divided these 20 tasks into three categories: phoneme segmentation, phoneme synthesis, and sound comparison. Phoneme segmentation tasks require the listener to count, delete, add, pronounce, or reverse individual phonemes within a word. For example, the clinician may ask the client to count the number of phonemes he hears in the word "dog," to say the word "dog" without the /g/, or to say the individual sounds in "dog" one at a time. Phoneme synthesis is a sound-blending task in which the clinician presents words one phoneme at a time and asks the client what the word is. Sound comparison requires the client to compare the sounds in different words. For example, the client may be asked to generate a list of words that begin with the same phoneme as a target word (Torgesen, 1999).

There are several commercially available assessments of phonemic awareness, of which a few are listed below:

1. *The Rosner Test of Auditory Analysis.* (Rosner, 1975) A brief test, the Rosner contains only 13 items and is the oldest test of phonemic awareness. It is appropriate for use with the K–5th grade population. This test can be found in *Helping Children Overcome Learning Difficulties* (Rosner, 1975). (Torgesen, 1999)

2. *Lindamood Auditory Conceptualization Test* (Lindamood & Lindamood, 1979). The LAC requires the client to manipulate colored blocks to indicate number, identity, and order

TABLE 22–4 Protocol for assessment of reading and spelling disorders used at the University of Florida Speech and Hearing Clinic

Assessment Area	Test	Subtest
Phonemic awareness	Lindamood Auditory Conceptualization Test	Entire test
	Comprehensive Test of Phonological Processes in Reading	Entire test
Single word recognition and decoding	Woodcock-Johnson Reading Mastery Test—Revised	Word identification Word attack
Spelling	Wide Range Achievement Test—3	Spelling
Reading fluency	Gray Oral Reading Test—3	Passage score
Reading comprehension	Gray Oral Reading Test—3	Comprehension score
	Woodcock-Johnson Reading Mastery Test—Revised	Passage comprehension
Rapid naming	Clinical Evaluation of Language Fundamentals—III	Rapid naming

Adapted from "Linguistic Deficits in Children with Reading Disabilities," by L. J. Lombardino, C. A. Riccio, G. W. Hynd, and S. B. Pinheiro, 1997, *American Journal of Speech-Language Pathology, 6,* pp. 71–78. Copyright 1997 by *American Journal of Speech-Language Pathology.* Adapted with permission.

of phonemes in a series of nonsense words. It has two sets of "recommended minimum scores": one set for children in grades K–6 and a second set for individuals from seventh grade to adulthood. The test is based on the premise that individuals who score below the recommended minimum score most likely will have difficulties in acquiring decoding skills. (Torgesen, 1999)

3. *Test of Phonological Awareness* (Torgesen & Bryant, 1993). *The Test of Phonological Awareness* (TOPA) contains two subtests based on sound comparison activities. The TOPA is a group-administered test appropriate for children in kindergarten and first grade. In the kindergarten version, the children are asked to compare the first sounds in words; in the first-grade version, they are asked to compare final sounds in words. The test is nationally normed.

4. *Yopp-Singer Test of Phoneme Segmentation* (Yopp, 1995). Like the TOPA, the *Yopp-Singer Test of Phoneme Segmentation* is for use with kindergarten and first-grade children. The test consists of 22 items that require the child to pronounce the individual phonemes in words that contain two and three phonemes. It was published in a volume of *The Reading Teacher* in 1995. (Torgesen, 1999)

5. *The Phonological Awareness Test* (Robertson & Salter, 1995). *The Phonological Awareness Test* is an individually administered test that is standardized for children in kindergarten through fifth grade. It consists of six different subtests that assess the child's ability to "(1) discriminate and produce rhymes; (2) segment sentences, compound words, syllables, and phonemes; (3) pronounce separately the beginning, ending, or medial sound in short words; (4) delete a syllable or a phoneme from a word and pronounce the word that remains; (5) use colored blocks to show the number and order of phonemes in words; and (6) blend together separately presented syllables or phonemes to make words" (Torgesen, 1999, p. 135).

6. *The Comprehensive Test of Phonological Processes in Reading* (Wagner & Torgesen, 1997). This individually administered test is standardized on children from kindergarten through high school. The children in kindergarten and first grade are asked to complete sound comparison tests as well as measures involving phoneme blending and segmentation. Children in second and higher grades are assessed based on phoneme segmentation and blending tests. In addition to the previously mentioned subtests, the test contains "four measures of rapid naming ability (objects, colors, digits, and letters) and two measures of short-term memory for phonological information" (Torgesen, 1999, p. 135).

Another area of interest in the assessment of individuals with reading disorders is word recognition. According to Ehri (1992), words in text can be identified in five different ways:

1. By identifying and blending together the individual phonemes in words;

2. By noticing and blending together familiar spelling patterns (i.e., *pre, in*), which is a more advanced form of decoding;

3. By recognizing words as whole units or reading them "by sight";

4. By making analogies to other words that are already known;

5. By using clues from the context to guess a word's identity (Torgesen, 1999, p. 139).

Each of these methods plays a different role in the developmental process of learning to read.

Phonetic decoding is particularly important in the early stages of learning to read.

> To use this method, readers must know the sounds that are usually represented by letters in words, then they must blend together the individual sounds that are identified in each word. This method is important to early reading success because it provides a relatively reliable way to identify words that have not been seen before. (Torgesen, 1999, p. 139)

As children mature, they become able to process groups of letters in larger chunks, called spelling patterns. Then, as children reread a word several times, it gets stored in memory and is read as a sight word without decoding the individual letters.

Various researchers (Glushko, 1981; Laxon, Coltheart, & Keating, 1988) have found that children also read by creating analogies to known words. For example, a child may notice the similarity between "pocket" and "locket" and make the adjustment needed for the initial phoneme. The use of analogies requires developed decoding skills.

Finally, children may make use of surrounding context and/or contextual pictures to guess at words they do not know (Biemiller, 1970). However, the use of context to guess at words is typically used by poorer readers who cannot rely on the other methods of word identification (Briggs, Austin, & Underwood, 1984; Simpson, Lorsback, & Whitehouse, 1983). It should be noted that good readers will often use contextual cues as a check system to determine reading accuracy, correcting their reading if the mispronounced word does not fit with the context (Adams, 1990).

Children with reading deficits are most impaired in their ability to identify and blend together individual phonemes in words. They have difficulty "in both the ability to apply alphabetic strategies in reading new words (phonetic decoding) and in the ability to retrieve sight words from memory (orthographic processing)" (Torgesen, 1999, p. 141). Additionally, when they learn these skills, they frequently have difficulty using them for fluent reading.

Assessment of a child's word recognition ability should be based on measures that test word recognition out of context, phonetic decoding, and word recognition fluency. Torgesen (1999) lists several tests that are often used to measure word recognition ability:

1. Tests of sight-word reading ability: Sight-word reading can be assessed using the *Word Identification Subtest of the Woodcock Reading Mastery Test—Revised* (Woodcock, 1987) and the reading subtest of the *Wide Range Achievement Test—3* (Wilkinson, 1995). The words on these lists increase in complexity and length and decrease in frequency of occurrence in the English language. Both of these tests are standardized nationally, and neither one has a time limit.

2. Tests of phonetic decoding ability: Phonetic decoding is best assessed using non-words to minimize the use of sight-reading. The *Word Attack Subtest on the Woodcock Reading Mastery Test—Revised* (Woodcock, 1987) is an example of a decoding test using non-words.

3. Tests of word recognition fluency: *The Gray Oral Reading Test—3rd edition (GORT-3)* (Wiederholt & Bryant, 1992) is a test that is frequently used to assess word fluency. The test consists of 13 reading passages of increasing difficulty, with five comprehension questions for each passage. The amount of time the child requires to orally read the

passage is documented. "The test provides procedures to combine the rate score with a score for word reading accuracy to form a Passage score. The Passage score reflects the combination of reading speed and accuracy, and typical normed reference comparisons are available for this score" (Torgesen, 1999, p. 143). Torgesen identifies a potential problem with the GORT-3 in that it is too difficult for beginning readers and disabled readers through the second grade.

To address this difficulty with the GORT-3, Torgesen and Wagner (1997) developed a test to assess fluency and accuracy in word recognition skills. These tests are the *Test of Word Reading Efficiency* and the *Nonword Reading Efficiency Test*. Each test is composed of a list of words or non-words (depending on the test) that increase in complexity as the test progresses. The child is asked to read as many words as he can in 45 seconds. The score is the average number of words read on both tests. There are two forms for each test.

It should be noted that word recognition fluency becomes more of a factor after second or third grade, after which children have developed word recognition skills that they can use with reasonable accuracy.

Another critical component of reading that needs to be assessed is narrative schema knowledge. Traditionally, this is tested in one of two ways: (1) use of comprehension-based measures such as asking questions about a story or (2) productive measures such as requiring the student to generate a story (Westby, 1999). As cited by Westby, Tough (1981) lists four types of questions to use when assessing children's comprehension of a narrative:

1. Reporting: What was the boy doing here? What happened here? Tell me about this picture.

2. Projecting: What is the boy saying to the big frog? What is the frog thinking? How does the boy feel?

3. Reasoning: Why is the frog thinking that? Why does the boy feel angry? Why did the big frog bite the little frog? Why did the tree fall down?

4. Predicting: What will happen next? What will the big frog do now? (Westby, 1999, pp. 170–171)

Another way to assess a child's narrative skills is to give a wordless picture book and ask the child to tell you a story about the book. The child should be reminded that the clinician cannot see the book, so he needs to make up the story like a story in a book. Students can also be asked to tell a story about an event in their lives, or to make up a story without any visual prompts (Westby, 1999).

One of the challenges in the assessment of reading and spelling disorders is differential diagnosis of dyslexia co-occurring with central auditory processing disorders, from dyslexia co-occurring with attention deficit disorder. All three disorders may present with very similar symptomology, even though they are three distinct diagnostic entities. Certainly, there can be a co-occurrence of any of the three disorders.

Individuals with central auditory processing disorders have normal intelligence and hearing acuity, but they are unable to process auditory information effectively. Most authorities report that central auditory processing disorders cause difficulties in detection, interpretation, and categorization of sounds and that these problems may be caused by some type of dysfunction in lower or higher level cortical processes (Schow & Nervonne, 1996).

Children who exhibit signs of language-based learning disabilities or reading and/or spelling disorders are often referred to audiologists to rule out central auditory processing disorders prior to further testing. Children who have poor academic achievement, behavior problems, phonological deficits, ADD/ADHD, or problems with oral language also should be referred for central auditory processing testing (Wallach & Butler, 1994).

> It is sometimes difficult to separate a central auditory processing disorder from a language deficit, owing to the underlying role of language in processing and learning. Young (1985) proposed that two types of central auditory processing disorders may be present in children. The first is related to attentional deficits, whereas the second includes both attentional problems and language deficits. (Vinson, 1999)

At the University of Florida Speech and Hearing Clinic, all children who are referred for dyslexia evaluations undergo central auditory processing testing, and vice versa. The role of the speech-language pathologist is to determine, through comprehensive testing, why the child is having academic difficulties (Dempsey, 1983). The role of the audiologist is to determine the site of the lesion (if there is one) within the auditory pathway and to assess the child's ability to understand speech in a variety of conditions (Wallach & Butler, 1994).

In summary, children should be screened for phonological awareness skills during the pre-kindergarten and kindergarten years as a means of predicting children who might have a reading disability. Assessment should focus on word recognition and word comprehension and on the skills necessary to recognize and comprehend language. These areas include reading and listening comprehension, vocabulary testing, decoding, spelling, reading speed, dependency on context, and metacognition. In addition, a comprehensive history should be taken. Examples of case history forms for children and adults can be found in Appendices 22–A and 22–B.

TREATMENT

There are a variety of treatment protocols for individuals with reading disabilities. A brief review of these protocols follows:

The Orton-Gillingham Method

The Orton-Gillingham method is based on a philosophy of teaching reading, spelling, and writing using an integrated curriculum of language skills. At the core of the method is the alphabetic principle that governs the orthographic structure of many languages, including English. "Alphabetic-phonic associations are trained from the first lesson and reinforced through phonetically controlled reading and spelling activities to form the foundation of reading and writing an alphabetic language" (Vinson, 1996, p. 211). This method also focuses on the role of cognition in reading, spelling, and writing. Clients are taught to think about the rules they have learned, and then to apply these rules in varying contexts (e.g., syllabication). Finally, the Orton-Gillingham method encourages the use of old information to make inferences, which is a skill required for continued independent learning (Lombardino, unpublished paper, 1998).

The Auditory Discrimination in Depth (ADD) Program

The ADD program was developed by the Lindamoods in 1975 for children in pre-kindergarten to 12th grade. The program consists of several levels, with the first three levels being recommended for kindergarten children to be used in a preventive manner as a foundation for successful reading and spelling. These three levels are also recommended for older students and adults who have language-based learning disabilities. The stimuli include syllable construction and reading charts, mouth-form cards, depicting the oral production plus the label and corresponding phonemes, the vowel circle, letter tiles, and colored blocks.

> The ADD program was developed to facilitate the acquisition of reading and spelling skills through a multimodality approach that uses auditory, visual, tactile, and kinesthetic information to train the conceptual elements of phonemes and the corresponding graphemes. (Vinson, 1999, pp. 211–212)

The auditory conceptual elements of consonant sounds are taught first, then the vowel sounds. The following tenets apply:

1. Sensory input is required to pair the basic auditory element with the oral motor activity.

2. Conceptualization of the distinctive features of each phoneme is mandatory.

3. Perception of same and different, number, and order of speech sounds in isolation is followed by perception of minimal changes between syllable units.

4. Storage and retrieval of the agreed upon representations for phonemes and graphemes are required for reading and spelling (LeGrand, unpublished paper, 1997).

Project Read

Project Read was developed by Greene and Enfield in 1991. It is a modification of the Orton-Gillingham method and also stresses the use of auditory, visual, and tactile stimuli. Goldsworthy (1996) described the method as "a systematic, structured, developmental approach based on the links of the language" (p 184). The method uses practice and generalization to move from part to whole and concrete to abstract.

The program consists of three parts: the phonology component, the comprehension component, and the written expression component. The phonology component is designed for children in grades 1 through 3. This component focuses on sound-symbol relationships, segmenting words into sounds, and learning syllabication patterns. The comprehension component is designed for children in grades 4 through 12. The comprehension component focuses on the acquisition and organization of information that uses specifically designed report forms. The written expression component addresses syntax in written language and includes clustering related information and editing procedures (Goldsworthy, 1996).

Montessori Reading Instruction

The Montessori method of reading instruction uses self-paced, multisensory input to teach the letters and their sounds. Visual-motor activities that are used to teach letter recognition are modified to teach reading and writing. This method uses alphabet cards to construct words. These alphabet cards are known as phonograms. The children participate in a variety of activities, including tracing sandpaper letters with their eyes open and closed, and tracing over the letters. A unique feature of the Montessori method is that it does not permit oral reading. Reading comprehension is checked by writing questions, then eliciting the answers to the questions (Buchanan, Weller, & Buchanan, 1997).

The Whole Language Approach

The Whole Language Approach is an informal, discovery-based method of integrating curricular goals, cognitive skills, and language skills (Goldsworthy, 1996). Hegde (1996) described the Whole Language Approach as follows:

> Language teaching should not be broken down into speaking, reading, and writing; instead, all aspects of literacy including speaking, listening, reading, and writing should be taught simultaneously as an integrated whole. (p. 189)

Writing on a daily basis is encouraged, with many teachers keeping a dialogue journal to monitor the child's progress in integrating knowledge and writing. Invented spellings are considered to be a normal process, and spelling is rarely corrected. The basic premise of integrating the curriculum with reading and writing skills is a sound one. However, the lack of phonological instruction has caused some children to have difficulty with reading and/or spelling.

The Laubach Method

The Laubach method operates on the basic principle of teaching sound-symbol associations. Consonant sounds are taught first, followed by the short vowels, then the long vowels. The program then addresses irregular spelling, followed by writing, reading, and grammar exercises of increasing complexity. The Laubach method was developed as a means of group instruction to high school dropouts, illiterate adults, and individuals learning English as a second language. It uses picture-association cards to teach sounds, letters, and key vocabulary words. The letters are taught in alphabetic sequence, with instruction on lowercase letters preceding that of uppercase letters (Buchanan, Weller, & Buchanan, 1997).

The Brody Reading Method

The Brody method of reading instruction is also a structured, sequential approach for students who need assistance in learning patterns in print. Extensive multisensory practice that progresses from one-syllable words to longer words in demanding text forms the foundation for teaching students decoding, comprehension, spelling, and writing (Goldsworthy, 1996).

The Wilson Reading System for Older Students (Grade 6–adulthood)

The Wilson Reading System is based on the Orton-Gillingham principles and on the research addressing phoneme/syllable segmentation skills. Wilson (1989) based his program on the belief that some individuals need to be directly taught syllable types and word construction rules. The program uses 12 steps and 56 substeps that are presented sequentially and cumulatively. "The structure of words in the English language are taught directly, thereby enabling students to master the underlying phonological coding system for use in reading and spelling" (Goldsworthy, 1996, p. 185).

The J & J Reading Materials

Goldsworthy (1996) recommends the J & J reading materials, which consist of a series of books "incorporating vocabulary, oral language expansion, written expression, spelling, comprehension, and higher level thinking skills with readability extending from primer through the end of fourth grade. . . . The J & J series presents the alphabetic code of English orthography in a sequential, cumulative format" (Goldsworthy, 1996, p. 183). These materials can be used along with programs such as the Orton-Gillingham method and the Project Read method described previously.

All the preceding programs stress decoding and phonological awareness abilities as critical components of learning to read. However, there is a step beyond that—learning to comprehend what is read. Students need to be taught active strategies to assist in comprehension of materials they read. One such system is Visualizing and Verbalizing. In this program, the child is encouraged to visualize pictures that depict the text as he reads, then to recall those pictures in order to recall the text. Other strategies are expressed by Ekwall (1995), who believed that reading comprehension involves "both a word or vocabulary factor and a group of skills that might be referred to as 'other comprehension skills'" (p. 102). As listed in Goldsworthy (1996), these comprehension skills include the following: recognizing main ideas, recognizing important details, developing visual images, predicting outcomes, following directions, recognizing an author's organization, and doing critical reading.

APPENDIX 22-A: READING CLINIC CASE HISTORY— PEDIATRIC

University of Florida Speech & Hearing Clinic   File No: _____
435 Dauer Hall
Gainesville, FL 32611-7420
(352) 392-2041

General Background Information

Client's Name: _____   Date: _____

Birthdate: _____   Male _____   Female _____

Social Security Number: _____

Parent's Name(s): _____

Home Phone #: _____   Work Phone #: _____

Address: _____

_____

Do you have Medicaid?   Yes _____   No _____

If yes, please provide your 8-digit policy/card #: _____

Name of primary care/family physician: _____

Please describe the problem that brings you here: _____

_____

_____

Who referred you to this clinic? _____

Has there been a diagnosis of a reading, language, or learning problem?   Yes _____   No _____

If yes, what type of problem and when was it diagnosed? _____

_____

Has treatment been received?   Yes ____   No ____

If yes, what type? _____

_____

Which of the following professional services have been received: (Check those that apply)

__ Physical Therapy   where _____ when _____ why _____

__ Occupational Therapy   where _____ when _____ why _____

__ Speech/language Therapy   where _____ when _____ why _____

__ Behavioral Therapy   where _____ when _____ why _____

__ Psychological Counseling where _____ when _____ why _____

Have academic tutoring services been sought?   Yes ____   No ____

If yes, in what area(s)? _____

_____

where _____ when _____

When were you first concerned about a reading, language, or learning problem?

_____

_____

What reasons do you feel may help explain these reading or other academic difficulties?

_____

_____

Developmental Information

Client was the (1st, 2nd, etc...) _____ born of (number of) _____ children

Client's weight at birth: _____

Were there any problems during the pregnancy?   Yes _____   No _____

If yes, describe. _____

_____

Were any medications taken during the pregnancy?   Yes _____   No _____

List: _____

Explain any difficulties at the time of birth: _____

_____

If premature birth, please note length of term: _____

Was there a prolonged hospital stay?   Yes _____   No _____

When did child: Sit alone? _____   Button clothes? _____

Stand alone? _____   Tie shoes? _____

Walk alone? _____   Feed self? _____

Become toilet trained? _____

Did your child ever have trouble nursing, drinking,
or eating (for example, choking and/or gagging)?   Yes _____   No _____

If yes, explain: _____

_____

Handedness for writing: Right _____   Left _____   Both _____

Coordination: Good _____   Average _____   Clumsy _____

Activity level: Unusually active _____   Very active _____   Average _____   Poor _____

Medical History

General health conditions: Excellent _____   Average _____   Poor _____

Any serious illnesses?   Yes _____   No _____   If yes, explain: _____

_____

Any operations?   Yes _____   No _____   If yes, explain: _____

_____

Any injuries?   Yes _____   No _____   If yes, explain: _____

_____

Please check all that apply and provide clarifying information under "Comment":

ILLNESS	COMMENT	Y	N
Allergies			
Recurrent colds/flu/sore throat			
Dizziness			
Dental problems			
Frequent laryngitis/hoarseness			
Epilepsy/seizure disorder			
Reading and/or spelling problems			
Other academic problems			
Attention Deficit Disorder (ADD)			
ADD with Hyperactivity (ADHD)			
Vision problems			
High fevers			
Kidney problems			
Swallowing/digestive disorders			
Respiratory difficulties			
Heart/circulatory problems			

ILLNESS	COMMENT	Y	N
Neurological disorders			
Cancer			
Endocrine/metabolic disorders (thyroid problems, diabetes)			
Viruses (HIV, Herpes)			
Connective Tissue Disorders (Lupus, Rheumatoid Arthritis)			
Frequent and/or intense headaches			
Measles			
Mumps			
Chicken Pox			
Meningitis			
Unusual fatigue/stress			
Mental illness			
Congenital disorders (list please)			

Additional Comments: _____

_____

_____

Audiologic History

Please check the appropriate column:

	Y	N
My child had 3+ ear infections between birth and 12 months of age.		
My child has had at least one ear infection which lasted more than 3 months.		
My child has been evaluated by an audiologist who determined that his/her hearing is within normal limits. Date of visit: _____		

	Y	N
My child has failed a hearing screening in school. Date of screening: _____		
My child has passed a hearing screening in school. Date of screening: _____		
I suspect my child has a hearing problem.		
My child prefers one ear over the other. If yes, which ear? Right ____ Left ____		
My child has had tubes in his/her ears. If yes, when? _____		
My child wears hearing aids. If yes, what type and for how long? _____		

Additional Comments: _____

_____

_____

Speech and Language Development

At what age did your child:

Begin babbling? _____ Use first words? _____

Begin to combine words? _____ Begin to use sentences? _____

Please check the appropriate box:

	Y	N
Did the sounds in your child's speech ever interfere with his/her ability to be understood by you or by others?		
Does your child have problems being understood now?		
Does your child ever act like he/she is deaf and cannot understand what you say?		
Does your child often fail to give close attention to details or make careless mistakes in schoolwork or other activities?		

	Y	N
Does your child have difficulty organizing tasks and activities?		
Does your child often not seem to listen to what is being said to him or her?		
Does your child often not follow through on instructions and fail to finish schoolwork, chores, or duties at school or home (not due to oppositional behavior or failure to understand directions)?		
Does your child often have difficulty sustaining attention in tasks or play activities?		
Does your child often avoid or strongly dislike tasks (such as schoolwork or homework) that require sustained mental effort?		
Does your child often lose things necessary for tasks or activities (e.g., school assignments, pencils, books, tools, or toys)?		
Is your child often easily distracted by extraneous stimuli?		
Is your child often forgetful in daily activities?		
Does your child often fidget with hands or feet or squirm in seat?		
Does your child often leave his/her seat in the classroom or in other situations in which remaining seated is expected?		
Does your child often have difficulty in playing or engaging in leisure activities quietly?		
Does your child often blurt out answers to questions before the questions have been completed?		
Does your child often have difficulty waiting in lines or waiting turn in games or group situations?		
Does your child ever seem confused when you give instructions and/or show difficulty in understanding what you say?		
Does your child ever have trouble producing complete sentences that you think he/she should be able to produce?		
Did your child ever engage in excessive repetition of words or sentences that he/she heard other people say?		
Does your child ever have difficulty recalling a familiar word while he/she is speaking?		
Does your child ever repeat TV commercials or radio ads in a rote way that seemed strange to you (like he/she was reading a script?)		

	Y	N
Does your child have problems in learning to read or spell now?		
Does your child have problems in learning that certain letters correspond with certain sounds?		
Does your child have problems in learning the alphabet?		
Does your child ever sound like he/she is stuttering or hesitant with his/her speech?		

Additional Comments: _____

_____

_____

Family History

Mother: _____ Age: ____ Highest grade in school ____ Occupation _____

Father: _____ Age: ____ Highest grade in school ____ Occupation _____

Children: _____ Age: ____ Highest grade in school ____ Occupation _____

_____ Age: ____ Highest grade in school ____ Occupation _____

_____ Age: ____ Highest grade in school ____ Occupation _____

_____ Age: ____ Highest grade in school ____ Occupation _____

Has any blood relative had a history of

Mental illness: Yes ____   No ____

Epilepsy: Yes ____   No ____

Chronic or serious medical problems: Yes ____   No ____

Hearing difficulty: Yes ____   No ____

Speech & Language difficulty: Yes ____   No ____

Difficulty in learning to read or spell: Yes ____   No ____

If yes, explain: _____

_____

Number of languages spoken at home: _____

Educational History

Present school placement: _____

Grade or class: _____ Teacher: _____

Describe progress in school: _____

_____

_____

What do you hope to get from this evaluation? _____

_____

Reprinted with permission from the University of Florida Speech and Hearing Clinic.

APPENDIX 22-B: READING CLINIC CASE HISTORY— ADULT

University of Florida Speech & Hearing Clinic
435 Dauer Hall
Gainesville, FL 32611-7420
(352) 392-2041

File No: _____

General Background Information

Client's Name: _____ Date: _____

Birthdate: _____ Male _____ Female _____

Home Phone #: _____ Work Phone #: _____

Address: _____

_____

Social Security Number: _____

Name and address of parent, spouse, sibling (please specify): _____

_____

Who referred you to this clinic?: _____

Has there been a diagnosis of a reading, language, or learning problem? Yes _____ No _____

If yes, a) What type of diagnosis were you given? _____

b) Who provided you with this diagnosis? _____

c) How long ago was this diagnosis given? _____

Are you right or left-handed? _____

Which of the following professional services have been received: (Check all that apply)

___ Physical Therapy   where _____ when _____ why _____

___ Occupational Therapy   where _____ when _____ why _____

___ Speech/language Therapy where _____ when _____ why _____

___ Behavioral Therapy   where _____   when _____   why _____

___ Psychological Counseling   where _____   when _____   why _____

When were you first concerned about a reading, language, or learning problem? _____

_____

_____

Have you had or are you currently having difficulty in keeping up with your schoolwork?

_____

_____

Do you have difficulty reading out loud? _____

Do you have difficulty comprehending what you read? _____

Do you have a history of difficulty learning a foreign language? _____

If you are currently having difficulty with reading and/or spelling, what strategies do you use to help yourself read and/or spell more effectively?

_____

_____

_____

_____

What reasons do you feel may help explain your reading or other academic difficulties?

_____

_____

Medical History

General health conditions: Excellent _____   Average _____   Poor _____

Any serious illnesses?   Yes _____   No _____   If yes, explain: _____

_____

Any operations?   Yes _____   No _____   If yes, explain: _____

_____

Any injuries?   Yes _____   No _____   If yes, explain: _____

_____

Do you have a history of	Explain	YES	NO
High fever?			
Headaches?			
Seizures or convulsions?			
Dizziness, fainting spells?			
Eye problems?			
Memory problems?			
Is your hearing normal? If no, explain.			
Did you have 3 or more ear infections during the first year of life?			
Did you have an ear infection that lasted 3 months or more?			
Did you ever have tubes placed in your ears? If yes, when and for how long?			
Are any medications being taken at this time? If yes, please list.			

Speech and Language History

	YES	NO
Did you say your first words between 12 and 18 months of age? If no, please explain.		
Did you use short sentences by 2 to 3 years of age? If no, please explain.		
Do you ever have difficulty recalling familiar words while speaking? If yes, explain.		
Do you have difficulty remembering information such as phone numbers? If yes, explain.		
Did you have difficulty learning the alphabet? If yes, explain.		
Did you have difficulty remembering letter-sound associations? If yes, explain.		
Did you have difficulty learning to read and/or spell in the early grades? If yes, explain.		
Have you received speech therapy, reading tutoring or any other special assistance in elementary school, high school, or college? If yes, explain.		

Additional Comments: _____

_____

_____

Family History

Has any blood relative had any history of	YES	NO
Mental illness?		
Epilepsy?		
Chronic or serious medical problems?		
Hearing difficulty?		
Speech & Language difficulty?		
Difficulty in learning to read or spell?		

If yes, explain: _____

_____

_____

Educational and Work History

Present grade and major area of study if you are in school _____

Highest grade attained if you are not in school now _____

Type of employment if working. Please describe the nature of your work

_____

_____

_____

Career goals if applicable _____

What do you hope to achieve with this evaluation? _____

_____

_____

Reprinted with permission from the University of Florida Speech and Hearing Clinic.

CHAPTER TWENTY-THREE
Syndromes

Author's note: This chapter deviates from the standard format used for the other chapters. I believe it will be easier to look up information on the various syndromes if the information is presented in a list format. The syndromes included are those frequently associated with communication disorders, and they are listed alphabetically. For a complete listing of syndromes affecting speech, language, and hearing, the reader is referred to *Syndrome Identification for Speech-Language Pathology: An Illustrated PocketGuide* by Robert J. Shprintzen (Singular Publishing Group, 2000).

TERMINOLOGY ASSOCIATED WITH SYNDROMES

In 1979 and 1980, an international working group met to develop a glossary of terms to be used in identifying language related to basic genetics. The glossary it developed can be applied within a general framework to classify syndromes.

For years, the term *birth defect* was used to identify "abnormalities related to errors in embryogenesis that were found in children" (Shprintzen, 1997, p. 49). However, there are problems with the term *birth defect* as defined. First, some abnormalities are not readily identifiable at birth because of lack of complete development of some anatomical structures. Also, it does not take into account behavioral abnormalities. It is becoming recognized that some behavioral abnormalities are caused by abnormal genetic conditions. To this end, the term *anomaly* has been adopted to replace the term birth defect (Shprintzen, 1997).

Anomaly is defined as "any deviation from normal structure, form, or function that is considered to be abnormal" (Shprintzen, 1997, p. 50). According to Shprintzen (1997), there are two types of anomalies: malformations and deformations. Also, anomalies may be classified as major or minor. Anomalies may occur in multiples within one individual. Thus, there are three commonly recognized types of multiple anomaly disorders: syndromes, sequences, and associations. Each of these terms is defined in Shprintzen (1997) as follows:

malformations: "anomalies in which there is an intrinsic error in the development of a tissue, organ, structure, or function" (p. 50); frequently genetic in origin.

deformations: "anomalies in which the problem is extrinsic to the tissue, organ, structure, or function" (p. 51); frequently caused by intrauterine accident.

minor anomalies: "those that typically do not require treatment to enhance either the quality or quantity of life. Minor anomalies include missing teeth, abnormal fingernails, a small sinus tract near the ear (known as a branchial cleft), or a streak of white hair in otherwise uniformly dark colored scalp hair" (p. 52).

major anomalies: "those that do require treatment. If left untreated, life or health could be threatened, or the quality of life would be significantly impaired. Major anomalies include cleft palate, congenital heart anomalies, missing digits or limbs, or metabolic abnormalities such as phenylketonuria. There are also major behavioral anomalies such as mental retardation, profound deafness, or hypernasal speech" (p. 52).

syndrome: "the presence of multiple anomalies in the same individual with all of those anomalies having a single cause" (p. 53).

sequence: "a disorder where many of the anomalies are actually secondary disorders, caused by a single anomaly which sets off a chain reaction of changes in the developing embryo that result in other anomalies" (p. 75); there are three types of sequences: malformation, deformation, and disruption.

association: "a multiple anomaly disorder that has a recurrent pattern, but for which there is no evidence of a specific etiology or sequential cascading effect" (p. 80).

aneuploidy: "rearrangements of chromosome structure resulting in an abnormal amount or structure of the chromosomes" (p. 53).

karyotype: a chromosome analysis.

In 1982, Cohen divided syndromes into two broad types: those of known origin and those of unknown origin. There are four types of "known genesis" syndromes: chromosomal, genetic, teratogenic, and mechanically induced.

Chromosomal Syndromes

Chromosomal syndromes have "an abnormality in chromosome structure that can be seen under a light microscope" (Shprintzen, 1997, p. 53). There are several types of chromosomal syndromes, including the following: deletion of whole chromosomes (Turner syndrome), addition of extra whole chromosomes (Down syndrome), deletion of parts of chromosomes (Wolf-Hirschhorn syndrome), addition of parts of chromosomes, restructured chromosomes, and rearrangements of chromosomes known as unbalanced translocations (Shprintzen, 1997).

Typically, individuals who have chromosome disorders have severe problems, including craniofacial malformations, short stature, mental retardation, and a myriad of severe malformations (e.g., limb anomalies, brain anomalies, heart anomalies). Speech and language impairments caused by neurological and/or structural malformations are also common in chromosomal disorders (Shprintzen, 1997).

Genetic Disorders

Genetic disorders comprise the largest group of multiple congenital anomalies. Syndromes of chromosome genesis are genetically based. However, those who study the origin of multiple anomalies refer to syndromes that are chromosomally based as those that have microscopically visible chromosomal rearrangements. Genetic syndromes do not have visible abnormalities (Shprintzen, 1997).

Teratogenic Disorders

A teratogen is any environmental agent that results in abnormal development of an embryo. Timing of the exposure to a teratogen is critical in determining how vulnerable the embryo is to damage. Typically, exposure in the first trimester is the most devastating. Teratogens include prescription drugs, illicit drugs, chemicals, viruses, X-ray exposure, maternal disease, maternal metabolic disorders, and anything that affects the environment of the womb. Not all teratogen-related problems are immediately obvious. Some may appear as learning disabilities that are not diagnosed until a child is school-aged (Jung, 1989).

Mechanically Induced Syndromes

This is a relatively rare category of syndromes. The most predominant problem in this category would be amnion rupture syndrome in which the amniotic sack ruptures.

Following is a description of a few syndromes frequently seen by speech-language pathologists. The descriptive information was compiled from Jung (1989), Pore and Reed (1999), and Shprintzen (1997, 1999).

ANGELMAN SYNDROME

Type
chromosome deletion

Physical Characteristics
microcephaly
mandibular prognathism
large mouth and chin
tongue thrusting
ataxia
unusual, "puppetlike" gait
seizures
optic atrophy
muscular anomalies
scoliosis
failure to thrive in many children

Resonance, Articulation, and Voice
most do not have speech development

Language
most do not have language development
severe congenital mental retardation typical

APERT'S SYNDROME

Type
genetic mutation

Physical Characteristics
craniostenosis
hydrocephalus
midfacial hypoplasia
strabismus
syndactyly and/or stenosis of fingers and toes
short upper arms
upper airway obstruction

occasional cleft palate

severe occlusal anomalies

Resonance

hyponasality secondary to choanal stenosis or atresia

hypernasality secondary to cleft palate

mixed resonance common

abnormal oral resonance secondary to reduced pharyngeal dimensions

Articulation

compensatory articulation secondary to cleft palate

speech delayed secondary to cognitive impairment

Voice

hoarseness

breathiness

calcification of the larynx

Language

delayed and/or impaired secondary to cognitive impairment, hydrocephalus, and/or other brain anomalies

probable mental retardation

Hearing

conductive hearing loss secondary to middle ear effusion

reduced middle ear volume

fixation of stapes footplate

CRI-DU-CHAT SYNDROME

Type

chromosome deletion

Physical Characteristics

small stature

microcephaly

orbital hypertelorism

downslanting eyes

posteriorly rotated ears

ear tags

    failure to thrive with feeding difficulty

    small hands with joint contractures

    large bowel malrotation

    severe hypotonia

    heart anomalies

    dislocated hips

    prominent nasal root

    micrognathia

    occasional cleft palate ± cleft lip

    facial asymmetry

    hypersensitivity

    self-injurious behaviors

Resonance

    hypernasality if cleft is present

Articulation

    often absent speech

    if speech present, severe delay in onset

    gross neurologically based articulatory impairment

Voice

    high-pitched cry and voice common

Language

    severe cognitive impairment

    severe expressive and receptive language deficits

    echolalia when speech is present

Hearing

    conductive hearing loss secondary to chronic otitis media

CROUZON SYNDROME

Type

    genetic

Physical Characteristics

    craniostenosis

exorbitism

cleft lip/palate occasionally

maxillary hypoplasia

Resonance

often hyponasal secondary to small nasal capsule

Articulation

may be impaired secondary to cleft lip/palate, midface deficiency and maxillary hypoplasia

typically, normal onset and development

Voice

normal

Language

usually normal

Hearing

conductive hearing loss common due to reduced volume of middle ear and frequent middle ear effusion

DE LANGE SYNDROME

Type

genetic

Physical Characteristics

short stature

infantile posture

small extremities

contracted elbows

microcephaly

short neck

hypertonia

hirsutism

seizures

renal abnormalities

pyloric stenosis

gastro-intestinal disorders with reflux

cardiac malformation
intestinal anomalies
anomalous auricles
small and dysmorphic nose
thin, downturned upper lip
micrognathia (underdeveloped mandible)
cleft palate
lack of facial expression
self-injurious behaviors

Resonance

possibly hypernasal secondary to cleft palate

Articulation

usually severely delayed or absent
neurogenic speech disorders

Voice

low pitch
hoarse cry

Language

severely delayed, impaired, or absent secondary to mental retardation

Hearing

conductive loss secondary to middle ear effusion
sensorineural loss ranging from mild to profound in approximately 50% of cases

DOWN SYNDROME (TRISOMY 21)

Type

whole chromosome addition

Physical Characteristics

general hypotonia
short neck

brachycephaly

brachydactyly

short fifth finger

flat occiput

upslanting eyes

small ears

cardiac malformation (in approximately 40% of patients)

obesity

airway obstruction

small teeth

open mouth posture with tongue protrusion

mouth breathing

small oral cavity

maxillary hypoplasia

flat facial profile

occasional cleft palate ± cleft lip

Resonance

occasionally hypernasal secondary to clefting

frequently hyponasal secondary to lymphoid tissue obstruction

Articulation

delayed onset

uncoordinated articulation secondary to hypotonia and malocclusion

Voice

low pitch

hoarseness

Language

delayed and often severely impaired

cognitive impairment

the most common cause of genetically based mental retardation

Hearing

usually normal

conductive loss common secondary to chronic otitis

DYSAUTONOMIA

Type
> genetic

Physical Characteristics
> hypotonia
> progressive scoliosis
> absent reflexes
> digestive problems
> pulmonary compromise secondary to aspiration
> decreased pain sensation
> ataxia
> delayed motor milestones
> poor suck in infancy
> absent/hypoactive gag
> absent or decreased papillae on tongue
> drooling
> mild facial asymmetry
> sad facial expression

Resonance
> hypernasality secondary to dysarthria and rhythm problems

Articulation
> dysarthria

Voice
> monotone

Language
> normal

Hearing
> normal

FETAL ALCOHOL SYNDROME

Type
teratogenic

Physical Characteristics
low birth weight/failure to thrive
microcephaly
heart anomalies
digital anomalies
joint abnormalities
kidney and/or heart abnormalities
poor coordination
hypotonia
flat philtrum
short nose
micrognathia
cleft palate ± cleft lip
auricular abnormalities
maxillary hypoplasia
hyperactivity in childhood
irritability in infancy

Resonance
possible hypernasality secondary to cleft palate

Articulation
speech delay
articulatory impairment secondary to motor deficits
dyspraxia
compensatory articulation secondary to cleft palate

Voice
hoarseness

Language
leading cause of birth defects and the third leading cause of mental retardation in the United States

global cognitive impairment
delayed and impaired

Hearing

normal hearing
conductive loss due to chronic otitis media possible

FRAGILE X SYNDROME

Type

genetic

Physical Characteristics

delayed motor development
large head
prominent forehead
long and narrow chin
high arched palate
dental abnormalities
hypotonia
large ears
psychiatric and behavioral problems
tactile defensiveness
possible cleft palate

Resonance

normal
hypernasality of cleft is present

Articulation

delayed speech
breakdown in connected passages
cluttering possible
possibly nonverbal

Voice

normal

Language

second leading cause of genetically based mental retardation

possible autism

auditory processing disorder

echolalia and perseveration

Hearing

normal

MARFAN SYNDROME

Type

genetic

Physical Characteristics

abnormal skeletal growth pattern

arachnodactyly

tall stature

hyperextensive joints

mitral valve prolapse

dilation of the aorta

aortic dissection

dislocated ocular lens

prognathism

vertical maxillary excess

occasional cleft palate

temporomandibular joint disease

Resonance

hypernasality secondary to cleft palate if present

occasional velopharyngeal insuffiency

Articulation

occasionally disordered secondary to malocclusion, open bite, and limited oral opening

Voice

normal

Language
> normal

Hearing
> usually normal

MOEBIUS SYNDROME

Type
> genetic

Physical Characteristics
> inanimate face and oral structures
> facial paralysis
> limb defects
> high-arched palate
> paralysis of soft palate
> short or deformed tongue
> feeding and swallowing difficulties

Resonance
> muffled oral resonance

Articulation
> severely impaired secondary to lack of animation of articulators
> dysarthria

Voice
> normal

Language
> delayed development of expressive language

Hearing
> normal to problematic

NOONAN SYNDROME

Type

genetic

Physical Characteristics

small stature
low posterior hairline
webbed neck
pulmonary stenosis
vertebral anomalies
pectus excavatum or carinatum
ptosis
downslanting eyes
vertical maxillary excess
occasional cleft palate (often submucous)

Resonance

hypernasality if cleft is present

Articulation

delayed or impaired if cognitive disorder is present
impaired secondary to malocclusion

Voice

occasional hoarseness

Language

delayed or impaired if cognitive delay is present

Hearing

occasional sensorineural hearing loss and/or conductive impairment

PRADER-WILLI SYNDROME

Type

genetic

Physical Characteristics
obesity
hypoplastic gonads
hypotonia
cryptorchidism
small hands and feet
insatiable appetite

Resonance
hypernasality secondary to hypotonia, which resolves with age

Articulation
delayed speech onset
impaired secondary to hypotonia

Voice
may be high pitched

Language
delayed and impaired

Hearing
normal

RETT'S DISORDER

Physical Characteristics
apparently normal prenatal and perinatal development
apparently normal psychomotor development through the first 5 months after birth
normal head circumference at birth
deceleration of head growth between ages 5 and 48 months
loss of previously acquired purposeful hand skills between ages 5 and 30 months with the subsequent development of stereotyped hand movements (e.g., hand wringing or hand washing)
appearance of poorly coordinated gait or trunk movements

Resonance
may be affected by oral pharyngeal problems

Articulation

oral dyspraxia

dysarthria

Voice

abnormal breathing patterns

Language

severely impaired expressive and receptive language development with severe psycho-motor retardation

loss of social engagement early in the course (although often social interaction develops later)

delayed auditory processing

Hearing

normal

STICKLER SYNDROME

Type

genetic

Physical Characteristics

mild midfacial hypoplasia

micrognathia

submucous or overt cleft palate

palatopharyngeal valving problems

vitreoretinal degeneration

joint laxity

epiphyseal dysplasia

round face

cleft palate

maxillary deficiency

Robin sequence

Resonance

hyponasality secondary to small nasal capsule and small nasopharynx

hypernasality secondary to cleft palate and velopharyngeal insuffiency

Articulation

articulatory distortion secondary to malocclusion

possible compensatory articulation secondary to clefting

Voice

normal

Language

normal

Hearing

occasional high frequency sensorineural hearing loss

conductive hearing loss caused by middle ear effusion secondary to clefting

TREACHER-COLLINS SYNDROME

Type

genetic

Physical Characteristics

choanal atresia

micrognathia

absent or hypoplastic zygomas

defects of lower eyelids

malar clefts

cleft palate

Robin sequence

occasional cleft lip

ossicular malformation

small or absent external ears

airway obstruction

Resonance

hyponasality secondary to nasal obstruction and small nasopharynx

occasional mixed resonance with velopharyngeal insuffiency combined with nasal obstruction

Articulation

misarticulations secondary to malocclusion and anterior skeletal open bite

severe tongue backing secondary to severe micrognathia

Voice

normal

Language

normal

Hearing

conductive loss of varying degree depending on degree of microtia

fixation of stapes footplate

occasionally a sensorineural loss

middle ear cavity may be absent or abnormally small

USHER SYNDROME

Type

genetic

Physical Characteristics

retinitis pigmentosa with night blindness

visual deterioration in adult life

occasional ataxia

occasional mental illness

four subtypes based on severity of hearing loss and visual impairment

Resonance

may be impaired due to hearing loss

Articulation

degree of impairment related to hearing loss

Voice

normal

Language

affected by hearing loss

Hearing

variable severity of sensorineural hearing loss

usually sloping to most severe in high frequencies

WILLIAMS SYNDROME

Type
chromosome deletion

Physical Characteristics
short stature
heart anomalies
microcephaly
limited joint movement
scoliosis
strabismus
hypertension
hypercalcemia
hyperopia
large mouth
thick lips
microdontia
enamel hypoplasia

Resonance
normal

Articulation
normal

Voice
usually normal; hoarseness occasionally observed

Language
performance is not normal
sophisticated structure
overuse of cliches
echolalia and overtalkativeness
perseveration common
"cocktail party" speech

Hearing
hyperacusis

CHAPTER TWENTY-FOUR
Traumatic Brain Injury

DEFINITION/DESCRIPTION

Traumatic brain injury is not associated with any particular age; rather, it can occur at any time in one's life. Traumatic brain injury is often referred to as a closed head injury and is typically classified as mild, moderate, or severe.

In the infant and toddler age range, most head injuries are caused by falls or abuse. In the older preschool population, the most common cause of injuries is falls. Elementary school-aged children are most likely to acquire head injuries as a result of sports, bike accidents, skateboarding accidents, pedestrian accidents, or accidents in which they are passengers in a car. Adolescents are more likely to suffer head injuries as a result of car crashes, usually at high speeds (Reed, 1994). Traumatic brain injury (TBI) is the number one cause of death in children. Car accidents, bicycle accidents, child abuse, and gunshot wounds are leading contributors to the increase in the number of pediatric traumatic brain injury cases seen by speech-language pathologists.

The incidence of TBI is approximately 200 persons per 100,000 people. Approximately 100,000 of these injuries result in death, whereas another 100,000 persons survive with varying degrees of disability, including acquired aphasia (Hegde, 1996).

Historically, research has not supported the notion of aphasia associated with TBI in children, preferring to reserve the term aphasia for use in describing adults with acquired language disorders. However, the Individuals with Disabilities Education Act (IDEA) designates TBI as a diagnostic category and defines TBI as follows:

> An acquired injury to the brain caused by an external physical force, resulting in total or partial functional disability or psychosocial impairment, or both, that adversely affect a child's educational performance. The term applies to open and closed head injuries resulting in impairments in one or more areas, such as: cognition; language; memory; attention; reasoning; abstract thinking; judgment; problem-solving; sensory, perceptual, and motor abilities; psychosocial behavior; physical functions; information processing; and speech. The term does not apply to brain injuries that are congenital or degenerative, or brain injuries induced by birth trauma. (U.S. Federal Register, 1992)

The IDEA calls for the reintegration of children with traumatic brain injury into the classrooms, and the teachers report that language disabilities are the factors that cause the greatest interference with success in school.

Kay and the Mild Traumatic Brain Injury Committee of the Head Injury Special Interest Group of the American Congress of Rehabilitation Medicine (1993) have defined traumatic brain injury as follows:

> Traumatically induced physiological disruption of brain function, as manifested by *at least one* of the following:
>
> 1. any period of loss of consciousness;
>
> 2. any loss of memory for events immediately before or after the accident;
>
> 3. any alteration in mental state at the time of the accident (e.g., feeling dazed, disoriented, or confused); and
>
> 4. focal neurological deficit(s) that may or may not be transient; but where (sic) the severity of the injury does not exceed the following:
>
>   *   loss of consciousness for approximately 30 minutes or less;
>
>   *   after 30 minutes, an initial Glasgow Coma Scale (GCS) of 13–15; and
>
>   *   posttraumatic amnesia (PTA) no greater than 24 hours.

Individuals with mild TBI may have a functional disability due to physical, cognitive, behavioral, or emotional symptoms that may persist after the injury. Typically, three categories of symptoms are associated with TBI.

The first category consists of physical symptoms, including dizziness, headaches, nausea, and vomiting. Blurred vision and sleep disturbances may also occur. Unexplained lethargy, quickness to fatigue, and other sensory losses may also occur in individuals with TBI (Green, Stevens, & Wolfe, 1997).

The second category of symptoms relates to cognitive deficits. When examining and determining the cognitive deficits that have occurred as the result of a TBI, the clinician must be careful to ascertain that the cognitive deficits are not caused by emotional or other causes beside the traumatic brain injury. Cognitive deficits frequently observed include poor attention skills, difficulty in concentrating, perceptual and memory deficits, problems with speech or language or both, and difficulty with executive functions (Green et al., 1997).

Behavioral changes with or without alterations in the degree of emotional responsivity constitute the third category of symptoms. Again, these symptoms must exist in the absence of other psychological, physical, or emotional stresses. Behavioral changes include emotional lability, disinhibition, irritability, and quickness to anger (Green et al., 1997).

Types of Injuries

It is important to differentiate among the various terms frequently used to describe head injury. A closed head injury is a non-penetrating brain injury in which the skull may be intact or fractured but the meninges are intact (Hegde, 1996). It is possible, in these cases, to have a minor head injury without brain injury. A penetrating head injury, which is also known as an open head injury, results in a fracturing or perforation of the skull with the meninges becoming torn or lacerated (Hegde, 1996).

Two other terms that are frequently encountered when studying traumatic brain injury are *coup injury* and *contrecoup injury*. In a coup injury, the injury is at the point of impact. This type of injury occurs when a blow to the head results in the brain's moving and slamming against the point of impact.

A contrecoup injury is a brain injury opposite from the impact. In these cases, a second injury occurs as the brain "bounces from the point of impact to the opposite side of the skull" (Blosser & DePompei, 1994).

It is also important to know whether the client has a focal lesion or a diffuse lesion. In a focal lesion, the damage is limited to a small area of the brain. This is in contrast to a diffuse lesion, which causes widespread damage. In diffuse lesions, frequently a twisting movement occurs, which can force tissues together, pull tissues apart, or create a tearing of axonal fibers as the injury occurs (Blosser & DePompei, 1994). Depending on the site of the damage, a diffuse lesion would be expected to be much more devastating to the client's cognition and language than would a focal lesion.

Nelson (1993) advocates dividing brain injury into four etiological categories: "(1) focal acquired lesions, (2) diffuse lesions associated with traumatic brain injury, (3) acquired childhood aphasia secondary to convulsive disorder, and (4) other kinds of brain injury or encephalopathy" (p. 116). Focal acquired lesions frequently are caused by strokes in children. These strokes commonly are the result of embolisms associated with congenital heart disease. They may also be associated with vascular disorders caused by sickle cell anemia. The strokes often result in left hemisphere lesions, from which recovery usually is fairly complete. Nelson (1993) does warn of possible enduring effects on language development and learning, however. Diffuse lesions associated with TBI resulting from falls, vehicular accidents, or abuse are the primary focus of this chapter. In these cases, it is not unusual to see relatively good language recovery in young children; however, long-term sequelae in terms of linguistic processing and cognition are common (Satz & Bullard-Bates, 1981; Ewing-Cobbs, Fletcher, & Levin, 1985).

Acquired aphasia secondary to convulsive disorders often includes unknown etiological factors. The problems can be either sudden or gradual in onset. Landau-Kleffner syndrome is a convulsive disorder characterized by epileptic discharges and severe language comprehension deficits (Nelson, 1993). Finally, Nelson (1993) refers to encephalopathies that are secondary to infection or irradiation. These would include disorders caused by tumors, encephalitis, meningitis, and cancer treatments. The extent of the damage in these last two categories varies depending on the extent and location of tissues involved, the age of the child, and the general health of the child.

Aphasias in the pediatric population caused by deficits in categories one, three, and four are relatively uncommon. In 1989, the death rate for children under 15 years of age from cerebrovascular disease (which contributes to stroke) was 4 per 100,000, compared to 2,296 per 100,000 in adults. More than one-third of strokes in children occur in the first 2 years of life. Usual etiological factors are sickle cell anemia, cardiac disease, vascular occlusions or malformations, and hemorrhage (Reed, 1994). Reed summarized much of the research in this area as outlined in Table 24–1.

In the pediatric population, lesions causing language deficits may initially be limited to the surface structure of the brain. However, as the learning demands increase, as they do in

TABLE 24-1	Associated physical, cognitive, perceptual motor, behavioral, and social problems in children with acquired aphasia due to traumatic brain injury
Area	*Effect of Traumatic Brain Injury*
Gross and fine motor	• Severe TBI: spasticity, delayed motor milestones • Mild TBI: fine motor and visuomotor deficits, reduction in age-appropriate play and physical activity
Cognitive	• Problems with long- and short-term memory, conceptual skills, problem solving • Reduced speed of information processing • Reduced attending skills
Perceptual motor	• Visual neglect, visual field cuts • Motor apraxia, reduced motor speed, poor motor sequencing
Behavioral	• Impulsivity, poor judgment, disinhibition, dependency, anger outbursts, denial, depression, emotional lability, apathy, lethargy, poor motivation
Social	• Does not learn from peers, does not generalize from social situations • Behaves like a much younger child, withdraws • Becomes distracted in noisy surroundings and becomes lost even in familiar surroundings

Adapted from *An Introduction to Children with Language Disorders* (2nd ed.) (p. 368), by V. A. Reed, 1994, Boston: Allyn and Bacon. Copyright 1994 by Allyn and Bacon.

grades 3 and 4, the deficits become more apparent. It is critical that the clinician understand the relationship between cognition and language because impaired cognitive processes (i.e., perception, memory, reasoning, and problem solving) interfere with language processes (Russell, 1993).

Underlying Complications

Cognitive and language deficits caused by TBI are rarely related to a single factor. Many secondary mechanisms may exist, which can create complications after the immediate injury. For example, the patient may have seizure activity. In fact, many head injury patients are placed on seizure medications as a prophylactic measure to minimize or prevent the occurrence of seizures. Swelling of the brain tissues also may be present. In closed head injuries (CHI), when tissue swells, a tight cavity is created between the brain and the cranium, leaving no place for the excess fluid. Therefore, the intracranial pressure increases and results in a decline in the patient's status. Hypoxia (lack of oxygen), hemorrhage, and the development of blood clots can also contribute to increased damage following the actual accident.

Effects of CHI and TBI

The resultant sequelae of TBI should be evaluated in terms of the effects that occur immediately after the injury, those that are observed during the acute recovery period, and those that are long-term, or residual, effects.

Initial Effects

A frequent initial effect is coma. "Coma is a state of unresponsiveness brought on by intracranial causes (supratentorial and subtentorial), diffuse lesions, and metabolic disturbances. States of stupor and coma may be described with terms such as lethargic, obtundurate, stuporous, and comatose, but are best described by using a standardized rating scale" (Golper, 1998. p. 151). Confusion and posttraumatic amnesia also are observed frequently immediately after the injury. In mild injuries commonly associated with a concussion, a loss of consciousness occurs that lasts less than 30 minutes, and posttraumatic amnesia (PTA) lasts less than 1 hour. An injury is regarded as moderate if a loss of consciousness or posttraumatic amnesia is present for more than 30 minutes but less than 24 hours. In severe cases, the coma lasts for more than 6 hours, and the PTA lasts for 1 to 7 days. In very severe cases, the PTA lasts for more than 7 days (Russell, 1993). The status of the patient on the Glasgow Coma Scale and the length of the PTA can be predictors of how the patient will do with regard to recovering language and cognitive functions. However, in the pediatric population, this needs to be interpreted with much caution because the Glasgow Coma Scale was developed for use with adults.

The patient may also have *retrograde amnesia,* which is difficulty remembering events leading up to the accident. Abnormal behaviors such as irritability, aggression, anxiety, hyperactivity, lethargy, and withdrawal may also be observed in the immediate period after the injury. Motor dysfunctions such as rigidity, tremor, spasticity, ataxia, and apraxia also may occur.

Acute Recovery Period

During the acute recovery period, speech production deficits may occur, such as difficulty with the production of consonants and possible mutism. The patient also may have speech comprehension problems and word retrieval deficits during the acute recovery stages. When shown common objects, the patient may have difficulty describing them. Syntactic problems, including a limited mean length of utterance, difficulty in constructing sentences, and fewer utterances, may be observed. In patients old enough to write, deficits in this area may be noted.

Long-Term (Residual) Effects

Long-term effects may include persistent word retrieval problems and a reduction in spontaneous speech. When speech does occur, it may be characterized by reduced fluency, in part caused by the word retrieval difficulties. Pragmatic problems are common. Subtle comprehension problems may be present that result in reading problems, poor mathematic reasoning skills, and, in general, poor academic performance. Memory problems may persist. Behaviorally, hyperactivity, and impulsivity are frequently observed in post-TBI patients. An additional problem may involve residual confusion, in which the patient is unable to recognize his or her own deficits.

Language deficits occurring after closed head injury are outlined in Table 24–2. In addition to the language deficits, psychological difficulties, which include depression, anger, and behaviors inappropriate for the situation, are frequently noted.

According to National Institutes of Health criteria (1984), three types of personality changes exist. The first one is apathy, in which the patient does not care about what happens. He or she has reduced interest in the usual activities and challenges, which is often misinterpreted as compliance or absence of a behavior problem. However, that misinterpretation often reinforces the apathy. In other words, the caregivers treat the patient as if he or she has a behavior problem, and, since the patient may have trouble making them understand otherwise, the apathy is reinforced. The second personality change occurs when the patient is

TABLE 24-2 Language deficits in individuals with TBI
Concentration
Sustained attention
Memory
Nonverbal problem solving
Part or whole analysis and synthesis
Conceptual organization and abstraction
Processing
Reasoning
Executive functioning (formulating goals, planning to achieve goals, carrying out plans)

Adapted from *Mild Traumatic Brain Injury: A Therapy and Resource Manual,* by B. S. Green, K. M. Stevens, and T. D. W. Wolfe, 1997, San Diego, CA: Singular Publishing Group. Copyright 1997 by Singular Publishing Group. Adapted with permission.

overly optimistic regarding the extent of the disability. Although positive thinking can be a good trait, care should be taken to ensure that the patient has realistic expectations regarding the rate and degree of recovery. The third change entails a loss of social restraint and judgment. In these cases, the patient often becomes tactless and talkative. He or she can become hurtful, which frequently damages the relationship with the family members. He or she may also have rage outbursts of abnormal intensity in response to trivial frustration.

Pediatric versus Adult Aphasia

Pediatric patients usually exhibit nonfluent aphasia with mutism, effortful speech, and impaired repetition skills. Syntactic problems, auditory comprehension deficits, anomia, and reading and writing difficulties also may be present. Children are less likely than adults to show paraphasia, jargon, and fluent aphasia.

In fluent aphasia, the patient does not have difficulty initiating speech, but he or she typically uses few if any content words. Syntax and prosody frequently stay intact, so the person appears to be speaking in sentences, but the sentences cannot be understood with regard to content.

Associated deficits in pediatric acquired aphasia include attentional disturbances and language impairments. As already mentioned, these language impairments include anomia. Also included are trouble with figurative and abstract language, difficulty in organizing the production of language, and problems in comprehending language. Cognitive and communication deficits result in academic underachievement. In her examination of the long-term residual effects of pediatric aphasia, Lees (1997) observed that, with adequate treatment, some children may achieve a relatively normal language profile based on testing used to measure progress after intensive therapy. However, Lees cautioned that, for some children, these normal language profiles masked persistent high-level difficulties, such as auditory verbal processing and lexical recall, that interfered with successful progress in school. Organically based behavioral and emotional deficits interfere with social interactions and impede the social-emotional growth that normally occurs during the school-age years. The child also may have perceptual-motor deficits that result in visual-field cuts, motor apraxia, or both.

ASSESSMENT

Neuropsychological testing of an individual who has sustained a TBI should be completed by a multidisciplinary team that includes professionals from medicine, nursing, social work, psychology, physical therapy, occupational therapy, psychiatry, audiology, and speech-language pathology. A list of areas of assessment is given in Table 24–3.

In Tomblin, Morris, and Spriestersbach (1994), VanDemark lists the following reasons for doing a cognitive/communication assessment on an individual who has sustained a traumatic brain injury:

1. Establish the presence or absence of deficits and collect baseline information on them.

2. Make a prognosis or a prediction about the amount of recovery an individual might expect.

3. Determine readiness for transfer to a rehabilitation program.

4. Conduct an in-depth, comprehensive evaluation to be used in planning and implementing a rehabilitation program.

5. Assess a client's progress in a rehabilitation program.

6. Determine if a client's cognitive/communicative abilities will support returning to work or living safely alone in the community.

7. Do a follow-up evaluation to ascertain if a client has maintained progress made in the rehabilitation program. (pp. 329–330)

Steps one, two, and three may be addressed in a trauma center or acute care setting. However, evaluations done in these settings need to be considered carefully because the

---

Table 24–3   Areas of assessment in TBI

Mood and behavior changes

Cognitive abilities

Language abilities

Memory and learning skills

Intelligence

Executive functioning

Academics and achievement

Abstract reasoning and concept formation

Fine motor control and speech

Sensory and perceptual skills

Tests of dissimulation

Personality inventory and psychosocial factors

Adapted from *Mild Traumatic Brain Injury: A Therapy and Resource Manual* (pp. 21–22), by B. S. Green, K. M. Stevens, and T. D. W. Wolfe, 1997, San Diego, CA: Singular Publishing Group. Copyright 1997 by Singular Publishing Group. Adapted with permission.

client's status and behaviors may change rather quickly. Even in the rehabilitation setting, mood and behavior changes will be observed. They can be caused by the actual injury, or they can be an emotional reaction to the injuries. Not only do the client's status and behavior change in the acute care setting, but the client may have limited ability to focus on the tasks at hand and may not have the stamina for extensive testing.

> The standard bedside mental status interview includes tasks related to language functions (assessing naming, repeating, reading, writing, and comprehension of verbal directions); orientation (determining if they know where they are, who they are, and the date and time); memory (assessing short-term memory and recall of information after a brief delay); attention and calculation (asking the patient to subtract by 7s from 100); drawing; and abstract reasoning (assessing proverb interpretation). (Golper, 1998, p. 137)

In the rehabilitation setting, all seven purposes may be addressed through evaluation. The clinician will be interested in establishing a preintervention baseline in order to be able to measure progress in the rehabilitation program. Third-party payers are going to want documented evidence of the need for intervention and the progress once the client is in a rehabilitation program. Once a complete history has been obtained and the patient has stabilized enough for thorough testing, cognitive and communication testing can take place.

Cognitive and communication tests typically fall into one of four categories. The first category is rating scales. Rating scales are typically based on observations of the client and may be completed by the clinician with the help of the family and other professionals interacting with the client. An example of a rating scale is the *Rancho Los Amigos Scale of Cognitive Levels and Expected Behavior* (Hagen & Malkmus, 1979). This scale rates a client's responses from Level I (no response) to Level VIII (purposeful appropriate response). The *Ranchos Los Amigos Scale* can be used to rate "levels of cognitive responses following coma during stages of recovery" (Golper, 1998, p. 151).

Another commonly used scale is the *Glasgow Coma Scale* (Jennett, Shook, Bond, & Brooks, 1981). The *Glasgow Coma Scale* is based on the clinician's observations of the "degree of eye opening, the best verbal response, and the best motor response to describe the level of disability the client is experiencing" (VanDemark, 1994).

The second category consists of assessments of communication and cognitive competence. These tests are administered by the speech-language pathologist in the acute care (if the patient is stable) and/or the rehabilitation setting.

Testing of cognitive abilities includes assessment of auditory and visual processing skills and a determination of attention abilities, similar to those assessed in attention deficit disorder. Of particular interest are the client's abilities to sustain attention and to use selective attention, divided attention, and alternating attention (Sohlberg & Mateer, 1989). Sustained attention is the ability to maintain a consistent behavioral response during repetitive or continuous activity. Selective attention refers to the client's ability to maintain focus on what is important in the presence of competing, distracting stimuli. Divided attention is the ability to simultaneously respond to more than one stimulus at a time, and alternating attention refers to the ability to shift attention between tasks that have different cognitive demands.

Testing of language abilities should concentrate on the comprehension of single words and sentences, auditory discrimination skills, and expressive language abilities. Assessment of memory and learning should be done in conjunction with language testing and should focus on auditory and visual memory, immediate and delayed recall, and the ability to learn new information. Intelligence testing should analyze verbal intelligence, nonverbal intelligence, and general knowledge.

Executive functioning refers to setting and executing goals and the ability to self-evaluate. Many individuals who have suffered a TBI have trouble with motivation and personal drive. Accident-induced lethargy contributes to this problem, which may occur even in individuals who were highly motivated and self-directed prior to the accident. Tests of dissimulation that assess the patient's effort and motivation also should be completed (Green et al., 1997). Problems with executive functioning may be manifested as reduced deficit awareness, poor goal-setting skills, lack of initiation of tasks, poor self-monitoring, difficulty in making and keeping a schedule, and poor time efficiency.

Testing of academic skills and achievement should include subject-specific testing. This includes mathematics, vocabulary, reading, and spelling. Abstract reasoning and concept formation should address problem-solving skills and the ability to make appropriate judgments. Motor strength, coordination, and manual dexterity should be part of the assessment of fine motor control and speed. Orientation in space and time, visual and tactile perceptual abilities, and responses to varying sensations may have a negative effect on the testing of sensory and perceptual skills.

Examples of tests in the cognitive/communicative category include the *Western Neuro Sensory Stimulation Profile* (WNSSP) (Ansell, Keenan, & de la Rocha, 1989). The WNSSP is designed to assess the severely impaired head-injured patient who is slow to recover. The test assesses arousal, attention, responses to sensory stimuli (auditory, visual, tactile, and olfactory), and expressive communication. According to VanDemark (1994), the WNSSP is "particularly effective for gathering baseline data and tracking a client's recovery pattern; it is not intended to compare a client with TBI's performance to that of a 'normal' individual" (p. 333).

Another cognitive/communication test is the *Brief Test of Head Injury* (BTHI). The BTHI was developed by Helm-Estabrooks and Hotz in 1991. Administered in 20–30 minutes, the BTHI is also intended for patients with severe head injuries. The scale assesses orientation/attention, following commands, linguistic organization, reading comprehension, naming, memory, and visual spatial skills.

The *Scales of Cognitive Ability for Traumatic Brain Injury* were developed in 1992 by Adamovich and Henderson. The SCATBI consists of five subtests designed to measure orientation, perception and discrimination, organization, recall, and reasoning. The results on this test can be compared to those of "normal" individuals and can be used on patients who are very low functioning and very high functioning.

A fourth test of cognitive/communicative ability is the *Ross Information Processing Assessment* (RIPA), which was developed by Ross in 1986. The RIPA can be administered to adolescents and adults who have had a TBI. It assesses cognitive and linguistic deficits through the following subtests: immediate memory, recent memory, temporal orientation for recent and remote memory, spatial orientation, orientation to the environment, recall of general information, problem solving and abstract thinking, organization, and auditory processing and retention (VanDemark, 1994).

Assessments of hearing, speech, and dysphagia constitute the third category of tests frequently used with patients who have sustained a traumatic brain injury. The speech evaluation should include an assessment of the client's voice and his motor speech skills (i.e., testing for apraxia and dysarthria).

The final category of tests centers around assessments of functional performance. There is tremendous emphasis on functional outcomes in therapy, with attention being paid to how well the client is able to participate in home and community activities (VanDemark, 1994). VanDemark cites Beukelman, Yorkston, and Lossing (1984) in noting that functional performance centers around two aspects: the client's needs with regard to communication, and how well the client is able to meet and express those needs. Two tests, the *Communicative Ability in Daily Living* (CADL) and the *Functional Communication Profile*, assess how an individual communicates in daily life. These two tests focus primarily on the communication abilities of the patient instead of assessing language per se (Vinson, 1999).

When assessing the strengths and weakness of an individual who has suffered a TBI, the professionals involved must communicate frequently and regularly in order to follow the changes that occur as the patient's physical injuries resolve. It is important to keep in mind that the patient may fatigue easily, so testing should be done in several short sessions rather than one long session. Sensitivity to the patient's emotional state also is important so that the individual does not become overly frustrated or depressed by his or her performance on the varying tasks that are presented to him.

TREATMENT

Whether in adults or children, treatment for TBI must be a team approach. Rehabilitation specialists functioning as a multidisciplinary team must be involved in order to work toward a positive resolution of any residual deficits. Family counseling in which family members are assigned their own roles in the rehabilitation process also is critical.

Factors affecting treatment include the stage of recovery, etiological factors, and age at the time of injury. In children, age is important because the younger the child, the greater the plasticity of the brain. It is believed that the more plasticity the brain has, the better the chances for natural recovery of some function. Regardless, therapy is needed to help manipulate the plasticity to ensure that the child recovers his or her maximum abilities (Rose, Johnson, & Attree, 1997).

Environmental enrichment is a key to recovery. Recovery from a traumatic brain injury is a long-term process that will extend beyond the rehabilitation setting into the client's natural environment.

> A common consequence of traumatic brian injury in humans is a reduction in cerebral arousal-activation. In combination with other common neuropsychological impairments, for example, inattention, memory, and motivation, this can result in significantly reduced levels of interaction between the patient and his environment. Coexisting sensory and motor impairments can restrict interaction still further. Clinicians agree that to increase levels of interaction between brain damaged patients and their environments is a vital part of any rehabilitation process. (Rose et al., 1997, p. 4)

Rose et al. advocate the use of computerized virtual reality therapy to create real-life and imaginary situations as a method of facilitating environmental interaction in a safe environment. Since most individuals have access to computer games, this method of bringing a variety of environments into a safe therapeutic setting holds great promise in therapy (Rose et al., 1997).

Because many patients suffering from residual effects of TBI fatigue easily, it is usually recommended that initial therapy sessions be brief and frequent. In other words, four 15-minute sessions per day may be more productive than a single 1-hour session. Functional communication goals should be targeted in individual and group therapy. Determining readiness to return to school should be a prime consideration in pediatric therapy. Thus, it will be important to focus not only on functional goals but also on general compensatory strategies that can be used to minimize the deficits. It also will be critical for the rehabilitation team, including the parents, to work closely with the classroom teacher when it is time for the child to return to the classroom. Initially, an appropriate classroom setting may be a class specifically designed for children recovering from TBI or a classroom for students with learning disabilities (Iskowitz, 1997). Similarly, the speech-language pathologist and other team members, such as the social worker, may need to interface with a client's employer and fellow employees to facilitate the client's return to work.

During the acute phase, therapy is likely to focus on sensory stimulation and working closely with the family to encourage responses from the client. Although speech and language abilities are a concern, it is also likely that, during this stage, issues related to self-care, swallowing, and feeding may be paramount. However, as the client progresses, more attention can be focused on speech and language goals and preparing the client to return to his or her home, school, social, and/or vocational environment. This includes focusing on prospective memory, which is the ability to remember to do things at the appropriate time (such as taking prescribed medications), and functional memory. Functional memory includes those skills that are needed to learn new information, recall old information, remember situational details, and function independently (Green et al., 1997).

SUMMARY

Throughout the past several years, speech-language pathologists have carried out discussions regarding the need to establish medical tracks and school-based tracks in speech-language pathology. However, the population of students with TBI helps point out the need to have both types of education regardless of the professional's primary employment site. Those who work with the child in the medical setting need to understand the educational setting to which the child will return as soon as possible. Similarly, those in the educational setting need to be familiar with the long-term sequelae of TBI and understand the nature of the injury and recovery process. It is also clear that these children need to be followed closely throughout their academic careers to monitor possible residual deficits that may play a role in a child's educational and social progress.

It is also critical that the speech-language pathologist track the patient's progress and maintenance of skills once the client has been discharged from active therapy. Cognitive and communicative demands will increase as the client explores reentering different social and vocational aspects of his life, and the need for additional therapy may become apparent.

CHAPTER TWENTY-FIVE
Voice Disorders

DEFINITION/DESCRIPTION

As people progress through their lifespan, various anatomical and physiological changes normally take place in the vocal mechanism. Voice disorders may be organic or functional in etiology, but regardless of the etiological factors, changes in one's voice can produce lifestyle changes that are profound in their implications for the affected person. There are a variety of voice disorders, including disorders caused by inflammation, edema, and lesions such as nodules and polyps, laryngeal papilloma, and laryngeal ulcers. Cancer of the larynx is addressed elsewhere in this book. There are also vocal problems caused by vocal fold immobility, neurological disorders of the voice, and spasmodic dysphonia. A general framework for the assessment and treatment of voice disorders is presented in this book. For specifics on different disorders, refer to *Organic Voice Disorders: Assessment and Treatment* (Brown, Vinson, & Crary, 1996, Singular Publishing Group).

ASSESSMENT

The physician (otolaryngologist) and the speech-language pathologist need to work as a team in the assessment, diagnosis, and treatment of voice disorders. Haynes and Pindzola (1998) list four reasons the speech-language pathologist should be involved in discussing the findings of a laryngeal examination:

1. By viewing the laryngeal exam, the clinician can make note of any alterations to the vocal mechanism (e.g., polyps, nodules).

2. Documentation of the extent of the vocal pathology is needed to establish a baseline against which to document progress in therapy.

3. If surgical intervention is recommended, the speech-language pathologist, the physician, and the patient need to discuss issues related to the provision of therapy during the post-surgical period.

4. If organic deviations are ruled out, the clinician could make informed decisions regarding the provision of therapy for functional voice disorders.

There are at least five basic steps in voice assessment: interviewing, observing, describing the voice, comparing observations to normal values and standards, and integrating information to determine a treatment plan or to determine its effectiveness. The job of the clinician is to describe the voice as objectively as possible. In most instances, the diagnosis of the abnormality affecting the voice should be left to the medical doctors.

As with all disorders, the first step in the assessment process is to take a comprehensive case history. During the intake interview, the clinician should observe the patient and note any overt signs of a voice disorder. The clinician should observe the breathing patterns of the client and assess the coordination of breathing and speaking. Vocal quality can be assessed by observation, as well as any compensation methods the client may be using. Assessing the psychological factors associated with the voice can also be of benefit in the long-term evaluation and treatment planning for the client. The clinician should inquire as to how the voice disorder is affecting the person in terms of his vocation and social life. Is the patient experiencing financial loss caused by unemployment? Does the patient enjoy attention from friends? "The medical history, voice usage, family history, history of the voice problem, work history, psychological history (including current stressors), and the impact of the voice disorder on the patient's life must be investigated to determine the origins of the voice complaint and the best treatment" (Bless & Hicks, 1996). A sample history form for adults is in Appendix 25–A, and a pediatric case history is in Appendix 25–B.

It is sometimes difficult to separate the physical illness from the psychological problems, and vice versa. Thus, an understanding of the psychological state of the client is a critical component to the voice evaluation (Bless & Hicks, 1996). A Voice Profile that indicates how the client feels about his voice is in Appendix 25–C. The Checklist of Sensory Systems (Appendix 25–D) will also provide the clinician with insight into the patient's assessment of his voice disorder.

The testing environment should be as free from extraneous noise as possible to facilitate recording of the client's voice. A totally quiet environment is not necessary; in fact, a level of noise around 30–40 dB may even be desirable because it forces the patient to increase his volume to be heard over the ambient noise.

A hearing screening should be done to be sure that the client's hearing is within normal limits at the screened frequencies. This is particularly important in clients who are referred for talking "too loud."

Perceptual measures are frequently based on a scale that ranges from 1 to 7 in equal-appearing intervals. These scales may rank from high to low, or in comparison to normal. Loudness, pitch, quality, and tempo can be assessed using an auditory-perceptual rating. An example of an auditory-perceptual rating form is in Appendix 25–E.

Instrumentation is used to measure the physiologic and acoustic characteristics of the patient's voice and to aid in describing the voice. Some of the instrumentation that is available includes laryngeal imaging techniques (videofluoroscopy and videolaryngscopy), acoustic measures, aerodynamic assessment, and a variety of other direct and indirect means of observing the larynx. Evaluation and diagnosis of voice and resonance disorders requires the clinician to understand the anatomy and physiology of voice, as well as the organic, functional, and psychiatric causes of voice disorders.

Videoendoscopy can be done using a rigid or a flexible (nasal) scope. A light source in the scope illuminates the laryngeal area, enabling the clinician to view the vocal folds and determine whether there is any apparent pathology or differences. Videostroboscopy can be used to study the apparent movement of the vocal folds. It can be used to "visualize the superior surface of the vocal folds during a variety of phonatory and breathing maneuvers.

It allows clinicians to determine the vibratory characteristics of the vocal folds" (Bless & Hicks, 1996, p. 140). The term "apparent movement" is applied because the eye can process only five distinct images per second. With stroboscopy, the rate of the video recording is approximately 33 frames per second. The eye "fuses these rapidly presented images into what is perceived as a complete picture of cycle-to-cycle vibration" (Bless & Hicks, 1996, p. 140). The videostroboscopy permits the clinician to determine whether there is inappropriate movement or positioning of the vocal folds, and to determine the impact of any laryngeal disease that may be present. Clinicians should be careful about documenting the movement of the folds as an objective measure, because the visual image is subjectively analyzed (Bless & Hicks, 1996).

Electroglottography (EGG) is another method of measuring laryngeal movement. Compared to videostroboscopy, it is relatively inexpensive, noninvasive, and easy to do. A pair of electrodes are positioned on either side of the thyroid cartilage, and a high-frequency electric current is passed between the electrodes. The neck and laryngeal tissues serve as the conductor between the electrodes. The EGG measurements can then be used "as an indirect measure of vocal fold closure patterns that reflects the degree of contact between tissues in the neck" (Bless & Hicks, 1996, p. 145). As the folds adduct, the voltage increases; as they abduct, the voltage decreases. The resultant wave form can be used to differentiate subtle dysphonias from normal voice, or pathological laryngeal conditions from normal accumulations.

Measures of aerodynamics include the measurement of average air pressures, air volumes, and airflows that are produced as part of the peripheral mechanics of the laryngeal, respiratory, and supralaryngeal airways (Bless & Hicks, 1996).

Acoustic measures should also be done using non-speech and speech tasks. Some examples of each are in Table 25–1.

Table 25–1 Examples of non-speech and speech tasks for acoustic measures	
Non-speech tasks:	Sustained [a], [i], and [u] vowels
	Sustained [s] consonant
	Sustained [z] consonant
	Pitch glides
	Loudness glides
	Adductory glides [a] and [ha]
	Register glides
Speech tasks:	Counting from 1–100 at a comfortable pitch and loudness
	"Where are you going?" at soft, medium, and loud volumes
	"The blue spot is on the key again" at soft, medium, & loud volumes
	Oral reading of the Rainbow or Grandfather Passage
	Descriptive speech, "Cookie Theft" picture
	Parent-child speech, "Goldilocks and the 3 Bears"
	Dramatic speech involving deep emotions (fear, anger . . .)
	Singing "Happy Birthday to You" at modal and falsetto

From "Diagnosis and Measurement: Assessing the 'WHs' of Voice Function," by D. M. Bless and D. M. Hicks, 1996, in *Organic Voice Disorders: Assessment and Treatment* (p. 149), by W. S. Brown, B. P. Vinson, and M. A. Crary (Eds.), San Diego, CA: Singular Publishing Group. Copyright 1996 by Singular Publishing Group. Used with permission.

A variety of instrumentation is available for use by the speech-language pathologists with expertise in the area of voice disorders. Instrumentation includes the following:

1. Visi-Pitch (Kay Elemetrics): the Visi-Pitch can be used to evaluate intensity, fundamental frequency, frequency range, optimal pitch, and habitual pitch.

2. The Phonatory Function Analyzer (Nagashima Medical Instruments): the Phonatory Function Analyzer evaluates frequency, phonation, rate of airflow, intensity, and volume of air expired.

3. The Fundamental Frequency Indicator (Special Instruments, America): the Fundamental Frequency Indicator utilizes a VU meter to indicate a client's fundamental frequency.

4. Nasometer (Kay Elemetrics): the nasometer provides "a visual analysis of the oral-nasal resonance ratio" (Shipley & McAfee, 1992, p. 267).

5. MacSpeech Lab, CSpeech, Micro Speech Lab: all three of these are computer-based programs that can be used to analyze the voice and provide diagnostic and treatment information for the clinician (Shipley & McAfee, 1998).

The subglottal pressure changes with hyperfunctional and hypofunctional voices. Unfortunately, with regard to air pressures, there is little standard information about the normal air pressures, and the predicted values based on laryngopathology. Subglottal air pressure plays a critical role in changing fundamental frequency and intonation control. Subglottal pressure increases at lower frequencies, causing a lateral extension of the vocal folds in the vibratory cycles. This lateral extension results in an increase in the effective length of the vocal folds, which is accompanied by an increased tension and results in changing of the pitch.

Clinical procedures such as the s/z ratio (Boone & McFarlane, 1994) can also be used to assess respiratory and phonatory efficiency. The normal duration of each phoneme is approximately 20–25 seconds for adults and 10 seconds for children. The clinician asks the client to produce a sustained /s/ and times the production using a stopwatch. The procedure is then repeated with a sustained /z/. The procedure should be repeated a minimum of two trials. The longest /s/ duration is then divided by the longest /z/ duration to produce an s/z ratio. The premise is that an s/z ratio will provide some indication of respiratory sufficiency and the presence or absence of vocal pathology. The interpretations of the ratios are as follows:

1. A ratio of 1.0 with normal duration is a normal duration of production and indicates that the respiratory ability is normal and there is no vocal fold pathology.

2. A 1.0 ratio with reduced duration is indicative of possible respiratory inefficiency.

3. A ratio of 1.2 or greater with normal duration of the /s/ is indicative of possible vocal fold pathology. Since the /z/ is voiced, an imbalance between the production of the /s/ and /z/ indicates a possible vocal pathology. The higher the ratio, the greater the likelihood of pathology (Shipley & McAfee, 1992).

Of course, this method should be followed up with videolaryngoscopy to confirm the suspected results.

"To make appropriate recommendations following assessment, the clinician should be familiar with various forms of phonosurgery, palatal surgery, and vocal fold physiology" (Golper, p. 4). The evaluation report should include a description of the testing environment, and the protocol used in the assessment process. This would include listing all tests and measurements taken and the client's performance on each one. The clinician should include a description of the instrumentation used since there are no standard protocols for voice assessment.

TREATMENT

Increased knowledge about the vocal system has led to an increase in physiologically based treatments for voice disorders.

> This change in clinical orientation has resulted in clinicians from different professional orientations working together to determine the most effective treatment based on (a) what the patient is capable of doing with his or her existing laryngeal mechanism; (b) knowledge of what can be changed with behavioral exercises; (c) knowledge of what is possible to surgically change; (d) recognition of the complex nature of voice production, and (e) incorporation of modern technology to increase therapeutic efficiency or improve outcome. (Hicks & Bless, 1996, p. 171)

Because different pathologies can present the same vocal symptoms, and because different symptoms can be caused by the same pathologies, it is critical to have a good understanding of vocal physiology and anatomy.

Depending on the vocal pathology, one or both of the following therapy interventions should occur: behavioral therapy or medical management.

Behavioral therapy should include the following steps:

1. *Patient education:* Include review of laryngeal structure and function; explanation of mechanical basis of the voice symptoms; review of the role that various contributing factors (i.e., abuse of voice, caffeine consumption, etc.) play in the voice disorder; clarification of recommendations; and explanation of therapy goals and time frame.

2. *Voice monitoring:* Adequate and appropriate voice monitoring is an "essential prerequisite for optimal behavioral change rather than a true therapy technique" (Hicks & Bless, 1996, p. 173). Voice monitoring, also referred to as ear training, is critical if the patient is to self-monitor the use of his voice and note when changes are occurring in the voice. Steps to achieve good voice monitoring skills are as follows:

   - Educating the patient about relevant voice performance parameters that cause the dysphonia

   - Asking the patient to demonstrate the various parameters and identify which ones are problematic

   - Using physiological measurements (acoustic analysis, etc.) to compare and contrast the normal and pathological voices

   - Shifting from a gross difference to the more subtle differences as the client's self-monitoring improves (Hicks & Bless, 1996).

3. *Improved breath support for speech:* The patient should progress to the point that he can sustain phonation for 10–12 seconds. He should also have proper breath pausing. This can be developed through reading passages with the pausing marked, to reading unmarked passages, then progressing to conversation.

4. *Identification and elimination of vocal abuse(s):* Abuse is composed of misuse and overuse. Although a client may demonstrate one or the other, it is often that both are a part of the client's voice profile. "Misuse is intuitively what patients and clinicians think of when referring to 'abuse.' It involves pushing the larynx beyond its physiologic limits and is commonly illustrated by severe coughing, throat clearing, yelling, or screaming. Overuse, in contrast, involves a wearing down or fatiguing process. It can be conceived of as using the larynx within appropriate physiologic boundaries, but for extensive, uninterrupted periods of time" (Hicks & Bless, 1996, p. 175). Therapy steps involved in this component of behavioral therapy are as follows:

   • Assist the patient in developing a voice use profile over a period of 1 week to identify instances of misuse or overuse.

   • The clinician and the client should each generate a list of 5–10 of the worst abuses of the voice.

   • Combine the two lists into a ranking of the five worst abuses.

   • Negotiate strategy options for eliminating, reducing, or modifying the abuses of the voice.

   • Implement and monitor a compliance with the identified strategy options.

   • As targets are obtained, adjust or include other targets until the voice misuse and overuse are extinguished (Hicks & Bless, 1996).

5. *Direct vocal/laryngeal manipulation:* The underlying principle to direct vocal/laryngeal manipulation is that it alters specific vocal aspects (pitch, loudness, laryngeal quality) to create the desired changes in the voice. It is appropriate for use in the following situations: irritative factors, immobility, spasmodic dysphonia, nodules/polyps, or neurologic dysphonias. There are three primary methods of providing direct vocal/laryngeal manipulation:

   • Reduction of vocal fold medial compression: Many vocal lesions are the result of overadduction (medial compression) of the vocal folds. These lesions include nodules, polyps, edema, inflammation, contact ulcers, and lesions of the lamini propria. One way of achieving the reduction is complete voice rest, although this is difficult for most clients to fully implement. Therefore, it is probably more productive to teach a soft glottal attack and a breathy quality to reduce the glottal compression. The strategies of reduced sustained phonation, increased breathy quality, and reduced loudness are short-term strategies until the voice has recovered. Common techniques include the "yawn-sign" approach, using /h/-initiated words, soft phonation, and purposeful breathy phonation. Another technique is resonant voice therapy in which the client increases oral vibratory sensations while decreasing vocal adduction.

   • Laryngeal reposturing: Increased laryngeal tension often occurs as clients try to overcompensate for the laryngeal pathology (such as scarring, nodules, or paralysis).

The result is that the larynx is in an elevated position. The clinician should manually reposition the larynx to a lower position by kneading the circumlaryngeal area to reduce the tension.

- Increased vocal fold medial compression: For cases of underadduction, such as in paralysis or joint fixation, efforts should be made to increase the adduction. Patients should be taught the physiology of speech and the importance of using the voice to its maximum capacity. Isometric exercises such as pushing, pulling, and pressing with the arms increase thoracic and cervical tension. This tension generalizes to the larynx and results in increased adduction of the vocal folds and better voicing. "Typical voice gains include increased conversational and maximum loudness, improved stability of phonation, reduced aphonia and breathy phonation, reduced vocal fatigue, improved sustained phonation, and reduced vocal effort" (Hicks & Bless, 1996, p. 179). This technique can also be used for abductor spasmodic dysphonia and other neurological dysphonias such as those associated with Parkinson's disease.

- Voice care "prescription": Voice care "prescription" is applicable for all organic lesions that require phonosurgery. This is a period of controlled use of the voice following phonosurgery. Phonosurgery may be necessary if behavioral modifications alone do not result in complete improvement of the voice (e.g., vocal nodules). Typically, the voice needs to be "babied" for 6–12 weeks following the surgery. A typical "prescription" is outlined in Table 25–2.

7. *Lifestyle changes:* Lifestyle changes may be necessary to decrease the number and amount of irritants to the vocal folds. This is particularly necessary when the client has an irritated larynx or contact ulcers. Lifestyle changes may include reducing/eliminating smoking, which affects the larynx through the hot smoke and the chemical absorption. Reducing alcohol consumption will also reduce the amount of irritant to which the voice mechanism is exposed. Clients should be counseled as to the impact of smoking and drinking alcohol with regard to laryngeal cancer. Gastroesophageal reflux may require medical management, but there are several practical things the client can do to reduce the impact of reflux on the laryngeal area. These are outlined in Table 25–3.

Medical management of voice disorders encompasses the following:

1. *Pharmacology:* Medical management of voice disorders with pharmaceuticals can have a negative and positive effect, so the benefits must be weighed against the potential

TABLE 25-2 Voice care "prescription" following phonosurgery

Weeks Post-Op	Voice Use
7–10 days	Complete voice rest
2nd & 3rd weeks	Unrestricted quiet talking but only in subdued conversational settings
4th week	Normal conversational voice in controlled/recreational settings, avoiding any overt misuse or overuse
5th week	Normal voice use in social settings with some competing background noise
6th week	Unrestricted voice use in social settings with the exception of overt use

TABLE 25–3 Measurements to reduce acid reflux
Avoid large meals.
Avoid eating late at night, trying to restrict eating beyond the normal dinner hour.
Remain upright for at least 2 hours following meals.
Avoid alcohol and tobacco products.
Eliminate any food documented to contribute to the reflux.
Avoid aspirin and ibuprofen.
If overweight, lose weight.
Avoid the following foods: fatty or fried foods, citrus juices, tomato products, caffeinated coffee, tea, and soda, chocolate, and carbonated beverages.
Elevate the head of the bed at least 6 inches, or sleep on a pillow wedge.

From "Principles of Treatment," by D. M. Hicks and D. M. Bless, 1996, in *Organic Voice Disorders: Assessment and Treatment* (pp. 164–166), by W. S. Brown, B. P. Vinson, and M. A. Crary (Eds.), San Diego, CA: Singular Publishing Group. Copyright 1996 by Singular Publishing Group. Used with permission.

problems. For example, bronchodilators may be prescribed to improve breath support but can also cause tremor and nervousness in the voice (Hicks & Bless, 1996). Some drugs that the client is taking for nonvoice-related problems may produce a drying effect on the vocal cords, making them more susceptible to harm. For example, Detrol that is used to treat urinary incompetence may produce drying of the vocal mucosa.

Antibiotics may be used to reduce inflammation and edema; cough suppressants may be used to reduce vocal fold trauma from severe coughing; and mucolytic agents may be used to liquefy the natural secretions of the upper airway. Anti-reflux medications may help in controlling gastroesophageal reflux, in addition to the behavioral measures previously outlined. Decongestants will help reduce edema of the upper airway. Anti-inflammatory drugs can help to reduce edema and erythema of the upper respiratory system. These may be delivered via injection, tapering pills, and aqueous sprays. Anti-tremor drugs may help control tremor associated with spasmodic dysphonia and other neurological conditions. Myoneural junction faciliators may also help in certain neurological conditions such as myasthenia gravis. Finally, botulinum toxin (BOTOX) is used to treat spasmodic dysphonia by paralyzing the muscles into which it is injected. This promotes phonatory stability by reducing the neuromuscular contractions of the intrinsic laryngeal muscles (Hicks & Bless, 1996).

2. *Surgery:* There are six categories of phonosurgery that can be used to preserve the laryngeal mucosa and maintain the integrity of the vocal ligament.

   • Tissue excision: This is the removal of pathologic tissue either through microdissection or the laser.

   • Tissue injections: Gelfoam, Teflon, collagen, and autologous fat have all been used in injections "for repair of defects due to tissue loss, scarring, sulcus vocalis, reduction of medial edge bowing, or repositioning the immobile vocal fold closer to midline" (Hicks & Bless, 1996, p. 184).

   • Tissue vaporization: in tissue vaporization, a laser is used to remove unwanted tissue such as is found in papilloma and vocal fold varices.

- Framework procedures: The most common application of framework procedures is the medialization of an immobile vocal fold. This is accomplished by placing an implant into the larynx to move the immobile vocal fold toward midline where the functioning fold can adduct. Cricothyroid approximation has been used in abductory spasms to counteract vocal fold flaccidity. Anterior commissure advancement procedures are also used in these cases to stretch the vocal folds, thereby creating increased tension and improving vocal fold approximation.

- Neuromuscular adjustment: Outcomes data are not particularly promising on these techniques. One is nerve lysis to treat adductor spasmodic dysphonia. Another is reinnervation for vocal fold paralysis.

- Conservation: The use of partial laryngectomy procedures has increased in recent years, with management by chemotherapy and radiation being more common than in previous years.

APPENDIX 25–A: TYPICAL ADULT VOICE HISTORY FORM

History of the Voice Problem

Symptoms
- What is the chief complaint?
- What changes in voice have been noticed (e.g., hoarsness, breathiness, vocal fatigue, loss of vocal range)?
- Are there associated sensations or symptoms (e.g., pain in the throat when using the voice, tickling or choking sensation, breathing problems, swallowing difficulties, heartburn, weight loss, coughing)?

Onset
- When did the symptoms first begin?
- Was the onset sudden or gradual in nature?
- What did the client think was causing the problem?

Duration
- Is the problem acute (days or weeks) or chronic (months or years)?

Variability
- Is the problem constant or does it wax and wane?
- If it varies, what factors seem to aggravate or relieve the symptoms (e.g., weather, amount of speaking, coughing, episodes, time of day)?

Progression of symptoms
- Since the time of onset, have the symptoms worsened, improved, or remained the same?
- What development prompted evaluation?

Previous evaluations, treatments, results
- Have there been previous evaluations or treatments (voice therapy, radiation therapy, acupuncture, homeopathy)?
- What were the effects of treatment?

Past Medical History

Major illnesses
- Have there been previous physical or mental illnesses?
- What was the length of each illness, extent of incapacity, types and effects of treatments?

Surgeries
- What surgeries have been performed?
- Was intubation or tracheotomy required?
- Were there complications (e.g., recurrent laryngeal nerve section, airway obstruction, hemangioma)?

Accidents or injuries
- Have there been traumatic injuries to the head or neck?

- Blunt or penetrating traumas (e.g., sports injuries, strangulation, automobile accidents)?

- Foreign body aspiration (e.g., choking on foods or small objects)?

- Ingestion of caustic agents (e.g., acids, alkalines)?

- Inhalation injuries or burns?

- Iatrogenic injuries (from irradiation, prolonged intubation, or tracheotomy)?

Allergies
- Are there allergies to foods? drugs? environment?

Review of symptoms
- Are other symptoms present that might be associated with the voice disorder?

- Are there problems in general health, ear, nose, and throat, breasts, musculoskeletal, respiratory, cardiovascular, genitourinary, or neurologic systems?

- Is there an identifiable symptom complex or pattern?

Current Health Practices

Medications
- Are any drugs being used on a regular or intermittent basis? prescription drugs? non-prescription drugs (i.e., aspirin, laxatives, vitamins, cold tablets, over-the-counter sleeping pills or nerve pills)?

Recreational drugs
- Is there past or present use of street drugs such as marijuana (pot), speed (amphetamines, Dexedrine, Ritalin), LSD (acid), PCP (angel dust), cocaine, heroin, mushrooms, etc.?

Tobacco
- What type and amount of tobacco is used?

- How long has the patient been smoking or chewing tobacco?

- Is there exposure to second-hand smoke?

Alcohol
- How much and what types of alcoholic beverages does the patient drink?

- Are there beneficial effects on the voice from drinking?

Caffeine
- Is there use of caffeine-containing drinks (e.g., coffee, tea, soft drinks, hot chocolate)? foods (e.g., chocolate, cocoa), or medications (e.g., Excedrin,™ Anacin,™ Vanquish,™ Triaminicin,™ Coricidin,™ Sinarest,™ No-Doz,™ diet pills)?

Dietary patterns
- Is a special or restricted diet used?

- Would the present diet promote gastroesophageal reflux (e.g., spicy foods, high fat foods, caffeine)?

- Is there evidence of an eating disorder such as anorexia nervosa or bulimia?

Voice usage	• In what ways is the voice typically used (e.g., cheering at a child's hockey game, professional or public speaking, talking over noise in a factory, singing, yodeling, crying)?
Stress management	• In what ways is stress managed (e.g., exercise, medication, counseling, meditation, support groups, primal scream therapy)?

Family/Work History

Hereditary conditions	• What inheritance patterns are present in the family history?
	• Are there similar problems in parents, siblings, offspring?
Family dynamics/ Learning	• Do environmental influences seem to account for the voice problem (e.g., is the patient from a large family that "always talked too loudly")?
	• What current family interaction patterns exist (e.g., shouting matches, verbal competitions at the dinner table)?
Major life changes	• What events have happened in the past 12 months that might increase stress?
Emotional reactions to illness	• Is there a family history of "throat cancer"?
	• Is over-reaction to the current voice problem based upon past family experiences?

Psychological Considerations

Psychological history	• What is the patient's mental health history?
	• Does it include depression, mania, suicide attempts, alcohol abuse, an eating disorder, schizophrenia, "nervous breakdowns," sexual abuse, or other psychological problems?
	• What past or present treatments have been used (e.g., psychotherapy, pharmacotherapy, electroconvulsive therapy, in-patient hospitalization)?
Current stress levels	• Have recent problems or circumstances elevated stress levels at home or work (e.g., financial problems, divorce, an illness or death in the family, a change in jobs, moving to a new city)?
Voice disability index	• What impact is the voice problem having on daily living activities?

From "Diagnosis and Measurement: Assessing the 'WHs' of Voice Function," by D. M. Bless and D. M. Hicks, 1996, in *Organic Voice Disorders: Assessment and Treatment* (pp. 164–166), by W. S. Brown, B. P. Vinson, and M. A. Crary (Eds.), San Diego, CA: Singular Publishing Group. Copyright 1996 by Singular Publishing Group. Used with permission.

APPENDIX 25-B: PEDIATRIC VOICE HISTORY— CONTRIBUTIONS TO THE VOICE PROBLEM

History	Factors
Voice history	• Past and present symptoms
	• Onset and duration
	• Clinical course and variability
	• Previous evaluations and/or treatments
Medical history	• Major illnesses
	• Surgeries
	• Accidents and/or injuries
	• Allergies
	• Drug/medication use
	• Relevant medical problems
Voice usage	• Excessive loudness
	• Voice strain/tension
	• Abusive habits
	• Affective voice usage
Family history	• Familial diseases, illnesses, conditions
	• Family dynamics, learning, environment
Developmental information	• Hearing history
	• Gross and fine motor development
	• Associated speech/language delays or disorders
	• Cognitive development
Child's personal profile	• Personality
	• Social interaction patterns
	• Personal habits, behaviors, stresses

APPENDIX 25-C: VOICE PROFILE

Read each statement and then circle the number which best indicates how you presently feel about your voice.

1 = Almost Never   2 = Sometimes   3 = Often   4 = Almost Always

1. I have to alter daily activities because of my voice.	1 2 3 4
2. My voice interferes with communication.	1 2 3 4
3. My voice is distracting to others.	1 2 3 4
4. It is difficult for others to hear me in noisy environments.	1 2 3 4
5. My voice gets tired during the day.	1 2 3 4
6. It takes a lot of energy to produce voice.	1 2 3 4
7. I miss work because of my voice.	1 2 3 4
8. I think about my voice problem.	1 2 3 4
9. My voice sounds worse than other speakers.	1 2 3 4
10. People make comments about my voice.	1 2 3 4

11. On a scale of 1 to 7, where 1 = normal, 4 = moderate, and 7 = severe impairment, circle the number that best describes how bad your voice is.

1	2	3	4	5	6	7
Normal			Moderate			Severe

APPENDIX 25-D: CHECKLIST OF SENSORY SYSTEMS

Mark (X) all symptoms associated with the voice problem.

_____ 1. Frequent throat clearing

_____ 2. Frequent coughing

_____ 3. Vocal fatigue that progresses with use of the voice

_____ 4. Irritation or pain in the voice box or throat

_____ 5. Strain or bulging of neck muscles

_____ 6. Swelling of veins and/or arteries in the neck

_____ 7. Feeling of a foreign substance or "lump" in the throat

_____ 8. Ear irritation, tickling, or earache

_____ 9. Frequent sore throats

_____ 10. A tickling, soreness, or burning sensation in the throat

_____ 11. Scratchy or dry throat

_____ 12. Tension and/or tightness in the throat

_____ 13. A feeling that talking is an effort

_____ 14. Pain or difficulty swallowing

_____ 15. Pain or burning sensation at the base of the tongue

---

APPENDIX 25-E: AUDITORY-PERCEPTUAL RATING FORM

Name: _____   Clinician: _____

MR #: _____   Date of Eval: _____

D. O. B.: _____   AudioTape #: _____

Gender: _____   Diagnosis: _____

Loudness

Strong _____ Weak

Mono-loudness _____ Excess Loudness Variation

Pitch

Excessively Low Pitch _____ Excessively High Pitch

Unsteady/Timorous _____ Monotone

Quality

Hyperfunction/tone _____ Hypofunction/Lax

Clear _____ Breathy

Rough _____ Smooth

Muffled/Dampened _____ Resonant

Hypernasal _____ Hyponasal

Hard Glottal Attack _____ Breathy Attack

Shrill _____ Creaky Voice/Glottal Fry

Tempo

Staccato _____ Smooth Flowing

Rapid Rate _____ Slow Rate

Other

25 years old _____ 75 years old

Normal _____ Abnormal

THE GRANDFATHER PASSAGE

You wished to know all about my grandfather. Well, he is nearly ninety-three years old; he dresses himself in an ancient black frock coat, usually minus several buttons, yet he still thinks as swiftly as ever. A long, flowing beard clings to his chin, giving those who observe him a pronounced feeling of the utmost respect. When he speaks, his voice is just a bit cracked and quivers a trifle. Twice each day he plays skillfully and with zest upon our small organ. Except in winter when the ooze of snow or ice prevents, he slowly takes a short walk in the open air each day. We have often urged him to walk more and smoke less, but he always answers, "Banana oil!" Grandfather likes to be modern in his language.

THE RAINBOW PASSAGE

When the sunight strikes raindrops in the air they act like a prism and form a rainbow. The rainbow is a division of white light into many beautiful colors. These take the shape of a long round arch, with its path high above, and its two ends apparently beyond the horizon. There is, according to legend, a boiling pot of gold at one end. People look, but no one ever finds it. When a man looks for something beyond his reach, his friends say he is looking for the pot of gold at the end of the rainbow.

Throughout the centuries men have explained the rainbow in various ways. Some have accepted it as a miracle without physical explanation. To the Hebrews it was a token that there would be no more universal floods. The Greeks used to imagine that it was a sign from the gods to foretell war or heavy rain. The Norsemen considered the rainbow as a bridge over which the gods passed from earth to their home in the sky. Other men have tried to explain the phenomenon physically. Aristotle thought that the rainbow was caused by reflection of the sun's rays by the rain. Since then physicists have found that it is not reflection, but refraction by the raindrops which causes the rainbow. Many complicated ideas about the rainbow have been formed. The difference in the rainbow depends considerably upon the size of the water drops, and the width of the colored band increases as the size of the drops increases. The actual primary rainbow observed is said to be the effect of superposition of a number of bows. If the red of the second bow falls upon the green of the first, the result is to give a bow with an abnormally wide yellow band, since red and green lights when mixed form yellow. This is a very common type of bow, one showing mainly red and yellow, with little or no green or blue.

THE DECLARATION OF INDEPENDENCE

We hold these truths to be self-evident, that all men are created equal, that they are endowed by the Creator with certain unalienable rights, that among these are life, liberty and the pursuit of happiness. That to secure these rights, governments are instituted among men, deriving their just powers from the consent of the governed, that whenever any form of government becomes destructive of these ends, it is the right of the people to alter or abolish it, and to institute new government, laying its foundation on such principles and organizing its powers in such form, as to them shall seem most likely to effect their safety and happiness.

Prudence, indeed, will dictate that governments long established should not be changed for light and transient causes; and accordingly all experience has shown, that mankind are more disposed to suffer, while evils are sufferable, than to right themselves by abolishing the forms to which they are accustomed. But when a long train of abuses and usurpations, pursuing invariably the same object evinces a design to reduce them under absolute despotism, it is their right, it is their duty, to throw off such government, and to provide new guards for their future security.

WEB SITES FOR PATIENT RESOURCES

Aphasia, TBI, Dementia, Neurogenic Disorders

Info on stroke and inexpensive materials: http://www.stroke.org

Stroke Discussion Group: cnet_stroke_dem_head_injury@listserv.arizona.edu

National Center for Neurogenic Communication Disorders: http://cnet.shs.arizona.edu/childneuro.list.heml

Amyotrophic Lateral Sclerosis Association: http://www.alsa.org

National Parkinson Foundation: http://www. parkinson.org

National Multiple Sclerosis Society: http://www.nmss.org

Traumatic Brain Injury discussion group: tbi-sprt@maelstrom.stjohns.edu

Alzheimer's Discussion Group: alzheimer@wubios.wustl.edu

Attention Deficit Disorder/Attention Deficit with Hyperactivity Disorder

Children and Adults with AD/H Disorders: http://www.chadd.org

Audiology

Acoustical Society of America: http://www.acoustics.org

American Academy of Audiology: http://www.audiology.org

Augmentative and Alternative Communication

Barkley Augmentative and Alternative Communication Center: http://aac.unl.eo

AAC Topics: http://www.asel.udel.edu/at-online

Adaptive Technology Resource Centre, University of Toronto: http://www.utoronto.ca/atrc/

Autism

Autism Society of America: http://www.autism-society.org

Center for the Study of Autism: http://www.autism.org

Central Auditory Processing Disorders

CAPD Parents' Page: http://pages.cthome.net/cbristol/capd.html

Cerebral Palsy

Information on cerebral palsy: http://www.irsc.org/cerebral.htm

United Cerebral Palsy: http://www.ucpa.org

Cleft Palate and Cleft Lip

Cleft Palate and Lip Resources: http://www.widesmiles.org

American Cleft Palate-Craniofacial Association: http://www.cleft.com

Down Syndrome

http://www.irsc.org/down.htm

Fluency Disorders

Stuttering Foundation of America: http://www.stuttersfa.org

Head and Neck Cancers

Archives of Otolaryngology—Head and Neck Surgery:
http://www.ama-assn.org/public/journals/otol/about.htm

CDC's TIPS: Tobacco Information and Prevention Source: http://www.cdc.gov/tobacco

LARYNX-C: The Larynx Cancer Online Support Group: http://tile.net/tile/listserv/larynxc

Cancer Guide: Basic Information on Cancer: cancerguide.org/basic

Healthtouch—Speaking after Laryngectomy:
http://www.healthtouch.com/level1/leaflets/aslha/aslha051

American Cancer Society: http://www.cancer.org/frames.html

Motor Speech Disorders

http://www.ticeinfo.com/speech/index.html

Multicultural Issues

ASHA Multicultural Issues Board Fact Sheets:
http://www.asha.org/professionals/multicultural/fact_hp.htm

American Dialect Society: http://www.americandialect.org

Voice Disorders

http://www.bgsm.edu/voice/index.html

ORGANIZATIONS

AboutFace (support for families and patients with craniofacial anomalies)
P. O. Box 93
Limekiln, PA 19535
(800) 225-3223

Alexander Graham Bell Association for the Deaf
3417 Volta Place, NW
Washington, DC 20007

American Academy of Audiology
8300 Greensboro Drive
Suite 750
McLean, VA 22101-3611

American Cancer Society
777 Third Avenue
New York, NY 10017

American Cleft Palate—Craniofacial Association
1218 Grandview Avenue
Pittsburgh, PA 15211
(800) 24-CLEFT

American Cleft Palate Education Foundation
331 Salk Hall
University of Pittsburgh
Pittsburgh, PA 15261
(800) 232-5338

American Coalition for Citizens with Disabilities
1200 15th Street, NW, Suite 201
Washington, DC 20005

American Council of the Blind
1211 Connecticut Avenue NW
Suite 506
Washington, DC 20036

American Council of the Blind Parents
Route A Box 78
Franklin, LA 70538

American Foundation for the Blind
15 West 16th Street
New York, NY 10011

American Speech-Language-Hearing Association
10801 Rockville Pike
Rockville, MD 20852-3279
(888) 498-6699
http://asha.org

Arthritis Association
5400 Peachtree Road, NE
Suite 1106
Atlanta, GA 30326

Association for Children and Adults with Learning Disabilities
4156 Library Road
Pittsburgh, PA 15234

Association for Retarded Children
2709 Avenue E. East
P. O. Box 6109
Arlington, TX 76011

The Association for the Severely Handicapped
1600 West Armory Way
Garden View Suite
Seattle, WA 98119

Attention Deficit Disorder Association
P. O. Box 972
Mentor, OH 44061
(800) 487-2282

Children and Adults with Attention Deficit Disorder (C.H.A.D.D.)
499 NW 70th Avenue
Suite 308
Plantation, FL 33317
(305) 587-3700

Closer Look: National Information Center for the Handicapped
Box 1492
Washington, DC 20009

Council for Exceptional Children
1920 Association Drive
Reston, VA 20091

Cystic Fibrosis Foundation
3384 Peachtree Road, NE
Suite 875
Atlanta, GA 30326

Down Syndrome Congress
1640 W. Roosevelt Road
Room 156E
Chicago, IL 60608

Epilepsy Foundation of America
4351 Garden City Drive
Landover, MD 20785
(800) EFA-1000

Higher Education and the Handicapped (HEATH)
1 DuPont Circle, NW
Suite 800
Washington, DC 20036-1193
(800) 544-3284

International Institute for Visually Impaired 0-7, Inc.
1975 Rutgers Circle
East Lansing, MI 48823

International Society of Augmentative and Alternative Communication (ISAAC)
49 The Donway West, Suite 308
Toronto, Ontario
M3C 3M9 Canada

Learning Disabilities Association of America (LDA)
4156 Library Road
Pittsburgh, PA 15234
(412) 341-1515

The Learning Disabilities Network
72 Sharp Street
Suite A-2
Hingham, MA 02043
(617) 340-5605

March of Dimes Birth Defect Foundation
1275 Mamaroneck Avenue
White Plains, NY 10605

Mental Health Association, National Headquarters
1800 North Kent Street
Arlington, VA 22209

Muscular Dystrophy Association, Inc.
810 Seventh Avenue
New York, NY 10019

The National Alliance for the Mentally Ill
P. O. Box 1016
Evanston, IL 60204

National Association for Visually Handicapped
305 East 24th Street
New York, NY 10010

National Association of the Deaf
814 Thayer Avenue
Silver Spring, MD 20910

National Association of the Deaf-Blind
2703 Forest Oak Circle
Norman, OK 73071

National Association of the Physically Handicapped, Inc.
76 Elm Street
London, OH 43140

National Center for Law and the Handicapped
1233 North Eddy Street
South Bend, IN 46817

National Center for Learning Disabilities (NCLD)
381 Park Avenue South
Suite 1420
New York, NY 10016
(212) 545-7510

National Cleft Palate Association (NCPA)
906 Hillside Lane
Flower Mound, TX 75028
(800) 645-9854

National Committee for Citizens in Education
410 Wilde Lake Village Green
Columbia, MD 21044

National Deaf-Blind Program
Bureau of Education for the Handicapped
Room 4046, Donohoe Building
400 6th Street, SW
Washington, DC 20202

National Easter Seal Society for Crippled Children and Adults
2023 W. Ogden Avenue
Chicago, IL 60612

National Federation of the Blind
1800 Johnson Street
Baltimore, MD 21230

National Hospice Organization
1901 North Fort Meyer Drive
Arlington, VA 22209

National Information Center for Children and Youth with Disabilities (NICHY)
P. O. Box 1492
Washington, DC 20013-1492
(800) 695-0285

National Multiple Sclerosis Society
205 East 42nd Street
New York, NY 10017

National Network of Learning Disabled Adults
P. O. Box 3130
Richardson, TX 75080

National Society for Autistic Children
1234 Massachusetts Avenue, NW
Suite 1017
Washington, DC 20005

National Spinal Cord Injury Foundation
369 Elliot Street
Newton Upper Falls, MA 02164

National Spinal Cord Injury Hotline
2201 Argonne Drive
Baltimore, MD 21218
(800) 526-3456

National Tay Sachs Foundation and Allied Diseases Association
122 East 42nd Street
New York, NY 10017

Orton Dyslexia Society
8415 Bellona Lane
Suite 115
Towson, MD 21204

Physical Education and Recreation for the Handicapped:
Information and Research Utilization Center
1201 16th Street, NW
Washington, DC 20036

President's Committee on Employment of the Handicapped
Washington, DC 20210

Speech Foundation of America
152 Lombard Road
Memphis, TN 38111

Spina Bifida Association of America
343 South Dearborn Street
Room 319
Chicago, IL 60604

Stuttering Foundation of America
http://www.stuttersfa.org

Tourette Syndrome Association
40-08 Corporal Kennedy Street
Bayside, NY 11361

United Cerebral Palsy Association
66 East 34th Street
3rd Floor
New York, NY 10016
http://www.ucpa.org

United States Society of Augmentative and Alternative Communication (USSAAC)
c/o Theresa Saldana
Fountain Valley School District
1721 Oak Street
Fountain Valley, CA 92708

PUBLICATIONS

American Journal of Speech-Language Pathology
American Speech-Language-Hearing Association
10801 Rockville Pike
Rockville, MD 20852-3279
(301) 897-5700, ext. 4304

The ASHA Leader
American Speech-Language-Hearing Association
10801 Rockville Pike
Rockville, MD 20852-3279
(301) 897-5700, ext. 4304

The Journal of Speech, Language and Hearing Research
American Speech-Language-Hearing Association
10801 Rockville Pike
Rockville, MD 20852-3279
(301) 897-5700, ext. 4304

ASHA
American Speech-Language-Hearing Association
10801 Rockville Pike
Rockville, MD 20852-3279
(301) 897-5700, ext. 4304

Language, Speech, and Hearing Services in the Schools
American Speech-Language-Hearing Association
10801 Rockville Pike
Rockville, MD 20852-3279
(301) 897-5700, ext. 4304

CH.A.D.D.ER. and CH.A.D.D.ER
Children and Adults with Attention Deficit Disorder
499 NW 70th Avenue
Suite 308
Plantation, FL 33317

ADDendum (Designed for adults with ADD)
c/o C. P. S.
5041-A Backlick Road
Annadale, VA 22003

ADDult News
c/o Mary Jane Johnson
ADDult Support Group
2620 Ivy Place
Toledo, OH 43613

Augmentative Communication News (quarterly clinical newsletter)
Augmentative Communication, Inc.
1 Surf Way
Monterey, CA 93940

Journal of Augmentative and Alternative Communication
Decker Periodicals, Inc.
4 Hughson Street South
4th Floor, P. O. Box 620
LCD 1, Hamilton, Ontario
L8N 3K7 Canada

Learning Disabilities: A Multidisciplinary Journal
Learning Disabilities Association of America (LDA)
4156 Library Road
Pittsburgh, PA 15234

LDA News Briefs
Learning Disabilities Association of America (LDA)
4156 Library Road
Pittsburgh, PA 15234

AAC EQUIPMENT

AbleNet, Inc.
1081 10th Avenue, SE
Minneapolis, MN 55414
(SpeakEasy, BIGmack)

ADAMLAB
33500 Van Born Road
Wayne, MI 48184
(Wolf, Whisper Wolf, Scan Wolf, Hawk)

Attainment Company, Inc.
P. O. Box 930160
Verna, WI 53593
(Attainment Talkers)

Canon USA, Inc.
1 Canon Plaza
Lake Success, NY 11042
(Canon Communicator)

Crestwood Company
6625 N. Sidney Place
Milwaukee, WI 53209
(TalkBack)

Don Johnston, Inc.
1000 N. Rand Road
Building 115
P. O. Box 639
Wauconda, IL
(Talk:About software, Co:Writer software)

Dynavox Systems, Inc.
2100 Wharton Street
Suite 630
Pittsburgh, PA 15203-1942
(DynaVox2, DynaMyte, DynaVox Software, DigiVox)

Innocomp
26210 Emery Road
Suite 302
Warrensville Heights, OH 44128
(Say-It-All, Scan-It-All, Say-It-Simply)

IntelliTools, Inc.
55 Leveroni Court
Suite 9
Novato, CA 94949
(IntelliTalk Software)

Mayer-Johnson Company
P. O. Box 1579
Solana Beach, CA 94061
(Speaking Dynamically software)

Prentke Romich Company
1022 Heyl Road
Wooster, OH 44691
(AlphaTalker, DeltaTalker, WalkerTalker, Minspeak devices)

TASH, Inc.
91 Station Street
Unit 1
Ajax, Ontario
L1S 3H2 Canada
(Voicemate, Scanmate, Switchmate)

Words+, Inc.
40015 Sierra Highway
Building B-145
Palmdale, CA 93550
(EZKeys, MessageMates, System 2000)

Zygo Industries, Inc.
P. O. Box 1008
Portland, OR 97207
(LightWriter, Parrot, Macaw)

LARYNGECTOMY EQUIPMENT

Artificial Speech Aids
Westridge Acres
3001-8 12th Street
Harlan, IA 51537
Phone: (712) 755-2389
(Tokyo Artificial Larynx and accessories)

A. S. Telecom, Inc.
9915 Saint Vital Street
Montreal, Quebec
HIH 4S5 Canada
Phone: (514) 326-5423
(Romet, Cooper-Rand, Denrick, Nu-Vois, Vocaltech, batteries, accessories, repairs)

Band K Prescription Shop
601 East Iron
Salina, KS 67401
Phone: (913) 827-4455
(Servox, batteries, accessories)

Bivona, Inc.
5700 West 23 Avenue
Gary, IN 46406
Phone: (800) 348-6064
Web address: www.bivona.com/index.htm
(Bivona Colorado Voice Restoration System, Bivona Duckbill Prosthesis, Bivona Ultra-low
Resistance Voice Prosthesis, Optivox, Tracheostoma Vents, Tracheostoma Valves and Kits,
Provox, Voice Restoration System, Provox Stomafilter, Stom-vent/Stom-vent 2, accessories)

California Speech and Hearing Instruments
1930 Wilshire Boulevard #810
Los Angeles, CA 90057
Phone: (213) 483-4481
(Cooper-Rand, Neovox, Servox, Macrovox, Romet, Nu-Vois, batteries, amplifiers, repairs)

Communicative Medical, Inc.
P. O. Box 8241
Spokane, WA 99203-0241
Phone: (800) 944-6801
(Servox, Nu-Vois, Trutone, Solatone, Toneaire, Romet, chargers, batteries, intraoral adapters, amplifiers, repairs, reconditioned aritificial larynges, and more)

Lauder Enterprises
11115 Whisper Hollow
San Antonio, TX 78230-3609
Phone: (800) 388-8642
(Servox, Nu-Vois, Denrick, Romet, PO Vox, Trutone, batteries, chargers, amplifiers, repairs, and more)

Professional Hearing & Speech Aids
30 Salem Market Place
Salem, CT 06103
Phone: (203) 525-2131
(Servox, Romet, Cooper-Rand, Nu-Vois, and amplifiers)

The Therabite Corporation
4661 West Chester Pike
Newtown Square, PA 19073-2227
Phone: (610) 356-9500
(Therapy aids)

TESTS AND/OR MATERIALS

Company	Inventory
Academic Communication Associates, Inc. Publication Center, Department 919 4149 Avenida de la Plata P. O. Box 4279 Oceanside, CA 92052-4279 Phone: (760) 758-9593	Therapy materials
Alimed Therapy Division 297 High Street Dedham, MA 02026	Aphasia, stroke, TBI, dementia tests, therapy materials, reference books, dysphagia supplies
Allyn & Bacon 160 Gould Street Needham Heights, MA 02494-2315 Phone: (800) 852-8024 Web address: www.abacon.com	Books

Company	Inventory
American Academy of Pediatrics 141 Northwest Point Boulevard P. O. Box 747 Elk Grove Village, IL 60009-0747 Phone: (800) 433-9016	Patient information pamphlets
American Guidance Service 4201 Woodland Road P. O. Box 99 Circle Pines, MN 55014-1796 Phone: (800) 328-2560 Web address: www.agsnet.com	Diagnostic and therapy materials
American Speech-Language-Hearing Association 10801 Rockville Pike Rockville, MD 20852-3279 Phone: (888) 498-6699 E-mail: productsales@asha.org	Variety of professional materials
Applied Symbolix 800 N. Wells Street Suite 200 Chicago, IL 60610 Phone: (800) 676-7551 Web address: www.symbolix.com	Diagnostic and therapy materials
Attainment Company P. O. Box 930160 Verona, WI 53593-0160 Phone: (800) 327-4269 Web address: www.attainment-inc.com	Therapy materials, AAC devices (Attainment Five Talker, Attainment Fifteen Talker, Personal Talker, Memo Talker)
Paul H. Brookes Publishing Company P. O. Box 10624 Baltimore, MD 21285-0624 Phone: (800) 638-3775 Web address: www.brookespublishing.com	Books
Communication Skill Builders 555 Academic Court San Antonio, TX 78204-2498 Phone: (800) 211-8378 Web address: www.hbtpc.com	Diagnostic and therapy materials
Constructive Playthings 13201 Arrington Road Grandview, MO 64030-2886 Phone: (800) 448-4115 Web address: www.constplay.com	Therapy supplies, pediatric furniture

Company	Inventory
Crestwood Company 6625 N. Sidney Place Milwaukee, WI 53209-3259 Phone: (414) 352-5678 Web address: www.communicationaids.com	AAC devices, switches, adapted toys
Don Johnston, Inc. 26799 W. Commerce Drive Volo, IL 60073 Phone: (800) 999-4660 Web address: www.donjohnston.com	AAC devices, software, therapy materials
Kaplan P. O. Box 609 1310 Lewisville-Clemmons Road Lewisville, NC 27023-0609 Phone: (800) 334-2014 E-mail: CEC@Kaplanco.com	Therapy materials, positioning equipment
Kay Elemetrics Corporation 2 Bridgewater Lane Lincoln Park, NJ 07035-1488 Phone: (201) 628-6200	Laryngeal imaging equipment
Laureate 110 East Spring Street Winooski, VT 05404-1898 Phone: (800) 562-6801 Web address: LaureateLearning.com	Software
LinguiSystems, Inc. 3100 4th Avenue East Moline, IL 61244-9700 Phone: (800) 776-4332 Web address: linguisystems.com	Therapy materials
Mayer-Johnson Company P. O. Box 1579 Solana Beach, CA 92075-7579 Phone: (800) 588-4548 Web address: www.mayer-johnson.com	AAC instructional materials, Tech/Talk, Tech/Four, Tech/Speak
Medical Arts Press 8500 Wyoming Avenue North Minneapolis, MN 55445-1825 Phone: (800) 328-2179	Office essentials, books, sanitizers

Company	Inventory
National Health Supply Corporation P. O. Box 737 2 South Street Garden City, NY 11530 Phone: (800) 645-3585	CPR supplies, first aid kits, audiometers, otoscopes
Parrot Software P. O. Box 250755 West Bloomfield, MI 48325-0755 Phone: (800) 727-7681 Web address: parrotsoftware.com	Software
PCI Educational Publishing 2800 NE Loop 410 Suite 105 San Antonio, TX 78218-1525 Phone: (800) 594-4263 Web address: pcicatalog.com	Adult therapy materials
Pro-Ed 8700 Shoal Creek Boulevard Austin, TX 78757-6897 Phone: (800) 897-3202 Web address: www.proedinc.com	Tests and instructional materials, books
The Psychological Corporation 555 Academic Court San Antonio, TX 78204-2498 Phone: (800) 211-8378 Web address: www.PsychCorp.com	Diagnostic and therapy materials
Psychological & Educational Publications, Inc. P. O. Box 520 Hydesville, CA 95547-0520 Phone: (800) 523-5775 Web address: www.pep1.com	Tests
S & S Opportunities P. O. Box 513 Colchester, CT 06415-0513 Phone: (800) 523-5775 Web address: www.snswwide.com	Adaptive equipment and toys
Sammons Preston P. O. Box 5071 Bolingbrook, IL 60440-5071 Phone: (800) 323-5547	Adaptive equipment and furniture

Company	Inventory
Singular Publishing Group 410 West "A" Street Suite 325 San Diego, CA 92101-7904 Phone: (800) 521-8545 Web address: www.singpub.com	Books and journals
Slosson Educational Publications, Inc. P. O. Box 280 East Aurora, NY 14052-0280 Phone: (800) 756-7766 E-mail: slosson@slosson.com	Diagnostic tests, therapy reference materials
The Speech Bin 1965 Twenty-fifth Avenue Vero Beach, FL 32960 Phone: (800) 477-3324	Therapy materials
Super Duper Publications Department ASHA99 P. O. Box 24997 Greenville, SC 29616-2497 Phone: (800) 277-8737 Web address: www.superduperinc.com	Therapy materials
Thinking Publications P. O. Box 163 424 Galloway Street Eau Claire, WI 54702-0163 Phone: (800) 225-4769 Web address:www.ThinkingPublications.com	Therapy materials
Western Psychological Services 12031 Wilshire Boulevard Los Angeles, CA 90025-1251 Phone: (800) 648-8857 Web address: www.wpspublish.com	Diagnostic and therapy materials, books, software
The Wright Group 19201 120th Avenue, NE Bethell, WA 98011 Phone: (800) 523-2371 Web address: www.TeacherHelp.com	Language and reading materials

Adamovich, B. B., & Henderson, J. (1992). *Scales of Cognitive Ability for Traumatic Brain Injury (SCATBI).* Chicago: The Riverside Publishing Company.

Adams, M. J. (1990). *Beginning to read: Thinking and learning about print.* Cambridge, MA: MIT Press.

Albert, M., Sparks, R., & Helm, N. (1973). Melodic intonation therapy for aphasia. *Archives of Neurology, 29,* 130–131.

Alberto, P. A., & Troutman, A. C. (1986). *Applied behavior analysis for teachers.* Columbus, OH: Merrill Publishing Company.

Alzheimer's Association. (1993). *Stages of symptom progression in Alzheimer's disease.* Chicago: Alzheimer's Association.

American Cleft Palate-Craniofacial Association. (1993). *Parameters for evaluation and treatment of patients with cleft lip/palate and other craniofacial anomalies.* Pittsburgh, PA: ACPCA.

American Joint Committee on Cancer. (1988). *Manual for staging of cancer* (3rd ed.). Philadelphia: J. B. Lippincott.

American Managed Care and Review Association. (1995). *Managed care: Quality, choice, satisfaction.* Washington, DC: AMCRA.

American Psychiatric Association. (1994). *Diagnostic and statistic manual of mental disorders—Revised* (4th ed.). Washington, DC: American Psychiatric Association.

American Speech-Language-Hearing Association. (1985a, June). Clinical management of communicatively handicapped minority language populations. *Asha, 27,* 29–32.

American Speech-Language-Hearing Association. (1985b, June). 1985 National colloquium on underserved populations report. *Asha, 27,* 31–35.

American Speech-Language-Hearing Association. (1987, April). Ad hoc committee on dysphagia report. *Asha, 29,* 57–58.

American Speech-Language-Hearing Association. (1989, March). Competencies for speech-language pathologists providing services in augmentative communication. *Asha, 31,* 107–110.

American Speech-Language-Hearing Association. (1991, March). Report: Augmentative and alternative communication. *Asha, 33* (Suppl. 5), 9–12.

American Speech-Language-Hearing Association. (1993, March). Preferred practice patterns for the professions of speech-language pathology and audiology. *Asha, 35*(Suppl 11), 1–102.

American Speech-Language-Hearing Association. (1994, March). Code of ethics. *Asha, 36*(Suppl. 13), 1–2.

American Speech-Language-Hearing Association. (1994, March). Statement of practices and procedures. *Asha, 36*(Suppl. 13), 3–5.

American Speech-Language-Hearing Association. (1994, June). Let's talk #49. *Asha, 36,* 9–12.

American Speech-Language-Hearing Association. (1995, September). Speech-language pathology assistants. *Asha, 37,* 39–43.

American Speech-Language-Hearing Association. (1995, December). Guidelines for the training and credentialing, use, and supervision of speech-language pathology assistants. *Asha, 37,* 1–102.

American Speech-Language-Hearing Association. (1996). *Dementia grand rounds* (videotape). Rockville, MD: American Speech-Language-Hearing Association.

Ansell, B. J., Keenan, J. E., & de la Rocha, O. (1989). *The Western Neuro Sensory Stimulation Profile.* Tustin, CA: Western Neuro Care Center.

Applebaum, P. S., & Grisso, T. (1988). Assessing patients' capacities to consent to treatment. *The New England Journal of Medicine, 319,* 1635–2638.

Arms, R. A., Dines, D. E., & Tinstman, T. C. (1974). Aspiration pneumonia. *Chest, 65,* 136.

Aronson, A. E. (1990). *Clinical voice disorders* (3rd ed.). New York: Thieme Medical Publishers.

Aronson, A. E. (1991). *Neurology for the medical speech-language pathologist.* Workshop presented in Tampa, FL.

Arvedson, J. C. (1993). Oral-motor and feeding assessment. In J. C. Arvedson & L. Brodsky (Eds.), *Pediatric swallowing and feeding—assessment and management* (pp. 249–292). San Diego, CA: Singular Publishing Group.

Arvedson, J. C., & Brodsky, L. (Eds.). (1993). *Pediatric swallowing and feeding—assessment and management.* San Diego, CA: Singular Publishing Group.

Arvedson, J. C., Rogers, B., & Brodsky, L. (1993). Anatomy, embryology, and physiology. In J. C. Arvedson & L. Brodsky (Eds.), *Pediatric swallowing and feeding—assessment and management.* San Diego, CA: Singular Publishing Group.

Arvedson, J. C. & Rogers, B. T. (1998). Dysphagia in children. In A. F. Johnson & B. H. Jacobson (Eds.), *Medical speech-language pathology: A practitioner's guide* (pp. 38–64). New York: Thieme Medical Publishers.

Baken, R. J. (1987). *Clinical measurement of speech and voice.* Boston: College-Hill Press.

Baker, B. (1986). Using images to generate speech. *Byte, 3,* 160–168.

Bankson, N., & Bernthal, J. (1990). *Bankson-Bernthal Test of Phonology.* Chicago: Riverside Press.

Barr, D. (1972). *Auditory perceptual disorders.* Springfield, IL: Charles C. Thomas.

Bates, E., Camaioni, L., & Volterra, V. (1975). The acquisition of performatives prior to speech. *Merrill-Palmer Quarterly, 21,* 205–206.

Battle, D. E., et al. (1983). Social dialects. *American Speech-Language-Hearing Association, 25*(9), 23.

Bayles, K. A. (1986). Management of neurogenic communication disorders associated with dementia. In R. Chapey (Ed.), *Language intervention strategies in adult aphasia* (3rd ed.). Baltimore: Williams & Wilkins.

Bayles, K. A., & Tomoeda, C. (1993). *Arizona Battery for Communication Disorders of Dementia (ABCD).* Phoenix, AZ: Canyonland Publishing.

Benson, D. F. (1979). *Aphasia, alexia, and agraphia.* New York: Churchill Livingstone.

Berndt, R. S., & Mitchum, C. C. (1998). An experimental treatment of sentence comprehension. In Helm-Estabrooks & Holland, *Approaches to the treatment of aphasia* (pp. 91–112). San Diego, CA: Singular Publishing Group.

Berndt, R. S., Mitchum, C. C., & Haendiges, A. N. (1996). Comprehension of reversible sentences in "agrammatism": A meta-analysis. *Cognition, 58,* 289–308.

Bess, F. H., & Humes, L. E. (1995). *Audiology: The fundamentals* (2nd ed.). Baltimore: Williams & Wilkins.

Beukelman, D. R., & Mirenda, P. (1992). *Augmentative and alternative communication: Management of severe communication disorders in children and adults.* Baltimore: Paul H. Brookes.

Beukelman, D., Yorkston, K., & Lossing, C. (1984). Functional communication assessment of adults with neurogenic disorders. In A. Halpern & M. Fuhrer (Eds.), *Functional assessment in rehabilitation.* Baltimore: Paul H. Brookes.

Biemiller, A. (1970). The development of the use of graphic and contextual information as children learn to read. *Reading Research Quarterly, 6,* 75–96.

Bishop, K., Rankin, J., & Mirenda, P. (1994). Impact of graphic symbol use on reading acquisition. *Augmentative and Alternative Communication, 10,* 113–125.

Blakeley, R. W. (1980). *Screening test for developmental apraxia of speech.* Austin, TX: Pro-Ed.

Bleile, K. (1991). *Child phonology: A book of exercises for students.* San Diego, CA: Singular Publishing Group.

Bleile, K. M. (1995). *Manual of articulation and phonological disorders.* San Diego, CA: Singular Publishing Group.

Bless, D. M. (1988). Voice assessment. In R. D. Kent & D. E. Yoder (Eds.), *Decision making in speech-language pathology.* Philadelphia: B. C. Decker.

Bless, D. M., & Hicks, D. M. (1996). Diagnosis and measurement: Assessing the "WHs" of voice function. In W. S. Brown, B. P. Vinson, & M. A. Crary (Eds.), *Organic voice disorders: Assessment and treatment* (pp. 119–171). San Diego, CA: Singular Publishing Group.

Bliss, C. K. (1965). *Blissymbolics.* Sydney, Australia: Semantography Publications.

Blood, G. W., Luther, A. R., & Stemple, J. C. (1992). Coping and adjustment in alaryngeal speakers. *American Journal of Speech-Language Pathology, 1*(2), 63–69.

Blood, G. W., Simpson, K. C., Dineen, M., Kauffman, S. M., & Raimondi, S. C. (1994). Spouses of individuals with laryngeal cancer: Caregiver strain and burden. *Journal of Communication Disorders, 27*, 19–35.

Bloomberg, K., Karlan, G. R., & Lloyd, L. L. (1990). The comparative translucency of initial lexical items represented in five graphic symbol systems and sets. *Journal of Speech and Hearing Research, 33*, 717–725.

Blosser, J. L., & DePompei, R. (1994). *Pediatric traumatic brain injury: Proactive intervention.* San Diego, CA: Singular Publishing Group.

Bondy, A. S., & Frost, L. A. (1993). Mands across the water: A report on the application of the picture-exchange communication system in Peru. *The Behavior Analyst, 16*, 123–128.

Boone, D., & McFarlane, S. C. (1994). *The voice and voice therapy* (5th ed.). Englewood Cliffs, NJ: Prentice-Hall.

Boone, D. R., & Plante, E. (1993). *Human communication and disorders.* Englewood Cliffs, NJ: Prentice-Hall.

Bountress, N. G. (1987). The Ann Arbor Decision. *American Speech-Language-Hearing Association, 25*(9), 55.

Briggs, A., Austin, R., & Underwood, G. (1984). Phonological coding in good and poor readers. *Reading Research Quarterly, 20*, 54–66.

Broder, H., & Strauss, R. (1989). Self-concept of early primary school age children with visible or invisible defects. *Cleft Palate Journal, 26*, 114–118.

Brown, L., Nietupski, J., & Hamre-Nietupski, S. (1976). The criterion of ultimate functioning and public school services for severely handicapped students. In M. A. Thomas (Ed.), *Hey, don't forget about me: Education's investment in the severely, profoundly, and multiply handicapped.* Reston, VA: Council for Exceptional Children.

Brown, R. (1973). *A first language.* Cambridge, MA: Harvard University.

Brown, W. S., Vinson, B. P., & Crary, M. A. (1996). *Organic voice disorders: Assessment and treatment.* San Diego, CA: Singular Publishing Group.

Buchanan, M., Weller, C., & Buchanan, M. (1997). *Special education desk reference.* San Diego, CA: Singular Publishing Group.

Buchholz, D. W. (1997). Neurologic disorders of swallowing. In M. E. Groher (Ed.), *Dysphagia: Diagnosis and management* (pp. 37–72). Newton, MA: Butterworth-Heinemann Publishers.

Bureau of Business Practice. (1988). *Personnel policy manual.* Englewood Cliffs, NJ: Prentice-Hall.

Burstein, F. D. (1999, October). *Overview of surgical options for VPI.* In Proceedings of the 12th Annual Symposium on Cleft Lip and Palate and Related Conditions. October 8–10, 1999. Atlanta, GA.

Bzoch, K. R. (1997a). Introduction to communicative disorders in cleft palate. In K. R. Bzoch, *Communicative disorders related to cleft lip and palate* (4th ed., pp. 3–44). Austin, TX: Pro-Ed.

Bzoch, K. R. (1997b). Etiological factors related to managing cleft palate speech. In K. R. Bzoch, *Communicative disorders related to cleft lip and palate* (4th ed., pp. 193–222). Austin, TX: Pro-Ed.

Calnan, J. S. (1971). Congenital large pharynx: A new syndrome with a report on 41 personal cases. *British Journal of Plastic Surgery, 24*, 263.

Campbell, D. (2000, Jan. 10). Comprehensive care. *Advance, 10.*

Cannito, M. P., & Marquardt, T. P. (1997). Ataxic dysarthria. In M. R. McNeil (Ed.), *Clinical management of sensorimotor speech disorders* (pp. 217–248). New York: Thieme Medical Publishers.

Cantwell, D. P., & Baker, L. (1992). Issues in the classification of child and adolescent psychopathology. *Journal of the American Academy of Child Adolescence, 27*, 532–533.

Carlson, F. (1986). *Picsyms categorical dictionary.* Unity, ME: Baggeboda Press.

Carlson, F. (1994). *Poppin's cut and paste with 1000+ DynaSyms.* Arlington, VA: Poppin & Company.

Carramazza, A., & Hillis, A. E. (1991). For a theory of remediation of cognitive deficits. Aphasia treatment: Current approaches and research opportunities. *Proceedings of a Workshop,* Bethesda, MD. U.S. Department of Health and Human Services, Public Health Service (NIH Publication No. 93-3424 Vol. 2). Rockville, MD: National Institutes of Health.

Caruso, A. J., & Strand, E. A. (Eds.). (1999a). *Clinical management of motor speech disorders in children*. New York: Thieme Medical Publishers.

Caruso, A. J., & Strand, E. A. (1999b). Motor speech disorders in children: Definitions, background, and a theoretical framework. In A. J. Caruso & E. A. Strand (Eds.), *Clinical management of motor speech disorders in children* (pp. 1–28). New York: Thieme Medical Publishers.

Case, J. L. (1991). *Clinical management of voice disorders* (2nd ed.). Austin, TX: Pro-Ed.

Casper, J. K., & Colton, R. H. (1993). *Clinical manual for laryngectomy and head/neck cancer rehabilitation*. San Diego, CA: Singular Publishing Group.

Casper, J. K., & Colton, R. H. (1998). *Clinical manual for laryngectomy and head/neck cancer rehabilitation* (2nd ed.). San Diego, CA: Singular Publishing Group.

Cassisi, N. J., Sapienza, C., & Vinson, B. P. (1996). Malignant lesions of the larynx. In W. S. Brown, B. P. Vinson, & M. A. Crary (Eds.), *Organic voice disorders: Assessment and treatment* (pp. 279–300). San Diego, CA: Singular Publishing Group.

Catts, H. W., & Kamhi, A. G. (1999). *Language and reading disabilities*. Boston: Allyn & Bacon.

Chall, J. (1983). *Stages of reading development*. New York: McGraw-Hill.

Cherney, L. R., Pannelli, J. J., & Cantiere, C. A. (1994). Clinical evaluation of dysphagia in adults. In L. R. Cherney (Ed.), *Clinical management of dysphagia in adults and children* (2nd ed.). Gaithersburg, MD: Aspen Publishers.

Cohen, M. M., Jr. (1982). *The child with multiple birth defects*. New York: Raven Press.

Coleman, T. J. (2000). *Clinical management of communication disorders in culturally diverse children*. Boston: Allyn & Bacon.

Cornett, B. S., & Davidson, T. L. (1999). Structuring clinical practice: Guidelines, pathways, and protocols. In B. S. Cornett, *Clinical practice management for speech-language pathologists* (pp. 53–80). Gaithersburg, MD: Aspen Publishers.

Crary, M. A. (1993). *Developmental motor speech disorders*. San Diego, CA: Singular Publishing Group.

Cregan, A., & Lloyd, L. L. (1990). *Sigsymbols: American edition*. Wauconda, IL: Don Johnston Developmental Equipment.

Crowe, T. A. (1997). *Applications of counseling in speech-language pathology and audiology*. Baltimore: Williams & Wilkins.

Crystal, D., & Varley, R. (1993). *Introduction to language pathology* (3rd ed.). San Diego, CA: Singular Publishing Group.

Dabul, B. (1979). *Apraxia battery for adults*. Tigard, OR: C. C. Publications.

Dabul, B. (1986). *Apraxia battery for adults*. Austin, TX: Pro-Ed.

Dahllof, G., et al. (1989). Caries, gingivitis, and dental abnormalities in preschool children with cleft lip and palate. *Cleft Palate Journal, 26*(3), 233–237.

D'Antonio, L. L., & Scherer, M. J. (1995). The evaluation of speech disorders associated with clefting. In R. J. Shprintzen & J. Bardach (Eds.), *Cleft palate speech management: A multidisciplinary approach* (pp. 176–220). St. Louis, MO: Mosby.

Davidhizar, R. (1997). Disability does not have to be the grief that never ends: Helping patients adjust. *Rehabilitation Nursing, 22*, 32–35.

Davis, G. A. (1993). *A survey of adult aphasia and related language disorders* (2nd ed.). Englewood Cliffs, NJ: Prentice-Hall.

DeCoste, D. C. (1997). Augmentative and alternative communication assessment strategies: Motor access and visual considerations. In S. L. Glennen & D. C. DeCoste (Eds.), *Handbook of augmentative and alternative communication* (pp. 243–282). San Diego, CA: Singular Publishing Group.

Dempsey, D. (1983). Selecting tests of auditory function in children. In E. Z. Lasky & J. Katz (Eds.), *Central auditory processing disorders: Problems of speech, language, and learning*. Austin, TX: Pro-Ed.

Dikengil, A. T. (1998). *Handbook for home health care for the speech-language pathologist*. San Diego, CA: Singular Publishing Group.

DiLima, B. N. (Ed.). (1995). *Stroke rehabilitation patient education manual*. Gaithersburg, MD: Aspen Publishers.

DiSimoni, F. G. (1989). *Comprehensive apraxia test*. Dalton, PA: Praxis House.

Donabedian, A. (1980). Explorations in quality assessment and monitoring. *Volume 1: The* definition of quality and approaches to its assessment. Ann Arbor, MI: Health Administration Press.

Dunst, C. (1980). *A clinical and educational manual for use with the Uzgiris and Hunt Scales of Infant Psychological Development.* Austin, TX: Pro-Ed.

Duvoisin, R. G., Golbe, L. I., Mark, M. H., Sage, J. I., & Walters, A. S. (1996). *Parkinson's disease handbook: A guide for patients and their families.* Staten Island, NY: The American Parkinson Disease Association.

Edelbrock, C., Costello, A. J., & Kessler, M. D. (1984). Empirical collaboration of attention deficit disorder. *Journal of the American Academy of Child Psychiatry, 23,* 285–290.

Ehri, L. C. (1992). Reconceptualizing the development of sight word reading and its relationship to recoding. In P. B. Gough, L. C. Ehri, & R. Trieman (Eds.), *Reading acquisition* (pp. 107–143). Hillsdale, NJ: Erlbaum.

Ehri, L. C., & Robbins, C. (1992). Beginners need some decoding skill to read words by analogy. *Reading Research Quarterly, 27,* 12–26.

Ekwall, E. E. (1985). *Locating and correcting reading difficulties* (4th ed.). Columbus, OH: Charles E. Merrill.

Enderby, P. M. (1983). *Frenchay dysarthria assessment.* Austin, TX: Pro-Ed.

Evans-Morris, S., & Klein, M. D. (1987). *Pre-feeding skills: A comprehensive resource for feeding development.* Tucson, AZ: Therapy Skill Builders.

Ewing-Cobbs, L., Fletcher, J. M., & Levin, H. S. (1985). In M. Ylvisaker (Ed.), *Head injury rehabilitation: Children and adolescents* (pp. 71–89). Austin, TX: Pro-Ed.

Feuerstein, R. (1979). *Dynamic assessment of the retarded performers: The learning potential assessment device, theory, instruments, and techniques.* Baltimore: University Park Press.

Field, T., & Vega-Lahr, N. (1984). Early interactions between infants with cranio-facial anomalies and their mothers. *Infant Behavior, 7,* 527–530.

Fischer, L., & Sorenson, G. P. (1985). *School law for counselors, psychologists, and social workers.* New York: Longman.

Fisher, H., & Logemann, J. (1971). *The Fisher-Logemann Test of Articulation Competence.* Boston: Houghton Mifflin.

Fleming, S., & Weaver, A. (1987). Index of dysphagia: A tool for identifying deglutition problems. *Dysphagia, 1,* 206–208.

Flower, R. M. (1984). *Delivery of speech-language pathology and audiology services.* Baltimore: Williams & Wilkins.

Fluharty, N. (1978). *Speech and language screening test for preschool children.* Bingingham, MA: Teaching Resources.

Fogel, A., & Thelen, E. (1987). Development of early expressive and communicative action: Reinterpreting the evidence from a dynamic systems perspective. *Developmental Psychology, 23,* 747–761.

Folstein, M. F., Folstein, S. A., & McHugh, P. R. (1975). Mini mental state: A practical method for grading the cognitive state of patients for the clinician. *Journal of Psychiatric Research, 12,* 189–198.

Foulds, R. (1980). Communication rates for nonspeech expression as a function of manual tasks and linguistic constraints. *Proceeding of the First International Conference on Rehabilitation Engineering.* Toronto, Canada.

Frattali, C. M. (1998). Clinical care in a changing health system. In N. Helm-Estabrooks & A. Holland, *Approaches to the treatment of aphasia* (pp. 241–266). San Diego, CA: Singular Publishing Group.

Frattali, C. M. (1999). Measuring and managing outcomes. In B. S. Cornett, *Clinical practice management for speech-language pathologists.* (pp. 29–52). Gaithersburg, MD: Aspen Publishers.

Fudala, B., & Reynolds, W. (1986). *Arizona Articulation Proficiency Scale.* Los Angeles: Western Psychological Services.

Galaburda, A. M. (1989). Ordinary and extraordinary brain development: Anatomical variation in developmental dyslexia. *Annals of Dyslexia, 39,* 67–79.

Gardner, W. (1961). Problems of laryngectomees. *Rehabilitation Record, 2,* 15–19.

Gauger, L. M., Lombardino, L. J., & Leonard, C. M. (1997). Brain morphology in children with specific language impairment. *Journal of Speech, Language, and Hearing Research, 40,* 1272–1284.

Glennen, S. L. (1997a). Introduction to augmentative and alternative communication. In S. L. Glennen & D. C. DeCoste (Eds.), *Handbook of augmentative and alternative communication.* (pp. 3–20). San Diego, CA: Singular Publishing Group.

Glennen, S. L. (1997b). Augmentative and alternative communication systems. In S. L. Glennen & D. C. DeCoste (Eds.), *Handbook of augmentative and alternative communication* (pp. 59–96). San Diego, CA: Singular Publishing Group.

Glennen, S. L. (1997c). Augmentative and alternative communication assessment strategies. In S. L. Glennen & D. C. DeCoste (Eds.), *Handbook of augmentative and alternative communication* (pp. 149–192). San Diego, CA: Singular Publishing Group.

Glennen, S. L., & DeCoste, D. C. (Eds.). (1997). *Handbook of augmentative and alternative communication.* San Diego, CA: Singular Publishing Group.

Glushko, R. J. (1981). Principles for pronouncing pring: The psychology of phonography. In A. M. Lesgold & C. A. Perfetti (Eds.), *Interactive processing in reading.* Hillsdale, NJ: Erlbaum.

Goldberg, S. A. (1997). *Clinical skills for speech-language pathologists.* San Diego, CA: Singular Publishing Group.

Goldman, R., & Fristoe, M. (1986). *Goldman-Fristoe Test of Articulation.* Circle Pines, MN: American Guidance Service.

Goldsworthy, C. L. (1996). *Developmental reading disabilities: A language-based treatment approach.* San Diego, CA: Singular Publishing Group.

Golper, L. A. C. (1998). *Sourcebook for medical speech pathology* (2nd ed.). San Diego, CA: Singular Publishing Group.

Gonzalez-Rothi, L. J. (1990). Transcortical aphasias. In L. L. LaPointe (Ed.), *Aphasia and related neurogenic language disorders* (pp. 78–95). New York: Thieme Medical Publishers.

Goodglass, H., & Kaplan, E. (1983). *The Boston diagnostic aphasia examination.* Philadelphia: Lea & Febriger.

Goosens, C. (1989). Aided communication intervention before assessment: A case study of a child with cerebral palsy. *Augmentative and Alternative Communication, 5*(1), 14–26.

Goosens, C. & Crain, S. (1986). *Augmentative communication intervention resource.* Lake Zurich, IL: Don Johnson Developmental Equipment.

Goosens, C., Crain, S., & Elder, P. (1992). *Engineering the preschool environment for interactive, symbolic communication.* Birmingham, AL: Southeast Augmentative Communication Conference.

Gould, W. J. (1988). The clinical voice laboratory: Clinical application of voice research. *Journal of Voice, 1,* 305–309.

Green, B. S., Stevens, K. M., & Wolfe, T. D. W. (1997). *Mild traumatic brain injury: A therapy and resource manual.* San Diego, CA: Singular Publishing Group.

Greene, V. E., & Enfield, M. L. (1991). *Project Read.* Bloomington, MN: Language Circle Enterprise.

Griffin, K. M., & Fazen, M. (1993). A managed care strategy for practitioners. In *Quality improvement digest.* Rockville, MD: ASHA.

Groher, M. E. (1984). *Dysphagia: Diagnosis and management.* Stoneham, MA: Butterworth Publishers.

Groher, M. E. (1997). *Dysphagia: Diagnosis and management.* Newton, MA: Butterworth-Heinemann Publishers.

Grunwell, P. (1986). *Phonological assessment of child speech.* Boston: College-Hill Press.

Guilmette, T. J. (1997). *Pocketguide to brain injury, cognitive, and neurobehavioral rehabilitation.* San Diego, CA: Singular Publishing Group.

Hageman, C. (1997). Flaccid dysarthria. In M. R. McNeil (Ed.), *Clinical management of sensorimotor speech disorders* (pp. 193–216). New York: Thieme Medical Publishers.

Hagen, C., & Malkmus, D. (1979). *Rancho Los Amigos Scale of Cognitive Function.* Downey, CA: Adult Brain Injury Service, Rancho Los Amigos Medical Center.

Hagery, R. & Howard, T. (1978). *How to make federal mandatory special education work for you.* Springfield, IL: Charles C. Thomas Publisher.

Haynes, S. (1985). Developmental apraxia of speech: Symptoms for the differential diagnosis of developmental apraxia. A seminar presented at the annual convention of the American Speech-Language-Hearing Association, Anaheim, CA.

Haynes, W. O., & Pindzola, R. H. (1998). *Diagnosis and evaluation in speech pathology* (5th ed.). Boston: Allyn & Bacon.

Hegde, M. N. (1996a). *Pocketguide to assessment in speech-language pathology.* San Diego, CA: Singular Publishing Group.

Hegde, M. N. (1996b). *Pocketguide to treatment in speech-language pathology.* San Diego, CA: Singular Publishing Group.

Hegde, M. N. (1998). *A coursebook on aphasia and other neurogenic language disorders* (2nd ed.). San Diego, CA: Singular Publishing Group.

Hegde, M. N., & Davis, D. (1995). *Clinical methods and practicum in speech-language pathology* (2nd ed.). San Diego, CA: Singular Publishing Group.

Helm-Estabrooks, N. (1992). *The test for oral and limb apraxia.* Austin, TX: Pro-Ed.

Helm-Estabrooks, N., & Albert, M. L. (1991). *Manual of aphasia therapy.* Austin, TX: Pro-Ed.

Helm-Estabrooks, N., & Holland, A. (1998). *Approaches to the treatment of aphasia.* San Diego, CA: Singular Publishing Group.

Helm-Estabrooks, N. & Hotz, G. (1991). *Brief Test of Head Injury (BTHI).* Chicago: The Riverside Publishing Company.

Helm-Estabrooks, N., Nicholas, M., & Morgan, A. (1989). *Melodic intonation therapy program.* San Antonio, TX: Special Press.

Henri, B. P., & Hallowell, B. (1999). Mastering managed care: Problems and possibilities. In B. S. Cornett, *Clinical practice management for speech-language pathologists* (pp. 3–28). Gaithersburg, MD: Aspen Publishers.

Hewitt, L. E. (1992, March). *Facilitating narrative comprehension: The importance of subjectivity.* Paper presented at the Conference on Pragmatics: From Theory to Therapy, State University of New York, Buffalo.

Heyer, J. L. (n.d.). *Programming for children with attention deficit disorders.* Purdue University Continuing Education. West Lafayette, IN: Purdue Research Foundation.

Hicks, D. M., & Bless, D. M. (1996). Principles of treatment. In W. S. Brown, B. P. Vinson, & M. A. Crary (Eds.), *Organic voice disorders: Assessment and treatment* (pp. 172–192). San Diego, CA: Singular Publishing Group.

Hirano, M. (1981). *Clinical examination of voice.* New York: Thieme Medical Publishers.

Hodson, B. W. (1986a). *The assessment of phonological processes* (Rev. ed.). Danville, IL: Interstate Printers & Publishers.

Hodson, B. W. (1986b). *The assessment of phonological processes—Spanish.* San Diego, CA: Los Amigos Association.

Hodson, B., & Paden, E. (1991).*Targeting intelligible speech: A phonological approach to remediation* (2nd ed.). San Diego, CA: College-Hill Press.

Holland, A. L. (1980). *Communication ability in daily living.* Baltimore: University Park Press.

Holston, J. T. (1992, February). *Assessment and management of auditory processing problems in children.* Paper presented at the Winter Conference of the Florida Speech-Language-Hearing Association, Gainesville, FL.

Huang, M. H. S. (1999). Velopharyngeal anatomy. In Proceedings of the 12th Annual Symposium on Cleft Lip and Palate and Related Conditions. October 8–10, 1999. Atlanta, GA.

Hubbell, R. D. (1988). *A handbook of English grammar and language sampling.* Englewood Cliffs, NJ: Prentice-Hall.

Hynd, G. (1991, March). *Brain morphology as it relates to learning disabilities.* Lecture at the 1991 G. Paul Moore Symposium, Gainesville, FL.

Hynd, G. W., Lorys, A. R., Semrud-Clikeman, M., Nieves, N., Huettner, M. I. S., & Lahey, B. B. (1991). Attention deficit disorder without hyperactivity (ADD/WO): A distinct behavioral and neurocognitive syndrome. *Journal of Child Neurology, 6,* 37–43.

Hynd, G., Semrud-Clikeman, M., Lorys, A., Novey, E., & Eliopulos, D. (1990). Brain morphology in developmental dyslexia and attention deficit disorder/hyperactivity. *Archives of Neurology, 47,* 919–926.

Irwin, E. C., & McWilliams, B. J. (1974). Play therapy for children with cleft palates. *Children Today, 3,* 18.

Iskowitz, M. (1997, June 16). Overcoming obstacles of pediatric TBI. *Advance, 7,* 5.

Jacobs, J. W., Bernard, M. R., & Delgado, A. (1977). Screening for organic mental syndromes in the medically ill. *Annals of Internal Medicine, 86,* 40–46.

James, S. (1989). Assessing children with language disorders. In D. Bernstein & E. Tiegerman (Eds.), *Language and communication disorders in children* (pp. 157–207). Columbus, OH: Merrill.

Johnson, A. F., & Jacobson, B. H. (Eds.). (1998). *Medical speech-language pathology: A practitioner's guide.* New York: Thieme Medical Publishers.

Johnson, D., & Myklebust, H. (1967). *Learning disabilities: Educational principles and practice.* New York: Grune and Stratton.

Johnson, D. J. (1997). Mental status and aging: Cognition and affect. In B. B. Shadden & M. A. Toner (Eds.), *Aging and communication* (pp. 67–96). Austin, TX: Pro-Ed.

Johnson, R. (1981). *The picture communication symbols.* Solana Beach, CA: Mayer-Johnson.

Jung, J. H. (1989). *Genetic syndromes in communication disorders.* Boston: College-Hill.

Kahmi, A. B., & Catts, H. W. (1989). *Reading disabilities: A developmental language perspective.* Austin, TX: Pro-Ed.

Kapp-Simon, K. (1986). Self concept of primary-school-age children with cleft lip, cleft palate, or both. *Cleft Palate-Craniofacial Journal, 23,* 24–27.

Kasten, S. J., Buchman, S. R., Stevenson, C., Berger, M. (1999, October). *A retrospective analysis of revision sphincter pharyngoplasty.* In Proceedings of the 12th Annual Symposium on Cleft Lip and Palate and Related Conditions. October 8–10, 1999. Atlanta, GA.

Kay, T., & the Mild Traumatic Brain Injury Committee of the Head Injury Special Interest Group of the American Congress of Rehabilitation Medicine. (1993). Definition of mild traumatic brain injury. *Journal of Head Trauma Rehabilitation, 8*(3), 86–87.

Kayser, H. (1994). Service delivery issues for multicultural populations. In R. Lubinski & C. Frattali, *Professional issues in speech-language pathology and audiology* (pp. 282–292). San Diego, CA: Singular Publishing Group.

Kearns, K. P. (1997). Broca's aphasia. In L. L. LaPointe, *Aphasia and related neurogenic language disorders* (2nd ed., pp. 1–41). New York: Thieme Medical Publishers.

Keith, R. W. (1988). Central auditory tests. In N. J. Lass, L. V. McReynolds, J. L. Northern, & D. E. Yoder (Eds.), *Speech, language, and hearing: Vol. 3. hearing disorders,* (pp. 1215–1236). Philadelphia: W. B. Saunders.

Kent, R. D. (1997). The perceptual sensorimotor speech examination for motor speech disorders. In M. R. McNeil (Ed.), *Clinical management of sensorimotor speech disorders* (pp. 27–47). New York: Thieme Medical Publishers.

Kent, R. D., & Adams, S. G. (1989). The concept and measurement of coordination in speech disorders. In S. A. Wallace (Ed.), *Perspectives on the coordination of movement* (pp. 415–449). Amsterdam: Elsevier Science Publishers.

Kertsz, A. (1982). *The Western Aphasia Battery.* New York: Grune & Stratton.

Khan, L., & Lewis, N. (1986). *The Khan-Lewis Phonological Analysis.* Circle Pines, MN: American Guidance Service.

Koegel, R., O'Dell, M., & Koegel, L. (1987). A natural language teaching paradigm for nonverbal autistic children. *Journal of Autism and Developmental Disorder, 2*(17), 187–199.

Kommers, M. S., Sullivan, M.D., & Yonkers, A. J. (1977). Counseling the laryngectomized patient. *The Laryngoscope, 87,* 1961–1965.

Kommers, M. S., & Sullivan, M. D. (1979). Wives' evaluation of problems related to laryngectomy. *Journal of Communication Disorders, 12,* 411–430.

Koop, E. (1987). *Surgeon General's report: Children with special health care needs.* Washington, DC: Office of Maternal and Child Health, U.S. Department of Health and Human Services, Public Health Service.

Koschkee, D. L., & Rammage, L. (1997). *Voice therapy in the medical setting.* San Diego, CA: Singular Publishing Group.

Krescheck, J. D., & Werner, E. O. (1989). *Structured photographic articulation test featuring Dudsberry.* Sandwich, IL: Janelle Publications.

Kubler-Ross, E. (1969). *On death and dying.* New York: Macmillan.

Lahey, B. B., Schaughency, E. A., Hynd G. W., Carlson, C. L., & Nieves, N. (1987). Attention deficit disorder with and without hyperactivity: Comparison of behavioral characteristics of clinic-referred children. *Journal of the American Academy of Child and Adolescent Psychiatry, 26,* 718–723.

Lahey, B. B., Schaughency, E. A., Strauss, C. C., & Frame, C. L. (1984). Are attention deficit disorders with and without hyperactivity similar or dissimilar disorders? *Journal of the American Academy of Child Psychiatry, 23,* 302–309.

Lahey, M. (1988). *Language disorders and language development.* New York: Macmillan.

Landes, T. L. (1999). Ethical issues involved in patients' rights to refuse artificially administered nutrition and hydration and implications for the speech-language pathologist. *American Journal of Speech-Language Pathology, 8*(2).

Lass, N. H., McReynolds, L. V., Northern, J. L., & Yoder, D. E. (1988). *Handbook of speech-language pathology and audiology*. Philadelphia: B. C. Decker.

Laxon, V., Coltheart, V., & Keating, C. (1988). Children find friendly words friendly too: Words with many orthograhic neighbours are easier to read and spell. *British Journal of Educational Psychology, 58*, 103–119.

Lees, J. (1997). Long-term effects of acquired aphasias in childhood. *Pediatric Rehabilitation, 1*(1), 45–49.

Leith, W. R. (1984). *Handbook of clinical methods in communication disorders*. San Diego, CA: Singular Publishing Group.

Leonard, C. M. (1998). Language. In H. Cohen (Ed.), *Neuroscience for rehabilitation* (2nd ed.). Philadelphia: Lippincott-Raven.

Leonard, J. R., Holt, G. P., & Maran, A. G. (1972). Treatment of vocal cord carcinoma by vertical hemilaryngectomy. *Annals of Oto-Rhino-Laryngology, 81*, 469.

Levin, H. S., O'Donnell, V. M., & Grossman, R. G. (1979). The Galveston Orientation and Amnesia Test: A practical scale to assess cognition after head injury. *Journal of Nervous System and Mental Disorders, 167*, 675–684.

Lindamood, C. H., & Lindamood, P. C. (1969). *Auditory discrimination in depth*. Boston: Teaching Resources Corporation.

Lindamood, C. H., & Lindamood, P. C. (1979). *Lindamood Auditory Conceptualization Test*. Austin, TX: Pro-Ed.

Lindamood, C. H., & Lindamood, P. C. (1984). *Auditory discrimination in depth*. Austin, TX: Pro-Ed.

Liss, J., Kuehn, D., & Hinkel, K. (1994). Direct training of velopharyngeal musculature. *National Center for Voice and Speech: Status Progress Report, 6*(5), 43–52.

Livesay, Y. (1995). Dyslexia and reading instruction: Presented to California educators, legislators, and advocates. *Answers, 1*, 1–8.

Logemann, J. A. (1998a). Dysphagia: Basic assessment and management issues. In A. F. Johnson & B. H. Jacobson, *Medical speech-language pathology: A practitioner's guide* (pp. 17–37). New York: Thieme Medical Publishers.

Logemann, J. A. (1998b). *Evaluation and treatment of swallowing disorders* (2nd ed.). Austin, TX: Pro-Ed.

Lombana, J. H. (1982) *Guidance for handicapped students*. Springfield, IL: Charles C. Thomas Publisher.

Lombardino, L. J., Ricco, C. A., Hynd, G., & Pinheiro, S. B. (1997). Linguistic deficits in children with learning disabilities. *American Journal of Speech-Language Pathology, 6*(3).

Lombardino, L. J., Stapell, J. B., & Gerhardt, K. J. (1987). Evaluating communicative behaviors in infancy. *Journal of Pediatric Health Care, 1*(5).

Longstreth, D. (1986). *The BELZ Dysphagia Scale*. Paper presented at the annual convention of the American Speech-Language-Hearing Association, Detroit, MI.

Losardo, A., & Coleman, T. J. (1996). *A framework for alternative and culturally appropriate assessment models*. South Carolina Speech-Language-Hearing Association Convention, Hilton Head.

Lowman, D. K., & Murphy, S. M. (1999). *The educator's guide to feeding children with disabilities*. Baltimore: Paul H. Brookes.

Lubinski, R., & Frattali, C. (1994). *Professional issues in speech-language pathology and audiology*. San Diego, CA: Singular Publishing Group.

Lund, N., & Duchan, J. (1988). *Assessing children's language in naturalistic contexts* (2nd ed.). Englewood Cliffs, NJ: Prentice-Hall.

Lyon, J. G. (1998). Treating real-life functionality in a couple coping with severe aphasia. In N. Helm-Estabrooks & A. Holland, *Approaches to the treatment of aphasia* (pp. 203–240). San Diego, CA: Singular Publishing Group.

Madell, J. R. (1994). Professional standards. In R. Lubinski & C. Frattali, *Professional issues in speech-language pathology and audiology* (pp. 52–60). San Diego, CA: Singular Publishing Group.

Maharaj, S. (1980). *Pictogram ideogram communication*. Saskatchewan, Canada: The Pictogram Centre.

Martin, F. N. (1994). *Introduction to audiology*. Englewood Cliffs, NJ: Prentice-Hall.

Martin, F. N. (2000). *Introduction to audiology* (6th ed.). Englewood Cliffs, NJ: Prentice-Hall.

Mason, R. M., & Grandstaff, H. L. (1971). Evaluating the velopharyngeal mechanism in hypernasal speakers. *Language, Speech, and Hearing Services in the Schools, 2*, 53–61.

Masterson, J., & Pagan, F. (1994). *The Macintosh interactive system for phonological analysis* [Computer program]. San Antonio, TX: The Psychological Corporation.

Mattes, L. (1993). *Spanish articulation measures*. Oceanside, CA: Academic Communication Associates.

McCormick, L., & Schiefelbusch, R. L. (1990). *Early language intervention: An introduction* (2nd ed.). Columbus, OH: Merrill Publishing Company.

McDonald, E. (1968). *Screening Deep Test of Articulation*. Pittsburgh, PA: Stanwix House.

McFarlane S. C., Fujiki, M., & Brinton B. (1984). *Coping with communicative handicaps*. San Diego, CA: College-Hill Press.

McKenna, J. P., Fornataro-Clerici, L. M., McMenamin, P. G., & Leonard, R. J. (1991). Laryngeal cancer: Diagnosis, treatment, and speech rehabilitation. *American Family Physician, 44*(1), 123–129.

McNeil, M. R. (Ed.). (1997). *Clinical management of sensorimotor speech disorders*. New York: Thieme Medical Publishers.

McNeil, M. R., Robin, D. A., & Schmidt, R. A. (1997). Apraxia of speech: Definition, differentiation, and treatment. In McNeil, M.R. (Ed.), *Clinical management of sensorimotor speech disorders* (pp. 311–344). New York: Thieme Medical Publishers.

McRury, M. (1998). *Clinical pathways: A quality improvement initiative* [unpublished document]. Columbus, OH: The Ohio State University Medical Center.

McWilliams, B. J., & Matthews, H. (1979). A comparison of intelligence and social maturity in children with unilateral complete clefts and those with isolated cleft palates. *Cleft Palate Journal, 16*, 363–372.

Miller, Robert M. (1984). Evaluation of swallowing disorders. In M. E. Groher (Ed.), *Dysphagia: Diagnosis and management*. Stoneham, MA: Butterworth Publishers.

Miller, Robert M. (1997). Clinical examination for dysphasia. In M. E. Groher (Ed.), *Dysphagia: Diagnosis and management* (pp. 169–190). Newton, MA: Butterworth-Heinemann Publishers.

Millikin, C. C. (1997). Symbol systems and vocabulary selection strategies. In S. L. Glennen & D. C. DeCoste (Eds.), *Handbook of augmentative and alternative communication* (pp. 97–148). San Diego, CA: Singular Publishing Group.

Million, R. R., Cassisi, N. J., & Mancuso, A. A. (1994). Larynx. In R. R. Million & N. J. Cassisi (Eds.), *Management of head and neck cancer: A multidisciplinary approach* (2nd ed., pp. 431–497). Philadelphia: J. B. Lippincott.

Mirenda, P. (1985). Designing pictorial communication systems for physically able-bodied students with severe handicaps. *Augmentative and Alternative Communication, 1*, 58–64.

Mirenda, P., & Locke, P. A. (1989). A comparison of symbol transparency in nonspeaking persons with intellectual disabilities. *Journal of Speech and Hearing Disorders, 54*, 131–140.

Mirenda, P., & Schuler, A. (1988). Augmenting communication for persons with autism: Issues and strategies. *Topics of Language Disorders, 9*, 24–43.

Mizuko, M. (1987). Transparency and ease of learning of symbols represented by Blissymbols, PCS, and Picsyms. *Augmentative and Alternative Communication, 3*, 129–136.

Moller, K. T., & Starr, C. D. (1993). *Cleft palate: Interdisciplinary issues and treatment*. Austin, TX: Pro-Ed.

Morgan, A. E., Hynd, G. W., Riccio, C., & Hall, J. (1996). Validity of DSM-IV ADHD predominant inattentive and combined types: Relationship to previous DSM diagnoses/subtype differences. *Journal of the American Academy of Child and Adolescent Psychiatry, 35*(3), 325–333.

Morris, H. L. (1973). Velopharyngeal competence and primary cleft palate surgery, 1960–1971: A critical review. *Cleft Palate Journal, 10*, 62.

Morris, H. L., & Smith, J. K. (1962). A multiple approach for evaluating velopharyngeal competency. *Journal of Speech and Hearing Disorders, 27*, 218–226.

Mueller, H. (1974). Speech. In N. R. Finnie (Ed.), *Handling the young cerebral palsied child at home* (pp. 133–140). London: William Heinemann Medical Books.

Mulholland, K. C. (1991). Protecting the right to die: The Patient Self-Determination Act of 1990. *Harvard Journal on Legislation, 28*, 609–630.

Murphy, S. M., & Caretto, V. (1999). Sensory aspects of feeding. In D. K. Lowman & S. M. Murphy (Eds.), *The educator's guide to feeding children with disabilities* (pp. 111–126). Baltimore: Paul H. Brookes.

Musiek, F. E., Geurkink, N. A., & Kietel, S. A. (1984). Test battery assessment of auditory perceptual dysfunction in children. *Laryngoscope, 92*, 251–257.

Nackashi, J. A., & Dixon-Wood, V. L. (1997). The craniofacial team: Medical supervision and coordination. In K. R. Bzoch, *Communicative disorders related to cleft lip and palate* (4th ed., pp. 169–192). Boston: College-Hill Press.

Naremore, R. C., Densmore, A. E., & Harman, D. R. (1995). *Language intervention with school-age children: Conversation, narrative, and text.* San Diego, CA: Singular Publishing Group.

Nation, J. E., & Aram, D. M. (1984). *Diagnosis of speech and language disorders.* San Diego, CA: Singular Publishing Group.

National Institutes of Health (1984). *Head injury: Hope through research.* (NIH Publication No. 84-2478, pp. 1–37). Bethesda, MD: National Institutes of Health.

Nelson, N. W. (1993). *Childhood language disorders in context: Infancy through adolescence.* New York: Macmillan.

Nelson, N. W. (1998). *Childhood language disorders in context: Infancy through adolescence* (2nd ed.). Boston: Allyn & Bacon.

Northern, J. L., & Downs, M. P. (1974). *Hearing in children.* Baltimore: Williams & Wilkins.

Northern, J. L., & Downs, M. P. (1991). *Hearing in children* (4th ed.). Baltimore: Williams & Wilkins.

Olswang, L., Stoel-Gammon, C., Coggins, T., & Carpenter, R. (1987). *Assessing prelinguistic and early linguistic behaviors in developmentally young children.* Seattle, WA: University of Washington Press.

Ourand, P. R., & Gray, S. (1997). Funding and legal issues in augmentative and alternative communication. In S. L. Glennen & D. C. DeCoste (Eds.), *Handbook of augmentative and alternative communication* (pp. 335–360). San Diego, CA: Singular Publishing Group.

Owens, R. E. (1995). *Language disorders: A functional approach to assessment and intervention* (2nd ed.). Needham Heights, MA: Allyn & Bacon.

Paris, S. G. (1991). Assessment and remediation of metacognitive aspects of children's reading comprehension. *Topics in Language Disorders, 12*, 32–50.

Patient Self-Determination Act, Pub. L. No. 101-508, S 4206, 1990 U.S. Code Cong. & Admin. News (104 Stat.) 29 (1990).

Paul, T., & Brandt, R. S. (1998). Oral and dental health status of children with cleft lip and/or palate. *Cleft Palate and Craniofacial Journal, 35*(4), 329–332.

Payne, J. C. (1994). *Communication profile: A functional skills survey.* Tucson, AZ: Communication Skills Builders.

Payne, J. C. (1997). *Adult neurogenic language disorders: Assessment and treatment.* San Diego, CA: Singular Publishing Group.

Pendergast, K., Dickey, S., Selmar, T., & Soder, A. (1969). *Photo Articulation Test.* Danville, IL: Interstate Publishers and Printers.

PennTech (1994). *Assistive technology statewide support initiative: Service delivery.* Unpublished paper. Harrisburg, PA: PennTech.

Perkins, J., & Olson, K. (1998, Winter). The threat of evidence-based definitions of medical necessity. *Health Advocate, 91*, 17.

Pierce, R. S. (1991). Apraxia of speech vs. phonemic paraphasia: Theoretical, diagnostic, and treatment considerations. In D. Vogel & M. P. Cannito (Eds.), *Treating disordered speech motor control: For clinicians by clinicians.* Austin, TX: Pro-Ed.

Pinder, G. L., & Faherty, A. S. (1999). Issues in pediatric feeding and swallowing. In A. J. Caruso & E. A. Strand (Eds.), *Clinical management of motor speech disorders in children* (pp. 281–318). New York: Thieme Medical Publishers.

Pore, S. G., & Reed, K. L. (1999). *Quick reference to speech-language pathology.* Gaithersburg, MD: Aspen Publishers.

Prather, R. J., & Swift, R. W. (1984). *Manual of voice therapy.* Boston: Little, Brown.

Prizant, B. (1983). Language and communicative behavior in autism: Toward an understanding of the "whole" of it. *Journal of Speech and Hearing Disorders, 46*, 241–249.

Prizant, B. M., & Duchan, J. F. (1981). The functions of immediate echolalia in autistic children. *Journal of Speech and Hearing Disorders, 11*, 5–16.

Prizant, B., & Wetherby, A. M. (1988). Providing services to children with autism (ages 0 to 2 years) and their families. *Topics in Language Disorders, 9*(1), 1–23.

Rao, P., & Goldsmith, T. (1994). Developing policies and procedures. In R. Lubinski & C. Frattali, *Professional Issues in Speech-Language Pathology and Audiology* (pp. 233–245). San Diego, CA: Singular Publishing Group.

Reed, V. A. (1994). *An introduction to children with language disorders* (2nd ed.) New York: Macmillan.

Reisberg, B., Ferris, S. H., DeLeon, M. J., & Crook, T. (1982). Global Deterioration Scale for assessment of primary degenerative dementia. *American Journal of Psychiatry, 139,* 1136–1139.

Retherford, K. (1993). *Guide to analysis of language transcripts* (2nd ed.). Eau Claire, WI: Thinking Publications.

Riski, J. E. (1999, October). *VCF: Neurological findings impacting speech.* In Proceedings of the 12th Annual Symposium on Cleft Lip and Palate and Related Conditions. October 8–10, 1999. Atlanta, GA.

Ritvo, E. R., & Freeman, B. J. (1978). National Society for Autistic Children definition of the syndrome of autism. *Journal of Autism and Childhood Schizophrenia, 8,* 162–167.

Robinson, C., & Salter, W. (1995). *Phonological Awareness Test.* East Moline, IL: LinguiSystems.

Roeser, R. J. (1988). Audiometric and immittance measures: Principles and interpretation. In R. J. Roeser & M. P. Downs (Eds.), *Auditory disorders in school children: Identification-remediation* (2nd ed., pp. 5–34). New York: Thieme Medical Publishers.

Roeser, R. J., & Downs, M. P. (1988). *Auditory disorders in school children: Identification-remediation* (2nd ed.). New York: Thieme Medical Publishers.

Romski, M. A., & Sevcik, R. (1992). Augmented language development in children with severe mental retardation. In S. Warren & J. Reichle (Eds.), *Causes and effects in communication and language intervention* (pp. 113–130). Baltimore: Paul H. Brookes.

Rose, F. D., Johnson, D. A., & Attree, E. A. (1997). Rehabilitation of the head-injured child: Basic research and new technology. *Pediatric Rehabilitation, 1*(1), 3–7.

Rosenbek, J. C., LaPointe, L. L., & Wertz, R. T. (1989). *Aphasia: A clinical approach.* Austin, TX: Pro-Ed.

Rosenbek, J. C., Lemme, M., Ahern, M., Harris, E., & Wertz, R. T. (1973). A treatment for apraxia of speech in adults. *Journal of Speech and Hearing Disorders, 38,* 462–472.

Rosner, J. (1975). *Helping children overcome learning difficulties.* New York: Walker and Company.

Ross, D. (1986). *Ross Information Processing Assessment (RIPA).* Chicago: The Riverside Press.

Ross, M., Brackett, D., & Maxon, A. B. (1991). *Assessment and management of mainstreamed hearing-impaired children: Principles and practices.* Austin, TX: Pro-Ed.

Ross, R. B. (1987). Treatment variables affecting facial growth in complete unilateral cleft lip and palate. *Cleft Palate Journal, 24,* 3–77.

Rothstein, L. F. (1990). *Special education law.* New York: Longman.

Rowland, C., & Schweigert, P. (1989). Tangible symbols: Symbolic communication for individuals with multisensory impairments. *Augmentative and Alternative Communication, 5,* 226–234.

Rowland, R. C. (1988, January). Malpractice in audiology and speech-language pathology. *Asha, 30.*

Rubens, A. B. (1976). Transcortical motor aphasia. In H. Whitaker & H. A. Whitaker (Eds.), *Studies in neurolinguistics* (Vol. I). New York: Academic Press.

Russell, N. K. (1993, April). Educational considerations in traumatic brain injury: The role of the speech-language pathologist. *Language, Speech, and Hearing Services in the Schools, 24,* 67–75.

Sabatino, C. P., & Gottlich, V. (1991). Seeking self-determination in the Patient Self-Determination Act. *Clearinghouse Review, 25,* 639–647.

Sandy, J., Williams, A., et al. (1998). The clinical standards advisory group (CSAG) cleft lip and palate study. *British Journal of Orthodontics, 25,* 21–30.

Sarno, M. T. (1969). *The Functional Communication Profile: Manual for directions* (Rehabilitative Monograph No. 42). New York: New York Institute of Rehabilitative Medicine.

Satz, P., & Bullard-Bates, C. (1981). Acquired aphasia in children. In M. T. Sarno (Ed.), *Acquired aphasia* (pp. 399–426). New York: Academic Press.

Scherer, R. C. (1990, September). Aerodynamic assessment in voice production in assessment of speech and voice production: Research and clinical applications. *Proceedings of a Conference.* NIH Publications, No 92-3236.

Schoenrock, L. D., King, A. Y., Everts, E. C. et al. (1972). Hemilaryngectomy: Deglutition evaluation and rehabilitation. *Trans American Academy of Ophthalmology and Otolaryngology, 76,* 752.

School Law Register. Capital Publications, Inc.

Schow, R. L., & Nerbonne, M. A. (1996). *Introduction to audiologic rehabilitation.* Needham Heights, MA: Simon & Schuster.

Schreibman, L. (1988). Autism. Vol. 15 in *Developmental Clinical Psychology and Psychiatry* series. Newbury Park, CA: Sage Publications.

Schuler, A., & Prizant, B. (1987). Facilitating communication: Prelanguage approaches. In D. Cohen and A. Donnellan (Eds.), *Handbook of autism and pervasive developmental disorders* (pp. 301–315). New York: John Wiley & Sons.

Scott, R. W. (2000). *Legal aspects of documenting patient care* (2nd ed.). Gaithersburg, MD: Aspen Publishers.

Secord, W. (1981a). *Test of Minimal Articulation Competence.* San Antonio, TX: The Psychological Corporation.

Secord, W. (1981b). *Clinical probes of articulation consistency.* San Antonio, TX: The Psychological Corporation.

Shames, G. H. (2000). *Counseling the communicatively disabled and their families: A manual for clinicians.* Boston: Allyn & Bacon.

Shaywitz, S. E., Shaywitz, B. A., Pugh, K. R., Fulbright, R. K., Constable, R. T., Mencel, W. E., Shankweiler, D. P., Liberman, A. M., Skudlarski, P., Fletcher, J. M., Katz, L., Marchione, K. E., Lacadie, C., Gatenby, C., & Gore, J. C. (1998). Functional disruption in the organization of the brain for reading in dyslexia. *Neurobiology, 95,* 2636–2641.

Shipley, K. G. (Ed.). (1992). *Interviewing and counseling in communicative disorders: Principles and procedures.* New York: Merrill Publishing Company.

Shipley, K. G., & McAfee, J. G. (1992). *Assessment in speech-language pathology: A resource manual.* San Diego, CA: Singular Publishing Group.

Shipley, K. G., & McAfee, J. G. (1998). *Assessment in speech-language pathology: A resource manual* (2nd ed.). San Diego, CA: Singular Publishing Group.

Shirley, J. C. (1999, October). *The orofacial examination: Normal and abnormal findings.* In Proceedings of the 12th Annual Symposium on Cleft Lip and Palate and Related Conditions. October 8–10, 1999. Atlanta, GA.

Shprintzen, R. J. (1989). Nasopharyngoscopy. In K. R. Bzoch, *Communicative disorders related to cleft lip and palate* (3rd ed., pp. 387–410). Boston: College-Hill Press.

Shprintzen, R. J. (1997). *Genetics, syndromes, and communication disorders.* San Diego, CA: Singular Publishing Group.

Shprintzen, R. J. (1999). *Syndrome identification for speech-language pathology: An illustrated pocketguide.* San Diego, CA: Singular Publishing Group.

Shriberg, L., & Kwiatkowski, J. (1980). *Natural process analysis.* New York: John Wiley.

Siegel, L. S. (1992). An evaluation of the discrepancy definition of dyslexia. *Journal of Learning Disabilities, 25,* 618–629.

Simpson, G. B., Lorsbach, T., & Whitehouse, D. (1983). Encoding and contextual components of word recogntion in good and poor readers. *Journal of Experimental Child Psychology, 35,* 161–171.

Skolnick, M. L., & McGall, G. N. (1972). Velopharyngeal competence and incompetence following pharyngeal flap surgery: Video fluoroscopic study in multiple projections. *Cleft Palate Journal, 9,* 1.

Sloan, C. (1991). *Treating auditory processing difficulties in children.* San Diego, CA: Singular Publishing Group.

Smit, A. B., & Hand, L. (1997). *Smit-Hand Articulation and Phonology Evaluation.* Los Angeles: Western Psychological Services.

Sohlberg, M. M., & Mateer, C. A. (1989). *Introduction to cognitive rehabilitation theory and practice.* New York: Guilford Press.

Spath, P. (Ed.). (1994*). Clinical paths: Tools for outcomes management.* Chicago: American Hospital Publishing.

Spath, P. (1995). Path-based patient care should build quality into the process. *Journal for Healthcare Quality, 17*(6), 26–29.

Stach, B. A. (1998). *Clinical audiology: An introduction.* San Diego, CA: Singular Publishing Group.

Stanovich, K. E. (1991). Discrepancy definitions of reading disability: Has intelligence led us astray? *Reading Research Quarterly, 26,* 1–29.

Stewart-Gonzalez, L. (2000). Service delivery in rural areas. In T. J. Coleman (Ed.), *Clinical management of communication disorders in culturally diverse children* (pp. 129–156). Boston: Allyn & Bacon

Stockman, I. (1986). Language acquisition in culturally diverse populations. In O. Taylor (Ed.), *Nature of communication disorders in culturally and linguistically diverse populations* (pp. 117–155). San Diego, CA: College-Hill Press.

Strand, E. A., & McCauley, R. J. (1999). Assessment procedures for treatment planning in children with phonologic and motor speech disorders. In A. J. Caruso and E. A. Strand (Eds.), *Clinical management of motor speech disorders in children* (pp. 73–108). New York: Thieme Medical Publishers.

Suzuki, T., & Ogiba, Y. (1961). Conditioned orientation reflex audiometry. *Archives of Otolaryngology, 74,* 84–90.

Swengel, K. E., & Marquette, J. S. (1997). Service delivery in AAC. In S. L. Glennen & D. C. DeCoste (Eds.), *Handbook of augmentative and alternative communication* (pp. 21–58). San Diego, CA: Singular Publishing Group.

Szeto, A., Allen, E., & Littrell, M. (1993). Comparison of speed and accuracy for selected electronic communication devices and input methods. *Augmentative and Alternative Communication, 9,* 229–242.

Tanner, D. C. (1980). Loss and grief: Implications for the speech-language pathologist and audiologist. *Asha, 22,* 916–928.

Tanner, D. C. (1999). *The family guide to surviving stroke and communication disorders.* Boston: Allyn & Bacon.

Templin, M. (1957). *Certain language skills in children: Their development and interrelationships.* (Institute of Child Welfare, Monograph, No. 26). Minneapolis, MN: The University of Minnesota Press.

Templin, M., & Darley, F. (1969). *The Templin-Darley Tests of Articulation.* Iowa City, IA: University of Iowa Bureau of Educational Research and Service.

Terrell, B., & Ripich, D. (1989). Discourse competence as a variable in intervention. *Seminars in Speech and Language Disorders, 24,* 77–92.

Tonkavich, J. L. (1988). Communication disorders in the elderly. In B. B. Shadden (Ed.), *Communication behavior and aging: A sourcebook for clinicians.* Baltimore: Williams & Wilkins.

Torgesen, J. K. (1999). Assessment and instruction for phonemic awareness and word recognition skills. In H. W. Catts & A. G. Kamhi (Eds.), *Language and reading disabilities* (pp. 128–153). Boston: Allyn & Bacon.

Torgesen, J. K., & Bryant, B. (1994). *Test of Phonological Awareness.* Austin, TX: Pro-Ed.

Torgesen, J. K., & Wagner, R. K. (1997). *Test of Word and Nonword Reading Efficiency.* Austin, TX: Pro-Ed.

Trace, R. (1996, January 8). Research links infantile autism, manic depression. *Advance for Speech-Language Pathologists and Audiologists,* 3,14.

Trace, R., & Breske, S. (1993, July 19). Legal issues in speech-language pathology documentation and communication are key safeguards. *Advance for Speech-Language Pathologists and Audiologists.*

Urdang, L. (1969). *The Random House dictionary of the English language: College edition.* New York: Random House.

VanDemark, A. A. (1994). Traumatic brain injury. In J. B. Tomblin, H. L. Morris, & D. C. Spriestersbach (Eds.), *Diagnosis in speech-language pathology* (pp. 327–338). San Diego, CA: Singular Publishing Group.

van Keulen, J. E., Weddington, G. T., & DeBose, C. E. (1998). *Speech, language, learning, and the African American child.* Boston: Allyn & Bacon.

Van Riper, C. (1979). *A career in speech pathology.* Englewood Cliffs, NJ: Prentice-Hall.

Van Riper, C., & Erickson, J. (1968). Predictive Screening Test of Articulation. *Journal of Speech and Hearing Disorders, 34,* 214-219.

Vinson, B. P. (1999). *Language disorders across the lifespan.* San Diego, CA: Singular Publishing Group.

Wagner, R. K., & Torgesen, J. K. (1997). *The Comprehensive Test of Phonological Processes in Reading*. Austin, TX: Pro-Ed.

Wallach, G. P., & Butler, K. G. (1994). *Language learning disabilities in school-age children and adolescents: Some principles and applications*. New York: Macmillan.

Weachter, E. (1959). *Concerns of parents related to the birth of a child with cleft of the lip and palate with implications for nurses*. Unpublished master's thesis, University of Chicago, Chicago, IL.

Weaver, A. W., & Fleming, S. M. (1978). Partial laryngectomy: Analysis of associated swallowing disorders. *American Journal of Surgery, 136,* 486.

Weed, L. L. (1972). The problem-oriented record. In J. W. Hurst & H. K. Walker (Eds.), *The problem-oriented system*. New York: Medcor.

Weiner, F. (1979). *Phonological process analysis*. Austin, TX: Pro-Ed.

Weiss, C. (1980). *Weiss Comprehensive Articulation Test*. Chicago: Riverside.

Wells, C. E. (1980). The differential diagnosis of psychiatric disorders in the elderly. In J. Cole & J. Barrett (Eds.), *Psychopathology in the aged*. New York: Raven Press.

Wertz, C., Dexter, M., & Moore, J. (1997). AAC and children with developmental disabilities. In S. L. Glennen & D. C. DeCoste (Eds.), *Handbook of augmentative and alternative communication* (pp. 395–444). San Diego, CA: Singular Publishing Group.

Wertz, R. T., LaPointe, L. L., & Rosenbek, J. C. (1991). *Apraxia of speech in adults*. San Diego, CA: Singular Publishing Group.

Westby, C. (1994). Multicultural issues. In J. B. Tomblin, H. L. Morris, & D. C. Spriestersbach (Eds.), *Diagnosis in speech-language pathology* (pp. 29–52). San Diego, CA: Singular Publishing Group.

Wetherby, A. M., & Prizant, B. (1990). *Communication and Symbolic Behavior Scales* (CSBS). Tucson, AZ: Communication Skill Builders.

Wiederholt, J. L., & Bryant, B. R. (1992). *Gray Oral Reading Tests—III*. Austin, TX: Pro-Ed.

Wiig, E. H., & Semel, E. (1984). *Language assessment and intervention for the learning disabled* (2nd ed.). New York: Merrill.

Wilkinson, G. S. (1995). *The Wide Range Achievement Test—3*. Wilmington, DE: Jastak Associates.

Willeford, J. A., & Burleigh, J. M. (1985). *Handbook of central auditory processing disorders in children*. New York: Grune & Stratton.

Wilson, B. A. (1989). *The Wilson reading system*. Millbury, MA: Wilson Language Training.

Wilson, W. F., Wilson, J. R., & Coleman, T. J. (2000). Culturally appropriate assessment: Issues and strategies. In T. J. Coleman (Ed.), *Clinical management of communication disorders in culturally diverse children* (pp. 101–128). Boston: Allyn & Bacon.

Wirz, S., Skinner, C., & Dean, E. (1990). *Revised Edinburgh functional communication profile*. Tucson, AZ: Communication Skills Builders.

Wolman, B. B. (1989). *Dictionary of behavioral science* (2nd ed.). New York: Academic Press.

Woodcock, R. W. (1987). *Woodcock Reading Mastery Tests—Revised*. Circle Pines, MN: American Guidance Service.

Woodcock, R. W., & Davies, C. O. (1969). *The Peabody rebus reading program*. Circle Pines, MN: American Guidance Services.

Wynder, E. L. (1978) The epidemiology of cancers of the upper alimentary and upper respiratory tracts. *Laryngoscope, 88*(Suppl. 6), 50–51.

Yopp, J. K. (1995). A test for assessing phonemic awareness in young children. *The Reading Teacher, 49,* 20–29.

Yorkston, K. M., Beukelman, D. P., & Traynor, C. (1984). *Assessment of intelligibility of dysarthric speech*. Austin, TX: Pro-Ed.

Young, M. (1985). Central auditory processing through the looking glass: A critical look at diagnosis and management. *Journal of Childhood Communication Disorders, 9,* 31–42.

Zaner, R. M. (1993). *Troubled voices: Stories of ethics and illness*. Cleveland, IL: The Pilgrim Press.

Zimmerman, I., Steiner, V., & Pond, R. (1992). *Preschool Language Scale 3*. Columbus, OH: Charles E. Merrill.

Zraick, R. I., & LaPointe, L. L. (1997). Hyperkinetic dysarthria. In A. J. Caruso & E. A. Strand (Eds.), *Clinical management of sensorimotor speech disorders* (pp. 249–260). New York: Thieme Medical Publishers.

INDEX

("t" indicates a table)

A

Abledata, AAC devices, 139
Accentuation, reflective listening, 56
Acceptance, in grief process, 49–50
Access barriers, ACC devices, 142
Accreditation
    graduate programs, 25
    speech-language professionals, 24
Achievement, ADD/ADHD assessment, 135
Acoustic (VIII) nerve, sensorineural hearing loss, 265
Acoustic measures
    hypernasality, 188
    voice disorder assessment, 411, 411t
    voice examination, 303
Acquired aphasia, convulsive disorders, 399
Activity, definition, 3
Activity-based therapy, language delays/disorders, 293
Acute inflammations, source of mechanical dysphagia, 239
Adaptive pointers, 147
Adult voice history form, 410, 418–420
Advance directives, 75
Advocacy, patient care, 13
Aerodynamics, laryngeal, 303
Affective control, ADD/ADHD, 132
African American children, language acquisition, 317
Agency for Health Care Policy and Research (AHCPR), outcomes
    management, 14
Aided Language Stimulation, use in autism, 178
Aided symbol systems, 153–154
Air conduction testing, hearing loss, 268
Alaryngeal speech, post laryngectomy, 306–307, 308t
Albert H. Wohlers and Company, liability insurance, 23
Alzheimer's disease
    assessment, 212–219, 213t, 215t, 216t
    description, 206–207
    DSM criteria, 210–211
    FOCUSED program, 220, 221t
    management strategies, 220
    medication, 220
    risk factors, 207t
    stage changes, 207–208, 208t, 209t
    treatment, 219–220, 221t
Ambulation, and ACC device use, 143
American Cleft Palate-Craniofacial Association, 179, 189, 191, 195
American English, consonants, diphthongs, vowel placement,
    117t
American Psychiatric Association (APA), 203
American Speech-Language-Hearing Association (ASHA)
    address, 430
    Code of Ethics, 13, 34–37
    counseling definition, 43
    critical pathways reference, 16
    dysphagia definition, 229
    malpractice complaints, 22
    non-speech communication demographics, 139

practices and procedures, 38–41
    publications, 434
    standards of care, 24–26
    stuffed bear with lip repair, 195
    support personnel, 27
Americans with Disabilities Act (ADA), 73, 77, 139
Amplification, interview function, 50
Amyotrophic lateral sclerosis (ALS), dysphagia, 235, 237
Aneurysm, definition, 82
Angelman's syndrome, 380
Anger, in grief process, 48
Ann Arbor Decision, dialect discrimination, 69
Anomia, 88
Apert's syndrome, 380–381
Aphasia
    definition, 81
    differentiated from dementia, 87t, 215t
    differentiated from motor speech disorders, 86t
    differentiated from right hemisphere disorders, 87t
    with/without dysarthria, 86t
    syndromes, 90–93
    from TBIs, 397
    treatment, 93–98
Appetite control, ADD/ADHD, 132
Apraxia
    assessment tasks, 104t
    assessment word imitation, 113
    clinical observations pre-evaluation, 103t
    definitions, 99, 100
    differentiated from dysarthria, 100t
    limb, oral and verbal assessment checklist, 109–112
    treatment, 105–107
Apraxia Battery for Adults, 102
Apraxia of speech (AOS). *See* Apraxia
Aracept, Alzheimer's disease medication, 220
Arizona Battery for Communication Disorders of Dementia, 218
Articulation disorder
    analysis of, 124t
    assessment, 119–120
    definition, 115
    treatment, 124–128
Articulatory substitutions, cleft lip/palate, 185t
ASHA's Functional Assessment of Communication Skills for
    Adults (ASHA FACS), 17
ASHA's Functional Communication Measure (FCM), 17
Asperger's Disorder, 171
Aspiration
    ALS risk, 237
    high risk evaluation, 244
    neuromuscular swallowing disorders, 231
    and non-oral feedings, 247, 248
    Parkinson's risk, 237
    pediatric feeding disorders, 320
    post laryngectomy risk, 240, 306
    PPS risk, 237